2025

医学考博阅读理解

高分全解 第⑪版

适用于全国统考和自主命题

环球卓越医学考博命题研究中心 / 组编

梁莉娟　张秀峰 / 主编

U0378947

机械工业出版社

CHINA MACHINE PRESS

本书作为已有良好市场声誉的"卓越医学考博英语应试教材"的单本,针对高校自主命题的医学院校的考生,重点讲解在医学考博英语考试中分值比重最大、难度值最高的阅读理解部分。本书分成基础篇、技巧篇、强化训练篇、真题篇、测试篇来循序渐进地夯实应试核心基础,提升应试技巧,掌握阅读理解命题规律,从基础篇的词汇、句子、篇章的学习过渡到全面提升解题的精确度和速度。本书的编排方式独特,重点突出,选材贴近命题题源,不仅是考博辅导的最佳帮手,而且是了解该行业最新发展及动向的便捷途径。

图书在版编目(CIP)数据

医学考博阅读理解高分全解 / 环球卓越医学考博命题研究中心组编 ; 梁莉娟, 张秀峰主编. -- 11版.
北京 : 机械工业出版社, 2024. 8. -- (卓越医学考博英语应试教材). -- ISBN 978-7-111-76621-6

　　Ⅰ. R
　　中国国家版本馆CIP数据核字第2024YU9845号

机械工业出版社(北京市百万庄大街22号　邮政编码100037)
策划编辑:孙铁军　　责任编辑:孙铁军　尹小云
责任校对:夏晓琳　　责任印制:单爱军
保定市中画美凯印刷有限公司印刷
2024年9月第11版第1次印刷
184mm×260mm·28.25印张·659千字
标准书号:ISBN 978-7-111-76621-6
定价:79.80元

电话服务　　　　　　　　　　　网络服务
客服电话:010-88361066　　　　机　工　官　网:www.cmpbook.com
　　　　　010-88379833　　　　机　工　官　博:weibo.com/cmp1952
　　　　　010-68326294　　　　金　书　网:www.golden-book.com
封底无防伪标均为盗版　　　机工教育服务网:www.cmpedu.com

丛书序
PREFACE

这是一套由全国知名医学博士英语统考培训机构"环球卓越"（优路教育旗下品牌）策划，联手医学博士英语资深辅导专家，为众多志在考取医学博士的考生量身定制的应试辅导用书。国家医学考试中心于2019年底修订了考试大纲，对全国医学博士外语统一考试的题型及各部分分值进行了局部调整。新大纲仍然设置了听力对话、听力短文、词语用法、完形填空、阅读理解和书面表达6种题型，但调整了具体命题形式，其中听力部分变化最大。"15个短对话+1个长对话+2个短文"的经典组合成为历史，从2020年开始，"5个短对话+5个小短文"的搭配将在很长一段时间内成为考生要面对的题型。考试时间为3个小时（含播放录音及收发卷时间）。

考纲的变化并未改变对考生能力的考查方向，因此为了帮助广大考生在较短的时间内系统备考，在听、说、读、写4个方面得到强化训练，全面提高英语应用和交际能力，顺利通过考试，本套"卓越医学考博英语应试教材"仍然是广大考生朋友们很好的选择。本丛书紧密结合最近几年卫生部组织的医学博士英语统一考试命题情况，针对最新考试大纲进行了修订，并针对新题型编写了大量针对性练习。本丛书包含《全国医学博士英语统考词汇巧战通关》《全国医学博士英语统考综合应试教程》《全国医学博士英语统考实战演练》三本传统综合分册，《医学考博阅读理解高分全解》《医学考博英语听力28天训练计划》两本专项分册，以及《18天攻克医学考博英语核心词》的单词小分册。传统分册从基础到综合再到真题实战，从模块详解到全套试题，高屋建瓴，逐步推进。阅读专项分册对分值较高的阅读理解进行字、词、句、语篇的详解和训练，从技术（语言知识）到技巧（做题方法），精讲多练。听力专项分册则根据听力训练的规律和考试考查目标，按天设置训练内容，分解目标，逐步达成最终目标。

本丛书的特点如下：

一、紧贴考试，实用性强

策划编写本丛书的作者常年在教学一线授课，从基础英语到医博考前辅导，积累了大量的应试辅导实战经验。丛书内容是他们多年辅导经验的提炼和结晶，实用性非常强，专为医学考博考生定制，是目前市面上较全面、系统的医学考博英语应试教材。

二、紧扣大纲，直击真题

本丛书紧扣最新大纲，体例设置与大纲保持一致；各部分考点紧密结合最新历年真题，还原真实考场环境，命题思路分析透彻，重点突出，讲解精确；各部分内容严格控制在大纲规定的范围之内，让考生准确把握考试的重点、难点及命题趋势。

三、内容精练，讲练结合

传统分册《全国医学博士英语统考词汇巧战通关》《全国医学博士英语统考综合应试教程》和《全国医学博士英语统考实战演练》简单精练，通过突破词汇基础关、学习各种题型应试方法以及在高质量实战中历练，考生可在有限的时间内进行全面复习，把握重点，比较系统地完成考前准备。阅读分册《医学考博阅读理解高分全解》则是根据考生的具体情况，分模块予以详解，提升基础，总结技巧，各个击破。听力专项《医学考博英语听力 28 天训练计划》则专练听力，循序渐进，按天分配学习任务，力争高分。核心词汇专项《18 天攻克医学考博英语核心词》在使用词频软件完整统计近十年全套真题的基础上，将该统计结果和大纲词汇进行比较，最后确定出记忆任务的内容和安排。按天设置，不断重复。

四、超值服务，锦上添花

本丛书附带赠送精品服务，由优路教育为每位购书读者提供专业的服务和强大的技术支持。具体为：

1. 《医学考博英语听力 28 天训练计划》附赠内容：优路教育"2025 年医学考博（统考）《英语听力 28 天训练计划》图书赠课英语（20 节）"网络视频课程。使用方法：刮开书籍封底的兑换码，扫描书籍封底二维码关注【优路医学考试】微信公众账号后，点击【兑换课程】-【点击这里兑换课程】的链接，输入兑换码，输入姓名手机号，将自动跳转至您的课程页，开始观看课程。后续看课路径：关注【优路医学考试】服务号，在底部菜单栏【我要学习】-【我的课程】查看课程。（可通过扫描文末二维码，关注后兑换课程）

2. 《18 天攻克医学考博英语核心词》附赠内容：优路教育"2025 年医学考博（统考）《18 天攻克医学考博英语核心词》图书赠课英语（20 节）"网络视频课程。使用方法：刮开书籍封底的兑换码，扫描书籍封底二维码关注【优路医学考试】微信公众账号后，点击【兑换课程】-【点击这里兑换课程】的链接，输入兑换码，输入姓名手机号，将自动跳转至您的课程页，开始观看课程。后续看课路径：关注【优路医学考试】服务号，在底部菜单栏【我要学习】-【我的课程】查看课程。（可通过扫描文末二维码，关注后兑换课程）

3. 《全国医学博士英语统考实战演练》附赠内容：优路教育"2025 年医学考博（统考）《实战演练》图书赠课英语（10 节）"网络视频课程。使用方法：刮开书籍封底的兑换码，扫描书籍封底二维码关注【优路医学考试】微信公众账号后，点击【兑换课程】-【点击这里兑换课程】的链接，输入兑换码，输入姓名手机号，将自动跳转至您的课程页，开始观看课程。后续看课路径：关注【优路医学考试】服务号，在底部菜单栏【我要学习】-【我的课程】查看课程。（可通过扫描文末二维码，关注后兑换课程）

4. 《全国医学博士英语统考综合应试教程》附赠内容：优路教育"2025 年医学考博（统考）《综合应试教程》图书赠课英语（10 节）"网络视频课程。使用方法：刮开书籍封底的兑换码，扫描书籍封底二维码关注【优路医学考试】微信公众账号后，点击【兑换课程】-【点击这里兑换课程】的链接，输入兑换码，输入姓名手机号，将自动跳转至您的课程页，开始观看课程。后续看课路径：关注【优路医学考试】服务号，在底部菜单栏【我要学习】-【我的课程】查看课程。（可通过扫描文末二维码，关注后兑换课程）

5.《全国医学博士英语统考综词汇巧战通关》附赠内容：优路教育"2025 年医学考博（统考）《词汇巧战通关》图书赠课【学习卡】英语（10 节）"网络视频课程。使用方法：刮开书籍封底的兑换码，扫描书籍封底二维码关注【优路医学考试】微信公众账号后，点击【兑换课程】-【点击这里兑换课程】的链接，输入兑换码，输入姓名手机号，将自动跳转至您的课程页，开始观看课程。后续看课路径：关注【优路医学考试】服务号，在底部菜单栏【我要学习】-【我的课程】查看课程。（可通过扫描文末二维码，关注后兑换课程）

6.《医学考博阅读理解高分全解》附赠内容：优路教育"2025 年医学考博（统考）《阅读理解高分全解》图书赠课【学习卡】英语（8 节）"网络视频课程。使用方法：刮开书籍封底的兑换码，扫描书籍封底二维码关注【优路医学考试】微信公众账号后，点击【兑换课程】-【点击这里兑换课程】的链接，输入兑换码，输入姓名手机号，将自动跳转至您的课程页，开始观看课程。后续看课路径：关注【优路医学考试】服务号，在底部菜单栏【我要学习】-【我的课程】查看课程。（可通过扫描文末二维码，关注后兑换课程）

优路教育技术支持及服务热线 400-8835-981，可以帮您解决兑换及观看课程中的技术问题。您也可以登录优路教育网站 www.youlu.com，在"医学博士英语"栏目下获取更多的学习资料和资讯。

编　者
2024 年 3 月于北京

扫码关注后兑换课程

前　言
FOREWORD

　　医学博士入学英语考试分成卫健委全国统考和高校自主命题两种方式。无论哪种考试方式，命题中的阅读理解部分都占据30%～45%的分值比例（卫生部统考分值比例为30%；自主命题则根据试卷情况，分值比例不等）。因此在各种形式的医博命题中，阅读部分占据了卷面成绩的半壁江山，是整个英语试卷的重心所在，真正体现了"得阅读者得天下"！

　　站在更深的层次上，医博英语虽然从形式上分为听力、词汇、完形填空、阅读理解和作文等几部分，但归根结底都是在考阅读理解能力。所谓完形填空题无非是在文中合适的地方留出信息空白，要求考生在正确理解上下文逻辑关系的基础上，结合语法知识进行填补；词汇题则是要求以句子为单位理解语篇，结合词汇的具体特点做出最佳选择；写作则是对阅读理解能力的反向考查——通过读别人的文章，积累内容素材和语言素材，否则笔下哪里来的好文章呢？但是，许多考生在做非阅读理解题的其他题型时，割裂地看待词汇和语法系统的考点，忽视了对语义的理解，这是这类题目解题准确率不高的原因之一。

　　为了帮助广大考生在较短的时间内系统备考，顺利通过考试，我们为广大考生量身定制了这本《医学考博阅读理解高分全解》。这是本书第11次修订。本次修订主要包含以下内容：1. 改写"技巧篇"阅读理解训练的解析，让考生更加明确解题的方式和过程；2. 增加了部分院校考博试题中的阅读理解部分。本书共分为六个部分：

　　第一部分为医学考博阅读理解的5大困惑，直击考生阅读理解疑问并进行答疑解惑。尽管寥寥数语，却一语中的，让考生清楚明了地定位自己的问题。同时该部分还提纲挈领地为考生制订了初步的复习计划。让考生在了解了自身水平和现状、知道了方法和步骤后，去执行计划。

　　第二部分为基础篇，从词汇、句子结构和阅读惯用十大句式等几个方面来夯实考生的必备基础能力。配套的练习文章亦从重点词汇、难句分析、文章翻译三个层面来进一步提升考生的能力。

　　第三部分为技巧篇，总结了解题流程与技巧，提供了多种阅读方法，并按文章结构类考题、主题类考题、态度类考题、局部细节类考题的顺序来分题型强化训练考生的解题能力。此外，本篇还用阅读理解经典文章详解的方式来综合展示解题步骤和方法。

第四部分为强化训练篇，为考生提供了20篇医学类阅读理解文章，帮助考生熟悉医学类文章的体裁，强化第三部分的解题技巧。

第五部分为真题篇，为考生提供了10套博士研究生入学考试英语真题中的阅读部分，帮助考生熟悉真题题型和考查点。

第六部分为测试篇。任何应试思维和能力的培养，都需要用考试来检验效果。因此该部分提供了五套严格按照医学博士入学考试命题难度设置的模拟试题，以供考生检测效果、强化能力、查漏补缺。

本书具备以下特点：

1. 编写体例独特。本书按照基础、技巧、强化训练三个阶段来设置，每个阶段的测试目标和应试能力一一对应，从词汇、句子结构、惯用句式，到分题型解题步骤，无论是基础性的讲解，还是技巧的总结，或是文章解析，都十分全面，总结性和针对性极强，与市面上其他同类图书有本质的区别。

2. 选材紧贴医学。本书所选的练习文章，绝大部分以医学为题材，这让考生自始至终处在专业学习和考试的氛围中。

3. 编写质量过硬。作者对医学博士英语考试的命题有比较深入的研究，对医学博士英语考试的材料来源有深入的追踪和分析。在这一背景下，作者进行了有效的选材，让本书完全适合医学博士英语考生的考前复习。

4. 附赠课程超值。一本书的容量有限，为了让考生全方位地提升应试能力，本书随书附赠环球卓越超值网络课堂，让考生有机会聆听名师的倾心讲解。此外，更有海量资料赠送，真正物超所值。知名教师与知名机构的强强联合，为考生提供了强大的考前后盾！

由于编者水平有限，且时间仓促，书中错误之处在所难免，敬请广大同行和考生批评指正！

编　者

2024年5月于北京

目 录
CONTENTS

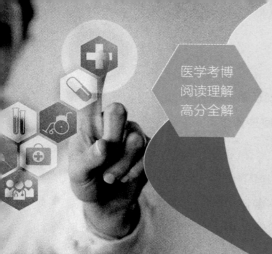

医学考博
阅读理解
高分全解

医学考博阅读理解的5大困惑

　　医博英语虽然从形式上分为听力、词汇、完形填空、阅读理解和写作等几部分，但归根结底都是在变相地考阅读理解。所谓完形填空题无非是在文中合适的地方留出信息空白，要求考生在正确理解上下文逻辑关系的基础上，结合语法知识进行填补；词汇题则是要求以句子为单位理解语篇，结合词汇的具体特点做出最佳选择；写作则是对阅读理解能力的反向考查——通过读别人的文章，积累内容素材和语言素材，否则笔下哪里来的好文章呢？但是，许多考生在做非阅读理解题的其他题型时，忽视了语义理解对词汇和语法考点的提示和限制，这是这类题目解题准确率不高的原因之一。

　　在各种形式的医博命题中，阅读部分占据了卷面成绩的半壁江山，是整个英语试卷的重心所在，真正是"得阅读者得天下"！

　　笔者根据多年的教学经验，总结出考生处理阅读理解题时面临的5大困惑并给予解惑。

　　困惑1：单词障碍使复习进展艰难，拿起文章一头雾水，满眼生词。

　　解惑1：

　　（1）单词是基本功，对解答整个试卷至关重要。但并不是说要把考纲要求的所有词汇都记得滚瓜烂熟，而是必须熟练掌握核心高频词汇，即在阅读中经常重现的词汇。医学专业文章中有不少专业术语，但这些词不会影响解题。在本书基础篇中，已为大家列出部分单词，在附赠的网络课堂中也有总结好的核心词汇。读者可在开始复习阅读的第1周集中背诵。不用会拼写，只要看到之后能认识就足够。大家会发现在接下来的阅读中会无数次地遇到它们。

　　（2）词汇的记忆是分层次的。有的考生拿着一本考纲，不分轻重缓急，一概全背，这是不科学的记忆方法。考生应该先背初高中词汇，因为它们的复现率最高；然后背大学核心词汇；至于一些复杂的专业词汇则可以忽略，因其对做题没有任何影响。

　　（3）积累非常重要。如果能在做完每篇阅读后花5分钟把认为最重要的几个词识记一下，经过一段时间的练习后，这种积累效果会非常惊人，大家不妨尝试一下。

困惑2：句子读不懂。有时候，一句话中的单词都认识，就是不知道这句话到底在说什么。有时候，英语句子那么长，根本分不清主谓宾到底是什么。

解惑2：

（1）这个问题出现在长难句的理解上。长难句是困扰广大考生的一个应试难点，要解决它，首先要对英语句型结构有所了解，因为读不懂句子的原因通常只是对几个固定的结构没有掌握，比如：并列、复合、倒装、多重否定等。将这几个难点单独挑出来集中攻破，会对读句子非常有帮助。考生可以参考本书基础篇来解决这个问题。

（2）此外，先找主、谓、宾，尤其是谓语动词，因为这是句子的核心，这是读句能力较差的考生可以使用的好方法。

（3）最后一点就是迎难而上，这是必要的。因为长难句是难点，而难点就是考点。考生英语阅读理解的不平衡性反映在复习和解题当中，其障碍所在就是难点，不断攻克难点就等于主动把握应试考点。

困惑3：做题速度慢，怎样才能提高速度？考试时10分钟要做完1篇阅读理解题目，每篇阅读理解含原文约40行，题目5道，怎么可能做得完？平时速度就如此慢，考试的时候怎么可能按时完成？

解惑3：

（1）多数考生做题速度慢的原因都是一样的：读原文花的时间太长了。所以应先快速阅读一遍原文，然后看题干，再回原文定位，读懂某个具体句子的意思，最后再做题。那么在阅读一篇新文章时，先快速阅读一遍原文是要达到什么目的呢？

● 答对主旨题和作者态度题。

● 关注并标记一些常考考点为定位所用。

（2）快速读了原文后能达到这两个要求就足够了，多读句子，或在某些句子、单词上多花时间都是浪费，这会导致做题速度慢。读原文应该读什么呢？参见本书技巧篇。

困惑4：读过原文后什么也记不住，花很多时间认认真真读了原文，结果是读了后面忘了前面，读完后脑子里一片空白，有时候甚至根本不知道它到底写了些什么。

解惑4：

（1）记不住的原因就是想记住的太多了，每句话都一样地去读，一样地去记，其结果就是什么都没记住，像没读一样。这样的话可试着挑选自认为最重要的话来记，比如主题句、首段、每段首句、全文末句、显示两者关系的句子（different、similarity、比较级关系、事件发生的顺序等）、事物的缺陷、作者的态度等。其余的可先放一放，体会一下记住这些句子对做题和定位效果是不是要好一点。下一步就是反过来推，根据做过的题目推断快速阅读原文时应该记住什么。

（2）经常小结需要记的东西。其实阅读理解中应该记忆和值得记忆的东西非常有规律，很好总结，长期坚持就可以抓住读原文和记忆的重点。一个很简单的道理：有10分力花到10个点上，每点只得1分力；花到5个点上，每点就有2分力，自然对这5个点的理解更深，记忆更清晰，把握得更好。

困惑5：做了很多篇阅读理解题，怎么没长进？词汇背了就认识，而阅读做了怎么和没做一样？毫无感觉不说，准确率还有所下降，越做越没信心，早知道就不练了！

解惑5：

提高阅读能力，其实就是提高几种具体的阅读技能：比如对文章结构的把握（这是做主旨题和态度题的关键），对常考考点的熟悉，对原文和选项之间的文字对应规律的掌握等。如果只是一味地做题，没有针对所需掌握的知识点和技能进行总结和积累，则对提高阅读技能没有任何帮助。故在运用正确阅读方法的同时做必要的总结，是提高阅读技能的关键。通过与考生的交流，我们为大家总结出了如下重要规律：

（1）掌握文章的结构类型及其标志词，以及文章结构类型和主旨题之间的关系。仔细分析主旨题的正确答案是怎样阐述原文篇章主旨和结构的，是帮助考生更深刻地理解原文结构的有效方法。（见本书技巧篇）

（2）根据题目反推原文考点。题目都考了原文哪些内容，这些内容有什么可总结的规律和特征词。这样总结非常重要，如果坚持下去，一段时间后，就会发现一些固定的原文出题点，日后再读原文的时候也就会自然而然地关注它们。（见本书技巧篇）

（3）分析错题。做错的题一定不能放过，检查其与正确答案的差别在哪，分析题中混淆项的写法，正确项对原文的改写形式，分析错题的同时更要关注正确答案与原文定位处的叙述之间的对应关系，尤其是词与词的对应关系。

除了这三点之外可总结的还有很多，比如词汇、难句等。总结是提高的关键，做阅读理解总是没有长进的考生，是不是很少总结呢？

阅读复习步骤

阅读复习大致可以分为三个阶段：基础阶段、技巧阶段和强化阶段。在这三个阶段，考生分别要解决不同层次、不同要求的问题，但从另一个层面来讲，这三个阶段又是不可分割、相互促进的。

（1）基础阶段　扫清基本的单词障碍，培养句子结构意识，能快速掌握长难句的准确含义。

（2）技巧阶段　了解并能快速准确地判断阅读文章的结构类型，掌握正确的阅读步骤（读题目—读原文—定位），熟悉考点、出题点，熟悉各类题型及相应的最便捷的解题方法。通过对一些经典文章整体、限时的练习，熟悉并完善自己的阅读方法，做到有详有略读原文，熟练掌握原文和正确答案之间的精确对应和改写。

（3）强化阶段　严格按照规定时间做题，分析并集中力量攻克自己的弱点，学会在规定时间内做对最多的题目，即不择手段多做对题。这个阶段为考前适应性练习阶段。

因此，根据复习步骤，本书也分成基础篇、技巧篇和强化训练篇，以便考生有规律地复习。下面，我们先从基础篇开始学习。

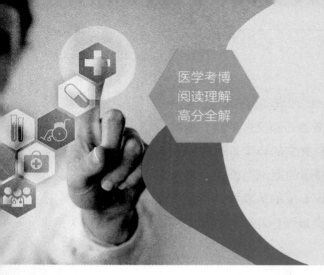

基 础 篇

第一节　基础能力之词汇

　　一般的初学者都会认为阅读生词太多，已经严重影响阅读的顺利进展。加之医学文章专业词汇频出，常用词难度较高，使得词汇成为阅读的最大瓶颈。完整的阅读过程多次被生词打断，这严重破坏了读者对篇章结构的理解。如果看每一篇文章，都还仅仅是停留在一个个小片断上面，那么对文章的整体思路、段落之间的联系怎能把握呢？所以说单词是攻克阅读的第一关。

　　很少有人能在做题之前，甚至在做题过程中，就已经解决了单词问题。大量考生甚至在考试前两周还在玩命地背单词。单词不可能提前准备好，阅读又要求连贯性，那怎么办呢？这里，我们要指出的是，背单词是有级别的，专业词汇是最后一个级别，即无须花精力去记忆的级别。本来考生的复习时间就很紧张，所以我们要把有限的时间用来记忆最重要的单词，即阅读中常见的、影响理解和解题的非专业词汇，而不是从字母A开始背起。从考试角度出发，我们将词汇分成了下列几个等级。

一、重点词

　　这类词汇本身并不难，也不偏，但是仅知道它们表面的意思却不够。它们通常在文章中起着举足轻重的作用：指示文章的结构、表明作者的态度、暗指出题点。了解这类词汇在阅读中深层次的含义，对于解题有着直接的帮助。

　　请先看下面的例题：

According to the author, the <u>conventional</u> notion of intelligence measured in terms of one's ability to read, write and compute _____.

　　A.　is a widely held but wrong concept

　　B.　will help eliminate intellectual prejudice

　　C.　is the root of all mental distress

D. will contribute to one's self-fulfillment

熟悉阅读理解出题规律的考生可能在没有查看原文的时候，就可以猜出正确答案。根据题干的重点词conventional（传统上的）和英文的行文规律——作者大都驳斥传统上的或过去的观点，可推断A项"广泛接受但是错误的观点"很有可能就是正确答案。其实，conventional就是引领转折结构和表明作者否定态度的重点词。

由这道例题可见，熟悉重点词所指明的文章结构和作者态度对于解题会起到至关重要的作用。类似的词汇还有：

alternative *n.* 二中择一；可供选择的办法、事物

【备注】该单词也可以解释为"可替换的选择"，通常是作者提出了另外一种解释。这个新提出的解释和上文论述过的解释应该是针对同一个对象，对新解释的评价应该是考生看到这个词后进一步关注的重点，例：the alternative explanation supposes that...（另一种解释则假定……）。alternative常常出现在"解释针对问题"型文章的主旨题的正确答案中。

compare *v.* 比较，相比；与……类似　*n.* 比较

【备注】通常表达两事物之间相似性和差异性的比较，有时候着重强调相似之处。

contrast *n.* （常与to连用）对照，对比；反差，差异

【备注】通常强调事物之间的差异。

controversy *n.* 争论，辩论，争议

【备注】该单词通常用于引出对立的观点，即不同人对同一事物的不同观点。这个词在观点对立的文章及其主旨题中较为常见，而不宜用来描述全文观点一致的文章。

counterpart *n.* 副本；极相似的人或物；配对物

【备注】很多人看到counter-这个前缀，很容易猜测这个词的含义是对比物。实际上，这个词用于表示可以比较、对照的对应物，在对照的同时有相似的含义，有点类似古诗词中对仗的写作手法，也有点像对联的上下联。

match *n.* （足球、棒球、篮球等）比赛，竞赛；匹配　*v.* 相配，相称

【备注】注意"匹配"的意思，是指两事物之间相似且有可比性，而不是完全相同，有counterpart的含义。

neutral *n.* 中立者，中立国；（机器或汽车的）空挡位置　*adj.* 中立的，中立国的；中性的，无确定性质的；（颜色等）不确定的

【备注】该单词常常在态度题中出现，表示一种不偏不倚、不赞扬也不批评、完全客观的态度。

对于这些词汇，大家要十分重视。根据历年真题分析，带有这些单词的句子经常就是考点所在。所以，大家要相当熟练地掌握这些词汇。根据以往成功通过考试的考生经验，这些

单词他们都背过2～3遍。因此大家要在整个复习过程中，利用零散时间不停地重复记忆。同时，在阅读中出现这些词的时候，回来再看一遍它们的确切含义，进行复现。

表示态度、逻辑关系的重点词汇

序 号	单 词	词 义	含 义
1	abandon	*vt.* 放弃，抛弃 *n.* 放任，放纵	否定。特别注意"放任，放纵"的含义。
2	accessible	*adj.* 易接近的；可被利用的；易受影响的；可理解的	通常表达作者对某事物的态度。
3	accommodate	*v.* 提供住处（或膳宿等）	主要是"提供便利，满足需要"的意思。
4	acute	*adj.* 敏锐的；剧烈的	多为褒义
5	additional	*adj.* 另外的，附加的，额外的	通常用这个词引出对上文观点和事物的追加叙述。因为是顺承关系，又是进一步阐述，所以引出的下文可以不用太关注。
6	adequate	*adj.* 适当的，足够的	反映作者的正面态度，表达作者对某观点、某事物的褒扬。
7	admitted	*adj.* 被承认的，被确认无疑的	正面态度词
8	advocate	*n.* 提倡者，鼓吹者 *vt.* 提倡，鼓吹	对某原因或者提议进行辩护，在阅读中引申为"拥护，支持"的意思。
9	alter	*v.* 改变	这个改变如果发生在观点上，就非常值得关注，因为观点是顺承还是转折对整篇文章的结构至关重要，例：alter accepted views of ancient literary works
10	amused	*adj.* 愉快的，好玩的，开心的	通常为褒义词
11	appropriate	*adj.* 适当的	正面态度词
12	approval	*n.* 赞成；承认；正式批准	不仅停留在许可的表面，还表达了赞同、认可、嘉奖的正面态度。
13	arguable	*adj.* 可论证的，可争辩的	表示观点可以通过证据来支持
14	assert	*v.* 断言，声称	没有正负面态度的倾向性，用于提出观点、理论。
15	assertion	*n.* 主张；断言，声明	确认的观点
16	assess	*vt.* 评定，评估	提出观点
17	associate	*vt.* 使发生联系，使联合	产生联系
18	attack	*vi.* 攻击 *n.* 进攻，攻击	这个词常被用于提出与上文对立的观点。
19	attribute	*v.* 把……归因于 *n.* 属性，品质	表示因果关系。
20	available	*adj.* 可用到的，可利用的	比较明显的褒义词，反映作者的正面态度。对于这个词本身及其修饰的主语一定要给予重点关注。
21	background	*n.* 背景；后台	有个别文章的第一段并没有直指focus，而是作为一种引子，引出下文，这样的段落常被问及作用，它们的作用就是提供了一种background。
22	barrier	*n.* 障碍物；栅栏；屏障	这个词常常引出事物的缺陷，因为缺陷是必考点，引出缺陷的这个词也就当然值得关注了。

（续）

序　号	单　词	词　义	含　义
23	besides	adv. 此外，除……之外	注意，besides有together with的含义，它虽然用于引出新事物，但是却暗含新事物和上文事物有着同样的特征，即上下文所述观点一致，是对顺承关系的叙述。
24	bias	n. 偏见，偏爱	持否定的态度
25	blame	n. 过失，责备 vt. 责备，谴责	表达事物缺陷的特征词。
26	cease	v. 停止，终止	
27	challenge	n. 挑战 vt. 向……挑战	在阅读中，这个词用得更多的是表达一个新事物对旧事物的背叛和挑战，表达新旧观点的对立。
28	charge	n. 负荷；费用；掌管 vt. 控诉；责令，告诫；指示；收费	
29	chief	adj. 主要的，首要的；首席的 n. 首领，领袖	最高级的特征词
30	coexist	vi. 共存	
31	coherent	adj. 黏在一起的；一致的，连贯的	
32	collide	vi. 碰撞；抵触	相反观点
33	community	n. 社区，团体，大众	常表示一个生物群落或人类社会群体。
34	compensate	v. 偿还，补偿，付报酬	
35	competition	n. 竞争，竞赛	
36	complicate	v.（使）变复杂	
37	component	n. 成分 adj. 组成的，构成的	
38	compose	v. 组成；写作	
39	concern	vt. 涉及，关系到	
40	condemn	vt. 声讨，谴责；宣判	这是一个常在态度题中出现的单词，表达负面态度。
41	confirm	vt. 确定，批准；使巩固；使有效	这个词关系到一个观点或证据是否有效，如果一个观点被confirm了，那的确是件欢欣鼓舞的事情，因为它必然是作者所支持的观点。
42	conflict	n. 斗争，冲突 vi. 抵触，冲突	常常用于引出对立的观点，表达事物之间的对立关系。

（续）

序 号	单 词	词 义	含 义
43	confront	vt. 使面临；对抗	这个词常常用于引出对立的观点，同时也表达一种贬义的色彩，即遭遇不好的事情。
44	confused	adj. 困惑的；难懂的	负面态度词
45	consistent	adj. 一致的，调和的；坚固的	正面态度词
46	contemporary	n. 同时代的人 adj. 当代的；同时代的	比较
47	contend	v. 斗争，竞争；主张	这个词常用于引出对立观点。
48	contest	n. 争论；竞赛 v. 争论，争辩；竞赛	提出观点
49	contradict	vt. 反驳，反对；否认；与……矛盾；与……抵触；与……相反	驳斥一种说法；否认……的说法；与……相矛盾；与……抵触
50	conventional	adj. 惯例的，常规的；习俗的，传统的	传统的、惯例的东西通常是作者反对的、要摒弃的，所以这个词引出的观点属于旧观点，之后必然有新观点取代它。
51	crash	n. 碰撞；坠落，坠毁 v. 碰撞；坠落，坠毁	贬义
52	critical	adj. 批评的，评论的，鉴定的；危急的；临界的	常在态度题中出现，表达作者的负面态度。
53	criticize	v. 批评，责备	表达一种负面态度。
54	debate	v. 争论，辩论 n. 争论，辩论	这是一个值得关注的单词，因为它的出现往往意味着有对立的观点，而观点的对立关系往往是考查的重点。
55	defect	n. 过失，缺点	表示事物缺陷的特征词，如果这个词出现，则后文值得关注，因为缺陷是一个重要的考点，表示缺陷的其他特征词：shortcoming, imperfection, deficiency。
56	definite	adj. 明确的，一定的	正面态度词
57	demonstrate	vt. 证明，论证	这个词如果在阅读中出现，就很值得关注，因为一个可被证明的观点是有效的观点，有效的观点也就是作者支持的观点。
58	depression	n. 沮丧，消沉	贬义态度词
59	descend	v. 下去，下来，下降	下降表示的是一种变化，因为变化在阅读中常常成为考点，所以出现这个词的句子值得关注。
60	destructive	adj. 破坏（性）的	在阅读中看到这个词应该首先想到它是个贬义词，有时候也引出某事物的缺陷，经常成为考点。

（续）

序 号	单 词	词 义	含 义
61	discouraging	*adj.* 令人气馁的	贬义词
62	distinct	*adj.* 清楚的，明显的；截然不同的，独特的	作为"截然不同的"讲时，是一个很值得关注的词，因为"事物的不同之处"经常成为考点。
63	drawback	*n.* 缺点；障碍	"缺陷"的特征词，值得重点关注，因为"缺陷"经常成为考点。
64	eliminate	*vt.* 排除，消除	表示"彻底消失"，常为考点。
65	embrace	*vt.* 拥抱；包含；接受；信奉 *vi.* 拥抱 *n.* 拥抱	正面态度词，表达欢迎、赞同之义。
66	enforce	*n.* 执行；强制	
67	enhance	*vt.* 提高，增强	表达事物的变化，值得关注。
68	evolution	*n.* 进展，发展；演变，进化	可能涉及达尔文的进化论。
69	exaggerate	*v.* 夸大，夸张	贬义词，时常引出事物的缺陷，值得关注。同义词有：overstate，overemphasize。
70	fruitful	*adj.* 果实累累的，多产的；富有成效的	褒义词
71	genuine	*adj.* 真实的，真正的；诚恳的	褒义词
72	identify	*vt.* 识别，鉴别；确定	当含义为to be or become the same 的时候表达两种事物的关系，经常成为考点，值得关注。
73	imitate	*vt.* 模仿，仿效；仿制，仿造	表示两者有联系。
74	impact	*n.* 碰撞；冲突，冲击；影响，效果	结果类命题的标志词
75	improper	*adj.* 不适当的，不合适的；不正确的；不合理的，不适宜的	表示事物缺陷的特征词，值得关注。
76	inaccuracy	*n.* 错误	表示事物缺陷的特征词，值得关注。
77	incomplete	*adj.* 不完全的，不完善的	负面态度词，表示事物缺陷的特征词，值得重点关注。
78	increase	*vt.* 增加，加大 *vi.* 增加；繁殖 *n.* 增加，增大，增长	表示事物变化的词，要予以足够关注，最好在读文章的时候给出标记，例如用一个向上的箭头表示变化的趋势。
79	incredible	*adj.* <口>难以置信的	表示惊奇的态度。
80	indifference	*n.* 不关心	通常出现在态度题中，充当混淆项。

（续）

序号	单词	词义	含义
81	inefficiency	*n.* 无效；无能；不称职	负面态度词，表示事物缺陷的特征词，值得重点关注。
82	initial	*adj.* 最初的，初始的；词首的 *n.* 词首大写字母	表示旧观点的特征词
83	innovative	*adj.* 创新的，革新（主义）的	表示新事物、新观点的特征词，新的东西总是作者支持的。
84	insight	*n.* 洞察力，见识	正面态度词
85	insufficiency	*n.* 不足	负面态度词，表示事物缺陷的特征词，值得重点关注。
86	interpret	*vt.* 解释，说明；口译，传译；认为是……的意思	这个词出现时，它能否有效地解释观点、现象是关键，也是应该关注的焦点。
87	invalid	*adj.* 无效的；无根据的 *n.* 病人，残疾者	负面态度词
88	investigate	*v.* 调查，研究	常常作为说明观点的论据，一般来说，调查的具体内容不必细看，关键是要看这个调查是否能有效支持证据。
89	justified	*adj.* 正当的；合法的；合理的	褒义词
90	merit	*n.* 优点；价值 *vt.* 有益于	褒义词
91	misunderstand	*vt.* 误解，误会	
92	modest	*adj.* 谦虚的，谦让的；适度的	表示一种适度的态度或情绪，常出现在态度题的正确选项里，和一个有感情色彩的词连用，例如：modest commendation（适度的赞扬），说得严谨客观，比较容易成为正确答案。如果modest所修饰的主态度词所表达的感情色彩正确，则无疑是正确答案。
93	negative	*n.* 否定；负数；底片 *adj.* 否定的；消极的；负的；阴性的 *vt.* 否定；拒绝（接受）	贬义词
94	neglect	*vt.* 忽视；疏忽 *n.* 忽视；疏忽	忽略了本应该在意、关注的东西，这个词本身就说明它忽略的对象读者应该给予足够的关注；同时"忽略"是个缺点，容易考查到，值得关注。
95	normally	*adv.* 正常地，通常	"通常"说明观点在阅读中总是成为旧观点和作者要摒弃的观点。

（续）

序 号	单 词	词 义	含 义
96	novel	*n.* 小说，长篇故事 *adj.* 新奇的，新颖的，异常的	当novel作为"新的"讲时，通常是作者支持、赞同的观点，也通常是作者想用大篇幅叙述的观点，所以值得重点关注。
97	objective	*n.* 目标，目的 *adj.* 客观的	经常作为态度词出现。
98	opposed	*adj.* 反对的，敌对的	负面态度词
99	opposite	*adj.* 相对的，对面的；对立的，相反的；对等的，对应的 *n.* 相反的事物	用于引出对立的观点，值得关注。
100	original	*n.* 原物，原作 *adj.* 最初的；原始的；独创的，新颖的	作为"新颖的，新奇的"讲时，值得关注，因为是新的，故通常是作者赞同的。
101	outline	*n.* 大纲，轮廓，略图；外形，要点，概要 *vt.* 描画轮廓；略述	整体的结构词
102	outstanding	*adj.* 突出的，显著的	褒义词
103	outweigh	*v.* 在重量（或价值等）上超过	常用于比较两个事物的重要程度，涉及常考查的事物之间的关系，值得关注。
104	overestimate	*vt.* 评价过高	表示缺陷、过失，经常考查到，值得关注。
105	overlook	*vt.* 俯瞰；远眺；没注意到	在阅读中值得关注的含义是"忽略"，即miss，ignore。
106	overwhelm	*vt.* 淹没；覆没；制服；压倒	表示"占绝对优势"，例如：overwhelming majority压倒性的多数。
107	partial	*adj.* 部分的，局部的；偏袒的，偏爱的	
108	passive	*adj.* 被动的	
109	persuasive	*adj.* 有说服力的	褒义词，通常用于作者赞同的观点及论据上，值得关注。
110	pessimism	*n.* 悲观，悲观主义	
111	positive	*adj.* 肯定的；积极的；绝对的；确实的	正面态度词
112	precious	*adj.* 宝贵的，贵重的，珍爱的	褒义词
113	precise	*adj.* 精确的，准确的	褒义词

（续）

序 号	单 词	词 义	含 义
114	predominant	adj. 卓越的；支配的；主要的，突出的，有影响的	褒义词
115	preference	n. 偏爱；优先选择	比较的含义
116	prejudice	n. 偏见，成见 v. 损害	常成为考点的表示缺陷的词
117	prevail	vi. 流行，盛行；获胜，成功	褒义词
118	previous	adj. 在前的，早先的	这个词常用于引出旧观点，也就是作者要摒弃的观点。
119	primitive	adj. 原始的，远古的；粗糙的，简单的	这个词有三个基本含义，当它作为"早期的"讲时，通常用于引出旧观点。
120	profoundly	adv. 深切地；深刻地；极度地	几个含义中，"深刻地"用得最多，褒义词，即having intellectual depth and insight。
121	prohibition	n. 禁止，阻止	
122	promptly	adv. 敏捷地，迅速地	
123	properly	adv. 适当地，完全地	褒义词
124	protest	n. 主张，断言；抗议	常用于引出对立的观点，值得关注。
125	puzzle	n. 难题，谜 v.（使）迷惑，（使）为难	常为"解释针对问题"类文章的特征词，尤其是当它出现在首段的时候，很可能意味着下文都在寻求对它的正确解释。
126	recruit	n. 新兵，新会员 vt. 组建；征募 vi. 征募新兵	有"新"的含义，故作者通常对其持正面态度。
127	refined	adj. 精制的；优雅的；精确的	褒义词
128	reform	n. 改革；改善，改良；改造 vt. 改革，革新，重新组成 vi. 革新，改过，重组	改良、革新都是作者一贯支持的观点。
129	reinforce	vt. 加强，增援；补充，增加……的数量；加固 n. 加固物	常用于表示事物之间的关系，值得关注，因为事物之间的关系常为考点。
130	reject	n. 不合格品 vt. 拒绝；排斥	表示否定了某事物、某观点。

（续）

序　号	单　词	词　义	含　义
131	relation	*n.* 关系，联系；亲戚	当该单词在阅读中出现时要予以足够的关注，因为事物之间的关系常常成为考点，而relation将引出对事物关系的直接叙述。
132	reliable	*adj.* 可靠的，可信赖的	褒义词
133	removal	*n.* 移动；免职；切除	否定某事物。
134	resemble	*vt.* 像，类似	这个词指的是两者相似，反映事物之间的关系，常常成为考点，所以值得关注。在阅读中，"相似"和"等于"几乎可以替换，因为相似的着眼点在共同之处，对不同之处和差异一般没有论述。
135	restate	*vt.* 重新叙述；重申	有"新"的含义，重申的理论、观点通常都是作者支持的。
136	revise	*vt.* 修订，校订，修改	修订多半是作者支持的，因为有推陈出"新"的意思。
137	revolution	*n.* 革命；旋转	这个词的英文解释的核心是change，因为有"革新"的含义，所以通常是作者所支持的。
138	rival	*n.* 竞争者，对手 *v.* 竞争，对抗，与……匹敌	这个词所体现的对手不只是单纯的竞争关系，还有一个"相匹配的"潜在含义，即one that equals another in desired qualities。
139	routine	*n.* 例行公事；常规；日常事务；程序	惯例、常规、习俗都有"旧的"这一含义，因此一般是作者将要摒弃的旧观点。
140	sanction	*n.* 批准；认可；同意；制裁 *v.* 批准；认可；同意；实施制裁	正面态度词
141	scheme	*v.* 计划，设计；图谋，策划 *n.* 安排配置；计划；阴谋；方案，图解，摘要	
142	segment	*n.* 段，节，片段 *v.* 分割	表示部分的标志词。
143	shortcoming	*n.* 缺点，短处	表示事物缺陷的特征词，值得重点关注，同义词：deficiency，defect。
144	similarity	*n.* 类似，类似处	一般用于表达事物之间的关系，经常成为考点，值得关注。
145	statistics	*n.* 统计学；统计表	这个词在阅读中出现时，通常引出一段论据以证明某观点。这个统计的具体内容、方式、数据等不必关注，它能否有效地支持其要说明的观点是关键，也是读者应当关注的焦点。
146	subject	*vt.* 使屈从于，使隶属 *n.* 主题，题目	当意思为"从属"的时候表达了两个事物之间的关系，容易成为考点，值得关注。

（续）

序号	单词	词义	含义
147	subordinate	*adj.* 次要的；从属的；下级的 *n.* 下属 *v.* 把……置于次要地位	
148	substituted	*adj.* 被取代的，被代替的	表达事物之间的关系，常成为考点，值得关注。
149	successive	*adj.* 连续的	注意与"成功的（successful）"区别开。
150	survey	*vi.* 测量 *vt./n.* 调查	看到这个词立刻想到它是论述某观点的论据，其内容并不重要，重要的是这个证据能否证明某观点有效。
151	suspect	*n.* 嫌疑犯 *adj.* 令人怀疑的，不可信的	负面态度词
152	tedious	*adj.* 单调乏味的，沉闷的，冗长乏味的	贬义词
153	tentative	*n.* 试验；假设 *adj.* 实验性的，试探的，尝试的；暂定的	它是论述某观点的论据，其内容并不重要，重要的是这个证据能否证明某观点有效。
154	transition	*n.* 转变，转换	表示事物变化的词，值得关注。
155	unavailable	*adj.* 难以获得的	贬义词，反映事物的缺陷，值得关注。
156	underestimate	*vt.* 低估，看轻	贬义词
157	undermine	*v.* 破坏	贬义词，表达对某事物、观点的否定。
158	undetermined	*adj.* 未确定的；未解决的	这个词出现有两种可能，一种是用于说明前面观点的无效性，另一种是引出下文的解决方案。
159	uniform	*adj.* 相同的，一致的；始终如一的 *n.* 制服	表示事物之间的关系，在遇到这个词的时候，最好用"="做个标记。
160	unique	*adj.* 唯一的，独特的	表明最高级的词汇，当它在阅读中出现时，最好做个标记，因为最高级常常能帮助判断正确选项，但这个词并不总代表"唯一"，有时候也有"独特的"这一含义，要注意分辨。例：They can make a unique contribution（特殊贡献）to society.
161	universal	*adj.* 普遍的；通用的；全体的	因为有"普遍的，通用的"这一含义，这个词常常引出一个旧观点，也就是作者通常反对的观点。
162	unrealistic	*adj.* 不切实际的	负面态度词
163	vague	*adj.* 含糊的，不清楚的	负面态度词

（续）

序　号	单　词	词　义	含　义
164	**validate**	*vt.* 使有效，使生效；确认，证实，验证	该词证明某观点有效，看到这个词，对它所支持的观点要予以足够关注，因为那一定是作者支持的观点。
165	**variety**	*n.* 变化，多样性；品种，种类	"变化"和"不同"常常成为考点，所以这类词无论谁出现，都值得关注。
166	**verify**	*vt.* 检验，校验；查证，核实	是个证明某观点有效性的词，看到这个词，对它所持的观点要予以足够关注，因为那一定是作者支持的观点。
167	**violate**	*vt.* 违犯；冒犯；干扰	引出对立观点，值得予以足够关注。
168	**whereas**	*conj.* 然而，反之；鉴于；尽管，但是	转折关系词
169	**while**	*conj.* 当……的时候；虽然	这是一个表达事物之间对比关系的连词，所引导的句子很值得关注。

二、高频词

　　本书对基础高频词汇和进阶高频词汇进行了分类整理，由于篇幅所限，我们将基础高频词按阶段总结在赠送的网络课堂中，大家可以下载复习。本丛书中有一本便携版词汇小书《18天攻克医博英语词汇核心词》，这本书中也有非常明确的指导，可直接参考。这些高频词汇是每位考生必须掌握的，因为它们在阅读中的重复率十分高。

　　1. 高中基础词汇：2 000个（见网络课堂）快速浏览一遍，在不熟悉的单词下面画一条横线，完成整体浏览后再查阅考纲（或者查看本套丛书的词汇分册，或是18天便携版词汇小书，用筛查—检测的方式唤醒记忆）弄清其意思。我们使用词频软件完整统计了近十年的全套真题，统计出了真题命题词汇的出现频率。从统计结果中发现，词频超过10次的，往往是初、高中词汇（甚至小学词汇），这部分高频词汇用上述办法复习即可。

　　2. 进阶高频词汇：1 000个（见《18天攻克医博英语词汇核心词》）通过研究真题发现，医学博士英语考试的词汇范围，在实际命题中并非严格以大纲为蓝本，考生认为不重要的，不一定是命题人不考的，比如antidioxide，即四六级的考试经验，未见得完全适用于医博英语考试，毕竟有"医学"这个限定词。基于这种现实情况，我们对词频3～10之间的词汇与大纲进行对照，删掉基础词汇，补充真题词汇，形成了18天便携版词汇小书的记忆主体。

经过实验，每天记忆50～60个单词（非完全陌生）是完全能够完成的。虽然我们不可能在如此短暂的时间内彻底记住这些单词，但我们可以无限次循环、重复，强化印象。即使不能很快记忆，也不必太过担心，因为在读文章、做真题的时候，你会无数次地遇到它们。通过阅读后的总结，你会发现它们就在我们所列的重点词汇和高频词汇表格之中，那时你的记忆就十分深刻了。同时需要提醒大家的是，背单词不需要背拼写，因为你只要认识它，它就不是你阅读的障碍了。

第二节　基础能力之句子结构

读懂句子结构是读懂一篇文章的基础，读懂居于重要位置的句子意义就更加重大。尽管医博考试阅读理解的文章一般都有一定的专业性，但考查点与普通文章完全一样。在读文章的时候，对句子的理解其实可以分为两个层面：第一层，就是我们简要分析句子的主谓宾，以及其所要表达的基本意思——为了让考生达到这个层面的要求，我们将给出常见的句子结构，并进行简要的分析，让大家了解出题人惯用的增加句子难度的方式和惯用的迷惑考生的方式，这是本章的重点；第二层是句子在阅读中扮演的角色，以及它的出现对文章整个篇章内容及结构的暗示作用——有着这种暗示作用的句子出现的位置和形式比较模式化，容易掌握。如果考生对句子的理解能达到这两个层次，对于做阅读理解题应该是足够了。

我们先来解决第一个层次的问题。大家可能常常会有这样的体会，一句话里面主要的词汇都认识，但是连在一起，就不知道它在说什么。在解决了单词问题之后，怎样读懂句子，或者说怎样读懂文章就成了最有待解决的问题。读懂句子的能力取决于两个方面：

> 第一，读句子的方法。
> 第二，对句子结构的理解和领悟。具体到阅读考试中，就是对句子惯用的结构组成方式的理解和领悟。

一、英语句式与汉语句式的区别

我们先来读一读最常见的汉语句子："许多夫妻因为错误的理由结了婚，结果在10年、20年或30年后才发觉他们原来是合不来的。他们在婚前几乎没有花时间去彼此了解，忽视了严重的性格差异，指望婚姻会自然而然地解决各种问题，我们希望避免重蹈覆辙。"如果我们要求大家将这一段汉语翻译成英语，你可能会写出若干个短句子，比如说：

> Many couples marry for the wrong reasons.

> They only find out ten, twenty, or thirty years later that they were incompatible.

> They hardly took the time to know each other before marriage.

> They overlooked serious personality conflicts.

> They expect that marriage was an automatic way to make everything work out right.

> We wanted to avoid the mistake.

英语是重逻辑的"形合"语言，即会采用多种连接手段将各自独立的小分句有逻辑地组合起来。用一个形象的比喻就是英语像"大树"，"树干"就是主句的"主谓宾"，而"枝条"就是其附加修饰成分，如定语从句、状语从句等。其实，上面那段中文翻译成英语可以用一句话来表示：

We wanted to avoid the mistake made by many couples of marrying for the wrong reasons, and only finding out ten, twenty, or thirty years later that they were incompatible, that they hardly took the time to know each other before marriage, that they overlooked serious personality conflicts in the expectation that marriage was an automatic way to make everything work out right.

这个长句我们可以这样来分析它：

We wanted to avoid the mistake（主句）

- made by many couples（过去分词短语做后置定语，修饰mistake）
- of marrying for the wrong reasons（介词短语做后置定语，修饰mistake）
- and only finding out ten, twenty, or thirty years later（finding out和marrying 并列）
    ✓ that they were incompatible（that引导find out的宾语从句）
    ✓ that they hardly took the time to know each other before marriage（that引导find out的宾语从句）
    ✓ that they overlooked serious personality conflicts in the expectation（that引导find out的宾语从句）
- that marriage was an automatic way to make everything work out right（that从句在名词后，做expectation的同位语）

这个句子大树般的逻辑关系图如下：

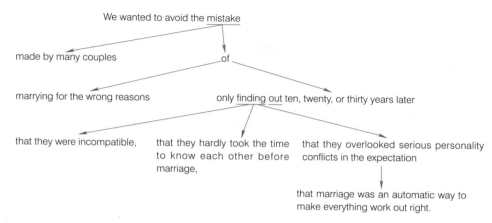

可以看出，对于英语句式的拆分，就像把大树的树干和枝条拆开的感觉一样。拆下枝条后，我们就可以把每一个小分句翻译成汉语，所以汉语就是竹节般的语言，是由一根一根竹节直线式地连在一起。每一根竹节就相当于英语的枝条，而英语的枝条则是长在树干上的。这就是英语句式和汉语句式的不同。

英语句子的阅读过程，从根本上说，就是将枝条拆离树干，并弄清楚枝条和树干的关系的过程。理解了汉语句子和英语句子的根本差别，就等于理解了英语句式分析的精髓。

二、如何找到英语句子的"树干"——句子的主谓宾

现在，我们就具体地说一说如何才能找到句子的"树干"。通常我们需要采用三个步骤。

第一步，把句子拆分为可以理解的较小的语言单位。

第二步，去掉修饰成分。

第三步，简缩出句子主干后，再逐层分析句式。

下面我们就对这三个步骤进行详细的讲解。

（一）把句子拆分为可以理解的较小的语言单位

由于英语语言是"形合"（结构、形式结合）起来的一棵大树，因此如果句子过长，考生就很难一下子理解整句话的意思。所以，我们要注意一边读一边拆分句子的语法结构。

在何处拆分呢？有的考生认为自己的英语基础知识比较差，对英语句子的语法结构不太理解。这没有关系，因为英语语法结构和逻辑结构比较明显，我们可以在"树干"和"枝条"的交界处拆分长句。那么这个"交界处"在哪儿呢？英语中有"信号词"来指示这个位置，在"信号词"处将句子分割，就可以更加有效地理解英语原文。这些"信号

词"如下。

名词后置定语：因为名词性主语后经常出现修饰成分，而使读者无法找到谓语，所以去掉名词后的后置定语是十分重要的。

连词：and，or，but，yet，for等并列连词连接并列句；when，as，since，until，before，after，because，since，though，although，so that等连接词连接状语从句。它们是理解英语句子的拆分点。

关系词：连接名词性从句的who，whom，whose，what，which，whatever，whichever等关系代词和when，where，how，why等关系副词；连接定语从句的who，which，that，whom，whose等关系代词和when，where，why等关系副词。它们也是理解英语句子的拆分点。

介词：on，from，with，at，of，to等介词常常引导介词短语做修饰语，它们也是理解英语句子的拆分点。

动词不定式符号to：动词不定式常常构成动词不定式短语做定语或状语修饰语，可以是拆分点。

分词：过去分词和现在分词可以构成分词短语做修饰语，可以是拆分点。

标点符号：标点符号常常断开句子的主干和修饰部分，也是一个明显的拆分点。

例如：A handful of them may be some of the wide-eyed enthusiasts who attended a meeting at the Royal Society of Medicine (RSM) earlier this year about why they should choose a career in medicine.（2018年全国医学博士英语统考阅读理解文章）

我们先进行句子的拆分：

★ A handful of them may be some of the wide-eyed enthusiasts

★ who attended a meeting at the Royal Society of Medicine (RSM) earlier this year

★ about why they should choose a career in medicine

1. 首先，我们在enthusiasts处分割，该词前面是主句，大意是"一部分人是热情的积极分子"，a handful of和wide-eyed都是名词的前置修饰语。

2. who引导的定语从句解释是什么样的enthusiasts——他们于年初在RSM参加了一次会议。at the Royal Society of Medicine (RSM) earlier this year是定语从句中的地点状语和时间状语。

3. about引导的介宾短语表示参与会议的原因，why引导的宾语从句做的是介词about的宾语，表示会议的主题，充当meeting的后置定语。

从上面的分析看出，合理地按照信息词来拆分长句，是理解长句的首要条件，这就是按照意群来理解句子。前期需要做刻意的分析，速度会较慢，假以时日地坚持练习后形成对意群的条件反射，速度自然也就快起来了。该句的意思是：其中一小部分人是今年早些时候参加皇家医学会（RSM）会议的一些热心人士，会议上讨论了他们为什么应该从医。

（二）去掉修饰成分

修饰成分主要有三类，分别是：定语结构、状语结构、插入结构。下面我们就给大家一一讲解这些修饰成分的组成以及用法。

1．定语结构

定语结构是修饰名词的扩展成分，当一个形容词修饰名词的时候，这个形容词通常会出现在名词的前面，例如a beautiful girl。还有部分定语是放在名词后面来修饰名词的。众所周知，汉语中的定语都在中心词的前面，而英语中较长的定语一般出现在中心词的后面，称为"后置定语"。

（1）后置定语的组成

英语语言浩瀚复杂，但是只要熟练掌握6种后置定语形式，就可以轻松地分析所有定语成分。考生只有牢牢地记住这些知识点才能在阅读和作文中灵活应用。

现将这6种后置定语形式总结在表格中，请考生注意举例和备注部分，这些都是往届考生经常出错或者不理解的地方。

序　号	形　　式	举　　例	备　　注
1	名词＋关系词＋定语从句	a boy whom China needs 中国需要的男孩	当先行词在从句中充当宾语的时候，关系词可以省略。
2	名词＋that＋同位语从句	the news that he died 他去世的消息	that引导的同位语从句的先行词在从句中不做任何成分，而that引导的定语从句的先行词要在从句中做主语或者宾语。
3	名词＋现在分词	a man shooting the bird 向小鸟开枪的男士	核心名词和分词的动词是主动的逻辑关系。
	名词＋过去分词	a man fancied by women 受女人喜爱的男士	核心名词和分词的动词是被动的逻辑关系。
4	名词＋不定式	a man to shoot the bird 将要向小鸟开枪的男士	在后置定语中，分词表示完成或经常性的动作，而动词不定式表示将来或一次性的动作。
5	名词＋介宾结构	threat of globalization 全球化的威胁	经常出现的介词有of、by等。of表示"……的"，by表示"通过"和"被"。
6	名词＋形容词短语	news available to Xiao Li 小李可获得的消息	积累常见短语中的形容词短语。

（2）后置定语的使用

首先，从理论上讲，一个名词后面可以跟很多个后置定语，而且这些后置定语的种类还可以是不一样的，比如第一个后置定语用定语从句，第二个后置定语用同位语从句。在实际写作中，一般一个名词最多跟2～3个后置定语，如果再多的话，就会显得十分冗长。没有后置定语结构的句子不是好的英语句子；同理，后置定语过多也不是十分漂亮的句子。那么，一个名词后面跟多个后置定语的结构就会带来下面的问题——逐层修饰还是递进修饰的问题。

①逐层修饰

【定义】第二个后置定语修饰的是第一个后置定语结尾的名词，而不是中心词。

【示例】a press conference/dominated by questions/on yesterday's election results

【讲解】dominated by questions这个过去分词短语是第一个后置定语，修饰前面的conference，而这后置定语又是以名词questions结尾的。on yesterday's election results是介宾结构。从理论上讲，它既可以修饰前面的名词conference，又可以修饰questions，这在语法上都是可以的。因为"昨天选举的结果"这个短语和"问题"的语义更近，所以它修饰的是questions，而不是conference，全句的核心词依旧是conference。这个词组我们可以翻译为"受昨天选举结果的问题所支配的记者招待会"。dominate是"支配"的意思，这里过去分词表示被动。

【逻辑关系图】

a press conference / dominated by questions / on yesterday's election results

②递进修饰

【定义】第二个后置定语不是修饰第一个后置定语结尾的名词，而是修饰中心词。

【示例】the great interest/in exceptional children/shown in public education

【讲解】in exceptional children是介宾短语，修饰前面的名词interest，指出interest（兴趣）是针对exceptional children（特殊孩子）的；shown in public education是一个过去分词短语，它既可以修饰exceptional children，也可以修饰interest。根据语义"被展示在公立教育部门"，我们可以知道，语义应该是"兴趣被展示在公立教育部门"，而不是"孩子被展示在公立教育部门"，所以第二个后置定语不是修饰"孩子"的，而是修饰"兴趣"的。本短语可以翻译为"公立教育显示出的对特殊孩子的兴趣"，核心词依旧是"兴趣"。

【逻辑关系图】

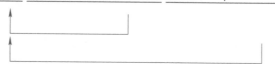

the great interest/in exceptional children/shown in public education

在后置定语的使用中，还有另外一种现象，就是谓语分割了名词和它的中心词，这主要是由于谓语太短，而后置定语部分过长的原因。如果后置定语由10个词组成，而谓语动词却只有两个词，那句子读起来就会给人一种头重脚轻的感觉。

例如：The day will surely come when all the people in the world enjoy freedom and live in happiness.（世界上所有的人都能享受自由并幸福地生活的那一天一定会到来。）

其中，day是中心词，后面的come为谓语动词，而when all the people in the world enjoy freedom and live in happiness是day的定语从句，是后置定语部分。由于它比谓语要长得多，所以就采取了先写谓语，再加后置定语的处理方式。

（3）后置定语结构在句式分析中的应用

后置定语在英语句式中使用频率相当高，所以能否合理有效地处理后置定语结构就是句式分析的重点所在。下面把对后置定语的处理方式总结如下。

序　号	方　式	原　因
1	在名词后进行分割	如果句子较长，则很有可能是后置定语较多，所以在名词处分割句子，是去掉后置定语的首要条件。
2	先把后置定语去掉，再寻找主干	后置定语看得再明白，它也是用来修饰名词的，是属于树枝的部分。所以我们只有找到中心词才可以找到主干，中心词才是句子的重点所在。
3	不论是逐层修饰还是递进修饰，中心词都是第1个名词	可以先不考虑是逐层修饰还是递进修饰，找到中心词是第一要务。
4	找到主干后，读后置定语，但不能调整语序	中文的定语在中心词前，而英语中的后置定语在中心词后，把后置定语提前势必会增加阅读的时间，并且也会使读者的大脑思维停留在中文上。要加快阅读速度，必须做到不调整语序。
5	根据语义判断是逐层修饰还是递进修饰	如果细节类题考到后置定语，则考生要把每个后置定语的意思弄清，再比较语义和哪个名词联系更紧密。
6	谓语分割中心词和后置定语	在词语题中有所体现，这是考生的盲点所在。

举一个具体的例子来说明上面表格的内容。

例如：It applies to traditional historians who view history as only external and internal criticism of sources and to social science historians who equate their activity with specific techniques.

这个句子看上去十分复杂，我们可以按照上一步的技巧先把它拆分，名词是拆分的一个重点。于是，上面的句子就被拆分成：

> It applies to traditional historians

> who view history as only external and internal criticism of sources

> and to social science historians

> who equate their activity with specific techniques

先把名词后面的后置定语去掉，就能够马上整理出句子的主干：It applies to traditional historians and to social science historians.（它既适用于传统历史学家，也适用于社会科学历史学家。）

然后再来阅读后置定语部分，who view history as only external and internal criticism of sources修饰前面的traditional historians。理解的时候，我们可以这样处理：先看到traditional historians，然后看到who引导的定语从句。于是我们就可以顺着语义理解为："这些传统的历史学家把历史仅看成对史料内部和外部的批评"，而不要把后面的定语从句翻译到中心词的前面，这样会影响阅读速度。

紧接着，我们看第二个定语从句："社会科学历史学家把科研看作具体的技巧。"于是，我们可以这样翻译整个句子："传统的历史学家把历史仅看成对史料内部和外部的批评，社会科学历史学家把科研看作具体的技巧，它适用于他们两者。"

2. 状语结构

和后置定语一样，状语结构也是修饰结构，只不过后置定语修饰的是名词，而状语结构修饰的是形容词、动词和整个句子的时间、地点等。比起后置定语结构来，状语比较简单，也是考生比较容易理解的地方，现将其在阅读中的考点总结如下。

序　号	形　式	用法及范例	备　注
1	副词	可以放在前面修饰形容词 exceedingly angry 可以放在前或后修饰动词 sharply distinguish A from B work hard 可以放在动词词组中间充当插入成分 refer only to	以-ly结尾的词一般为副词，起修饰作用。如果不是表示否定关系的副词，就可以忽略。

（续）

序　号	形　式	用法及范例	备　注
2	介宾结构	放在句首或句尾修饰句子 In 1997, I ...	介宾结构开头，一般为状语，可以先忽略。
3	分词	放在句子前或后修饰句子 Dancing, he comes to the classroom. His father gave him a lot of money, allowing him to lead a luxury life.	分词放在句首，与主语之间一般有逗号，可以先忽略；如果没有逗号，则可能是动名词做主语，就是阅读的重点了。
4	动词不定式	放在动词后做目的状语 I come here to help you.	目的状语是考点所在，不能忽略。
5	状语从句	重点依赖于状语从句的连词来判断主句和从句的逻辑关系，比如when引导时间状语从句，although引导让步状语从句	根据状语从句的类型，确定哪些句子可以忽略，哪些需要重视。比如，原因状语不能忽略，让步状语则可以忽略。具体讲解见"基础能力之阅读惯用十大句式"部分。

除了动词不定式结构和特定的状语从句外，其他状语部分都是起修饰作用的，是英语句式大树中的枝条部分，是考生理解句子主干的障碍物。因此，我们在阅读中首先要忽略状语，直接定位到句子的谓语动词部分，才能更快、更准确地理解句意。

例如：The President said at a press conference dominated by questions on yesterday's election results that he could not explain why the Republicans had suffered such a widespread defeat.

本句结构复杂，首先在"信号词"处分割句子，本句就被拆分为：

➢ The President said

➢ at a press conference dominated by questions on yesterday's election results（介宾结构拆分）

➢ that he could not explain（连词拆分）

➢ why the Republicans had suffered such a widespread defeat（关系词拆分）

在动词said后出现了介宾结构at a press conference，我们知道动词后的介宾结构一般为状语，所以我们首先忽略该部分。句子"The President said…that he could not explain"中，that引导said的宾语从句，从句是"说"的内容。因此这部分翻译为："总统说他不能解释为什么共和党遭到了如此的惨败。"

再阅读介宾结构at a press conference（在记者招待会上），是"说"这个动作发生的地点，接下来的内容是conference的后置定语。在逐层修饰部分，我们已经介绍了对它的分析，请大家参考。所以整句话可以翻译为："在主要问及昨天选举结果的记者招待会上，总统说他不能解释为什么共和党遭到了如此的惨败。"

通过上面的例子可以看出首先忽略状语结构的重要性。

3. 插入结构

（1）插入结构在句式分析中的作用

插入结构是书面语中经常出现的高级结构，尤其是在说明文和议论文中被高频率地使用。所谓"插入"，就是把紧密相连的两个语法成分分割开，这种分割为考生在阅读中设置了两个障碍。

第一，使考生无法形成连贯思维来理解句意。

当我们读完一个名词，接着就读到一个动词时，我们的思维是连贯的。而如果我们在读过一个名词后，马上看到的是后置定语，我们的思维就会被打乱，等读到谓语时，早已经不知其主语身在何处了。

例如："Scientific" creationism, which is being pushed by some for "equal time" in the classrooms whenever the scientific accounts of evolution are given, is based on religion, not science.

本来"Scientific" creationism和is based on religion是紧密相连的主语和谓语，而中间插入了which引导的非限制性定语从句，就使我们的思维发生间断，无法理解句子了。而如果我们不去阅读which从句的内容，那这句话就比较容易了。本句可以翻译为：所谓"科学的"造物主义理论的基础是宗教而不是科学，但在教学时每当对进化论进行科学论述时，有些人就用它来争得"同等数量的学时"。

当然考生也可以用忽略后置定语的方法来找到主谓，但是细心的读者会发现，which这个定语从句出现在两个逗号中间，这两个逗号其实就是插入语的标志，如果我们能直接略读则阅读速度就更快了。

第二，阅读插入成分会消耗考生很多时间，而真正留给做题的时间就变得有限。

例如：Nancy Dubler, director of Montefiore Medical Center, contends that the principle will shield doctors who insisted that they could not give patients sufficient mediation to control their pain if that might hasten death.

句中Nancy Dubler的谓语是contends（认为），而director of Montefiore Medical Center是插入结构，是Nancy的职位，属于无用信息，出题人用此来转移考生的注意力。本句的意思是：蒙特非奥里医疗中心主任南希·道布勒认为，这项原则将保护一些医生，他们直到现在还坚持说，在大量药物可能加速病人死亡的情况下，他们不能给病人开足够的药来帮助他们止痛。

通过以上分析可以得出如下结论：面对插入成分，首先要忽略其存在，直接把紧密相连的语法部分连接在一起。其次，如果细节类题涉及插入成分的内容，则我们再通过仔细阅读插入成分来解题。

（2）插入结构的组成及应用

那么，插入结构出现在句子中的哪些位置呢？什么结构可以做插入成分呢？插入结构的标志又是什么呢？请看如下的表格。

序　号	位　置	结　构	备　注
1	主谓之间	后置定语的6种形式充当插入成分	由于主语是名词，所以较长的后置定语就自然而然地将主谓分割开。
		同位语（表示职位、头衔、身份等）充当插入成分	
		状语结构充当插入成分	
2	谓宾之间	状语结构充当插入成分	插入结构多出现在两个逗号和两个破折号之间，但通常是两个逗号或破折号同时存在，缺一不可。否则的话，则可能是其他结构。
		"某人说"的结构（见第二组例句）	
3	短语之间	动词短语之间多是状语结构插入	
		名词短语之间多是后置定语插入	

下面我们再通过一系列例句来帮助考生体会忽略插入成分，找到句子的主干。

第一组例句：主谓之间插入成分，注意逗号和破折号的用法。

例1：This, *for those yet unaware of such a disadvantage*, refers to discrimination against those whose surnames begin with a letter in the lower half of the alphabet.

【句式解析】句子主干为：This refers to discrimination…，插入结构是for those…，是介宾短语，是整个句子的状语，在句中充当插入成分。

【译文】对于那些还没有意识到存在这种不公平待遇的人，这指的是歧视那些姓氏字母在字母表中排得靠后的人。

例2：Numerous other commercial enterprises, *from theaters to magazine publishers, from gas and electric utilities to milk processors*, bring better and more efficient services to consumers through the use of computers.

【句式解析】句子主干为：Numerous other commercial enterprises bring better and more efficient services…，两个from…to介宾短语是enterprise的后置定语，插入

在主语和谓语之间。介宾结构到底是状语还是定语，更多地需要从语义上来判断。注意与例1的区别。

【译文】许多其他商业企业，从剧院到杂志社，从燃气电力公司到牛奶加工厂，都通过计算机的使用给消费者带来更好、效率更高的服务。

例3：In the early industrialized countries of Europe the process of industrialization — *with all the far-reaching changes in social patterns that followed* — was spread over nearly a century, whereas nowadays a developing nation may undergo the same process in a decade or so.

【句式解析】句子主干为：the process of industrialization was spread over nearly a century，插入成分为with all the far-reaching changes...，是介宾短语，是process的后置定语，而不是句子的状语。

【译文】在先期实现工业化的欧洲国家中，其工业化进程以及随之而来的各种深刻的社会结构变革，持续了将近一个世纪之久，而如今一个发展中国家在10年左右就可能完成这个过程。

例4：Paul Ehrlich of Stanford University, *a pioneer of environmental studies,* argues the true enemies of science are those who question the evidence supporting global warming.

【句式解析】句子主干为：Paul Ehrlich argues the true enemies of science are those...，其中a pioneer of environmental studies是同位语充当插入成分，表明Paul的身份。在新闻报道体裁的文章中，引用某专家的言论，多采用这种句式结构，即人名＋职位＋动词（contend，maintain，hold，believe等）＋that引导的宾语从句。

【译文】作为环境研究的先驱者，斯坦福大学的保罗·埃利希认为，科学真正的敌人是那些对支持全球变暖的证据提出质疑的人。

例5：The emphasis on data gathered first-hand, *combined with a cross-cultural perspective brought to the analysis of cultures past and present*, makes this study a unique important social science.

【句式解析】句子主干为：The emphasis makes this study a unique important social science，插入成分为过去分词短语，是emphasis的后置定语，分裂了主语和谓语。

【译文】强调收集第一手资料，加上在分析过去和现在文化形态时采用跨文化视角，使得这一研究成为一门独特并且非常重要的社会科学学科。

第二组例句：谓语与宾语或谓语与表语之间插入

例1："I am not," he said, "a teacher."

【句式解析】he said分割了I am not a teacher。这种"某人说"在句子中间分割谓宾或系表的情况经常发生。

【译文】他说："我不是老师。"

例2：The existence of the giant clouds was virtually required for the Big Bang, *first put forward in the 1920s*, to maintain its reign as the dominant explanation of the cosmos.

【句式解析】句子主干为：The existence of the giant clouds was required for the Big Bang to maintain its reign...，插入语为first put forward in the 1920s，是过去分词短语做Big Bang的后置定语，分割了be required和其宾补to do sth.，连接在一起是be required to do sth.（被要求做某事）。

【译文】巨大的宇宙云的存在，实际上是20世纪20年代首创的大爆炸论得以保持其宇宙起源论主导地位所不可缺少的。

例3：The debate invited anyone with an opinion of the BBC — *including ordinary listeners and viewers* — to say what was good or bad about the Corporation, and even whether they thought it was worth keeping.

【句式解析】句子主干为：The debate invited anyone to say what was good or bad about...，插入结构是including分词短语，充当的后置定语，是递进修饰的结构，修饰anyone。它分割了invited sb. to do sth.中的动词和充当宾补的动词不定式。

【译文】该争论邀请所有对BBC持有见解的人——包括普通听众和观众——评说它的优劣，甚至讨论它有没有继续存在的必要。

第三组例句：短语之间插入

例句：Here is an example, *which I heard at a nurses' convention,* of a story which works well because the audience all shared the same view of doctors.

【句式解析】句子主干为：Here is an example of a story...，which引导的从句是example的后置定语，插在example of 这个短语中间。

【译文】下面举一个例子，它是我在一次护士大会上听到的。这个故事效果很好，因为听众对医生都有同样的看法。

综合长难句分析的第二个步骤可以看出，去掉修饰成分十分重要，这些修饰成分主要就是本节内所论述的后置定语结构、状语结构和插入结构。考生不仅要了解这些结构的组成和用法，同时还要达到十分熟练的程度，从而做到在阅读中形成条件反射，一看到这些结构就能明白出题人的意图所在，这是阅读取得高分的前提。

（三）简缩出句子主干后，再逐层分析句式

把长句在信息词处进行分割，然后再去掉所有的后置定语、状语、插入结构后，剩下的就是句子的主干。我们期望剩下的就是"名＋动＋名"的主谓宾结构，或者是主谓结构，再或者是"主＋谓＋宾＋宾补"结构，这种主干其实就是英语的简单句。

如果从句过多，那么就应该首先找到主句的主体部分（即主语、谓语和宾语），再确定从句的主体部分。如果从句中还有从句，则需要再确定下面一层从句的主、谓、宾。注意阅读时要一层一层地进行分析，先把同一层次的内容看完，再看下一层次的内容。

下面举例说明如何首先找到句子的主干，再来层层分析句子。

例1：A survey of new stories in 1996 reveals that the anti-science tag has been attached to many other groups as well, from authorities who advocated the elimination of the last remaining stocks of smallpox virus to Republicans who advocated decreased funding for basic research.

第一步，在信息词处分割。

➢ A survey of new stories in 1996 reveals

➢ that the anti-science tag has been attached to many other groups as well（从句连词处分割）

➢ from authorities（介宾处分割）

➢ who advocated the elimination / of the last remaining stocks / of smallpox virus（从句连词处分割）

➢ to Republicans（介宾处分割）

➢ who advocated decreased funding for basic research（从句连词处分割）

第二步，去掉修饰成分。

第一个that从句位于动词后，我们可以判断为宾语从句，属于主干部分，不能忽略；as well副词短语，是状语结构，可以忽略；from为介宾结构充当后置定语，修饰groups，可以忽略；第一个who引导定语从句，可以忽略；第二个who也引导定语从句，也可以忽略。

第三步，简缩出句子主干。

A survey reveals that the anti-science tag has been attached to many other groups. 这就是主句的主谓宾。然后我们再重点分析宾语从句中嵌套两个who引导的定语从句的情况。从句的主语是the anti-science tag（反科学标签），谓语是has been attached to（被贴到），宾语是many other groups（许多别的人群），后面用了一个from sb. who…to sb. who的结

构来举例解释这些groups包括什么人。

这句话的意思是：1996年进行的一次对新书的调查显示，"反科学"标签也被贴在了很多别的人群身上，包括提倡根除残余天花病毒的权威机构，以及提倡削减基础科学研究经费的民主党人。

例2：Today, stepladders carry labels several inches long that warn, among other things, that you might — surprise! — fall off.

第一步，在信息词处分割。

> stepladders carry labels several inches long

> that warn（从句连接that处分割）

> among other things（标点符号处分割）

> that you might（从句连接that处分割）

> — surprise! —（标点符号处分割）

> fall off（标点符号处分割）

第二步，去掉修饰成分。

首先读到：stepladders carry labels（梯子上贴着标签），主谓宾已经齐全，所以这就是主句的主谓宾。下面我们就要寻找枝条的结构。这个labels有两个修饰语：several inches long和一个that引导的从句，这两个后置定语是递进修饰的。among other things在两个逗号之间，是插入语，可忽略；"surprise!"在两个破折号间，也可忽略。

第三步，简缩出句子主干。

主句的主谓宾比较简单，而在that引导的定语从句中，主语是that（也就是labels），谓语是warn，宾语又是另一个that引导的从句，在warn和宾语从句中插入among other things，表示宾语的内容只是warn（警告）的众多内容中列举的一个。这个被列举的内容是fall off（摔下来），但在fall off之前又插入了一个"surprise！"。插入这个词是因为作者认为梯子警告fall off是一件令人吃惊的事，因为爬梯子本来就有摔下来的危险，但商家为了怕消费者控告，竟然将这么明显的事情也写进了警告语。

这个句子的阅读顺序应该是：

> 第一层stepladders carry labels several inches long that；

> 第二层是that warn that you might fall off；

> 最后看两个插入部分among other things和surprise。

综上所述，长句的分析理解需要综合运用后置定语、状语、插入结构以及我们高中时所熟悉的从句知识，这是考试的难点和出题人的热爱点，也是一切题目的基础。

考生经常发现，读懂带讲解的例句并不难，但是每当自己划分长句的时候，问题就出现了。这主要还是由于实践经验少，不能快速判断后置定语、状语、插入语和层层从句的结构。多做练习题会有助于句式分析能力的提高。

第三节　基础能力之阅读惯用十大句式

在了解了读英语长句的一般方法后，我们要详细为考生介绍在阅读考试中经常出现的十大惯用句式，这些惯用句式也是细节类题的命题点所在，在阅读中占有十分重要的地位。

这十大惯用句式包括：

- ➤ 定语从句
- ➤ 非谓语结构
- ➤ 状语从句
- ➤ 同位结构
- ➤ 并列结构
- ➤ 比较结构
- ➤ 分裂结构
- ➤ 倒装结构
- ➤ 强调结构
- ➤ 双否结构

下面，我们就为大家一一讲解这些结构的难点和考点。

一、定语从句

定语从句的简单标志是：名词＋连接词＋从句。一般连接词前是名词的为定语从句，因为它是后置定语的一种，用来修饰名词。

简单的定语从句的内容，比如先行词在从句中充当主语和宾语的情况，请参照本套丛书的语法分册进行学习。这里，主要为大家列举出定语从句的难点和考点所在。通常可以在定语从句上命题的，有如下5点。

序　号	难　点	考　点	阅 读 技 巧
1	属于树枝部分，不是句子主干	在寻找主句主谓宾时应当忽略，是第二个层次要考虑的内容，而不是首要考虑的内容。	在找到主句主谓宾后，可以将定语从句还原，即把先行词代入从句中，形成完整的句子。
2	省略连词的定语从句 the man (whom) I know	由于连词是我们分割句子的信息词，省略连词会给分割造成影响。	先行词只有做从句宾语时，其后才可以省略连词。所以一般当从句缺宾语，前面又有两个名词相连时，就属于这种情况。
3	which引导非限制性定语从句	要求考生判断which是指代一个词的意思，还是前面整个句子的意思。	如果看到"，+ which+谓语动词"结构，则多半就是非限制性定语从句。要依赖语义来判断其指代的部分。
4	介词提前的定语从句 the house in which we live	能否还原从句	用先行词替换which，然后把介词词组移至从句句末。这个介词词组要么和前面的动词构成搭配，要么就是其本身充当从句的状语。
5	when, where引导的定语从句 the house where we live	与when和where引导的状语从句进行区分	看到"n. +when/where+主谓宾"结构时，when/where多半是引导名词的定语从句，而不是整个句子的状语从句，考生会发现把when翻译成"当……的时候"，把where翻译成"在……地方"时，上下文不通。
		能否还原从句	把when/where替换成"介词+which"，再用中心词替换which，把介宾结构放到从句结尾，它多半是从句的时间或地点状语。

下面我们就举一些具体例子来解析其中的几个考点。

1. 非限制性定语从句，which指代名词

例句：The innovator will search for alternative courses, **which** may prove easier in the long run and are bound to be more interesting and challenging even if they lead to dead ends.

【句式解析】在这句话中，which引导非限制性定语从句，用来限定先行词courses，因为它和courses的语义连接得更为紧密。定语从句部分又带and连接的并列成分和even if引导的让步状语从句，使这个分句理解起来有一定的难度。其实我们只要找到句子的主干"The innovator will search for alternative courses."就可以解决问题了，不要让那些连词迷惑了你的视线。

【译文】即使这些方式可能会是死路一条，那些力求创新的人们也将寻找那些从长远来看更加浅显易懂、生动有趣、富于挑战的可替换方式。

2．非限制性定语从句，which指代主句

例句：Reducing the cost will tend to increase the supply offered by sellers and producers, which in turn will lower the price and permit more consumers to buy the product.

【句式解析】前半句我们去掉过去分词短语offered by sellers and producers这个后置定语的修饰成分，剩下的主干是Reducing the cost will tend to increase the supply。which引导的非限制性定语从句是我们第二层要分析的内容。从句的意思是会降低价格，我们发现，应该是主句的内容"降低成本会增加供应"会导致价格降低，所以which指代的是前面整个一句话的内容。

【译文】降低成本将会增加生产商和销售商的供货，这反过来就会降低价格，更多的消费者就能购买该产品。

3．介词提前的定语从句，介宾结构充当从句状语

例句：Indeed, there is evidence that the rate at which individuals forget is directly related to how much they have learned.

【句式解析】这句话的关键点不是对主句的理解而是对从句的理解，主句很清晰there is evidence，that引导同位语从句来解释evidence要说明的内容。而在这个同位语从句中，识别它的主干则是解决问题的关键：the rate is directly related to how much they have learned，句中的at which individuals forget是由"介词＋关系代词"引导的定语从句来修饰先行词rate，还原从句就变成了individuals forget at the rate，介宾短语充当从句的状语，看清楚这一点，句子也就变得十分简单了。

【译文】事实的确如此，那就是个人遗忘的速度与他们学习知识的多少密切相关。

4．介词提前的定语从句，介宾结构充当从句宾补，与动词构成搭配

例句：Now since the assessment of intelligence is a comparative matter we must be sure that the scale with which we are comparing our subjects provides a "valid" or "fair" comparison.

【句式解析】that引导的从句的主干是：the scale provides a "valid" or "fair" comparison，scale的定语从句是with which we are comparing our subjects，还原从句为we are comparing our subjects with the scale，介宾短语和动词compare形成词组，充当从句的宾补。这样分析了句子结构之后，我们就可以理解这句话了。

【译文】既然对于人的才智的评估是相比较得出的事实，所以我们必须确保当我们评价主体的时候所采用的标准是"有效的""公正的"。

5. 关系副词when和where引导的定语从句

例句：Or so the thinking has gone since the early 1980s when juries（陪审团）began holding more companies liable for their customers' misfortunes.

【句式解析】本句的主干清晰，即the thinking has gone，主语、谓语已经齐全；when引导的从句如果翻译为"当……的时候"（当陪审团开始认为更多的公司要对其客户的不幸负责的时候，自从20世纪80年代早期这种想法就不见了），上下文不通顺，可见when引导的是1980s的定语从句。我们首先将when变成in which，也就是in 1980s，再还原从句，将in 1980s放在从句的句末，juries（陪审团）began holding more companies liable for their customers' misfortunes in 1980s，介宾结构充当从句的时间状语。

【译文】自从20世纪80年代初期陪审团开始认为更多的公司要对其客户的不幸负责时起，这种想法就消失了。

二、非谓语结构

1. 非谓语结构和句子的完整性

我们都知道，句子最重要的特征就是有完整独立的主谓结构。什么样的词能构成独立的谓语部分？注意：do / does和is / am / are的各种时态变化都可以做谓语，但是单纯的to do / doing / done和to be / being的形式是不可以做谓语的。

通过"非谓语"这个称呼，我们可以知道：动名词、分词和动词不定式在改变动词形式的时候，把动词的词性也进行了转换。所以，一个看似句子的结构，如果没有独立的谓语部分，那它就不是句子，而是分词短语或者独立主格结构。

例如学生在作文中曾写出这样一句话：With as many as 120 varieties in existence, we discovering how cancer works.

with引导的是一个独立主格结构，在这个句子中做原因状语，也就是说"因为现存癌症有120种之多，所以……"。这句话的主语是we，因为单纯doing的形式是不可以做谓语的，所以在这个句子里，discovering就绝不可能是谓语。works虽然是谓语，但它是how cancer works这个从句的谓语，即discovering how cancer works，而不是主句的谓语。所以，这个句子的主句缺少谓语，是一个错句。

2. 动名词、分词和动词不定式的区别

实际上，这个词性的转换是两个系统，一个是动名词和分词，另一个是动词不定式。通过名称可知，"动名词"就是把动词转换为名词，"分词"就是把动词转换为形容词和副词；而"动词不定式"则是把动词转换为名词、形容词和副词，也就是除了动词之外的

实词词性。这两个系统的区别就在于：动名词和分词系统表示经常性或完成的动作；而动词不定式系统表示一次性或未来的动作。

我们可以通过下面的表格来理解它们三者的区别。

项　目	词　性	句子成分	例　子
不定式	名词	主语	*To die or not to die* is a question.（"要死"，表将来）
		宾语	I want *to come here*.
	形容词	定语	man *to shoot the bird*（将要开枪的人）
	副词	状语	I came here *to make money*.（目的状语）
		宾补	I expect you *to come*.
分词	形容词	定语	man *shooting the bird*（开枪的人）
	副词	状语	He came to the classroom, *singing*.（伴随状语）
		宾补	I saw him *coming*.（看的时候，他正前来）
动名词	名词	主语	*Forgetting* is adaptive.（表示经常性的动作）
		宾语	contribute to *doing the homework*（to为介词）

分词有现在分词（v.+ing）和过去分词（v.+ed），前者表示主动，后者表示被动。现在分词和动名词的形式一样，我们要从它充当的句子成分中来判断两者。因为动名词把动词变成了名词，所以在由名词充当的句子成分中（比如主语和宾语位置）出现了动词的-ing形式，那它就是动名词；在定语和状语位置的就是分词。

动名词的被动形式和过去分词的形式不同，前者是being + done的形式，后者是done的形式，无being。例如：Being beaten by him is her trouble.（被他打是她的苦恼。）动名词做主语，不可以写成：Beaten by him is her trouble.

3. 非谓语结构的考点及用法

了解非谓语结构的本质之后，我们为大家总结了非谓语结构在阅读中的8个重点。对于分词和动名词来说，最重要的就是要找到逻辑主语，即这个动词的施动者或被动者到底是谁。动词不定式的重点是要分清其句子成分，到底是主语、宾语、定语还是状语。请考生看如下表格。

序　号	项　目	考　点	阅读技巧
1	动名词	位于句首做主语	动名词做主语时，主谓之间无逗号，且只有一个动名词时，谓语动词永远是单数形式。而分词位于句首做伴随状语的时候，状语和主语、谓语之间有逗号相隔，且分词的逻辑主语为句子的主语。

（续）

序　号	项　目	考　点	阅读技巧
2	动名词	位于介词后充当宾语	做介词的宾语，只能使用动名词，不能使用动词不定式。特别是在介词to后，要用doing的形式，例如：contribute to doing sth.，这时to为介词，而不是动词不定式的符号。
3	分词	位于句首做伴随状语	一般与主语之间有逗号相隔，而且其逻辑主语就是主句主语；如果分词的逻辑主语与主句主语不一致，则要加上主语。
4		位于名词后做定语	分词的逻辑主语就是所修饰的名词。
5		独立主格	分词的逻辑主语与主句主语不一致，加上主语的形式。这是把两句话连接在一起的方法，即把某句话的谓语动词变成分词。
6		with + 名词+分词	这也是独立主格形式，表示伴随。
7	动词不定式	复合不定式	在不定式前加上疑问词，例如：how to do sth.。这只不过是给不定式加上了语义，其用法与动词不定式完全相同。
8		多重不定式套叠	want to do it to earn money to marry you这个例子中一共出现了3个动词不定式。第一个to do it为want的宾语，而后两个则为目的状语。在很多动词不定式出现的时候，多为目的状语。

下面举一些具体的例子来解析其中的几个考点。

（1）介词to后面的动名词用法

例句：To criticize it for such failure is roughly comparable **to criticizing** a thermometer for not **measuring** wind velocity.

【句式解析】本句话中动词不定式To criticize it做主语。谓语是is comparable to，是"和……进行比较"的意思，其中to是介词。criticizing是动名词，做介词的宾语。measuring也是动名词，做介词for的宾语。

【译文】因为这样的失败而批评它，就好像批评温度计不能测量风速一样。

（2）分词位于句末做状语

例句：At the same time these computers record which hours are busiest and which employees are the most efficient, **allowing** personnel and staffing assignments to be made accordingly.

【句式解析】本句的主谓语是computers record（计算机记录），其中record是动词。宾语为which引导的两个从句which hours are busiest（什么时段最忙）和which employees are the most efficient（哪些员工最有效率）。allowing是分词做状语，其逻辑主语是computer，用逗号与主干部分进行了分隔。

【译文】与此同时，这些计算机记录了最繁忙的时段和最有效率的员工，这样就使员工的工作任务得到了合理的分配。

（3）分词位于名词后做定语

例句：An invisible border divides those **arguing** for computers in the classroom on the behalf of students' career prospects and those **arguing** for computers in the classroom for broader reasons of educational reform.

【句式解析】句子主干为：An invisible border divides those...and those...（看不见的界限分割了那些……人和那些……人）。第一个arguing for在名词后，是定语，修饰those；第二个arguing for也是同样的句子成分。

【译文】一些人支持把计算机引入课堂是出于对学生就业前景的考虑，而另外一些人则是出于更广泛的教育改革的原因而支持这样做，一条并不明显的界限将这两派人分割开来。

（4）独立主格结构

例句：For a small group of students, professional training might be the way to go since well-developed skills, **all other factors being equal**, can be the difference between having a job and not.

【句式解析】句子的主干为professional training might be the way to go（职业化教育是前进的方向）。since引导原因状语从句，从句的主语是well-developed skills，谓语是can be the difference，其中all other factors being equal是独立主格结构，all other factors是逻辑主语，being是现在分词，做句子的状语。

【译文】对于一小部分学生来说，职业教育可能是可以选择的方向，因为在其他条件相同的情况下，完善的技术就是能否找到工作的关键。

（5）复合不定式

例句：**Where to** turn for expert information and **how to** determine which expert advice to accept are questions facing many people today.

【句式解析】句子的主语是两个复合不定式Where to turn for expert information和how to determine...，which expert advice to accept从句是determine的宾语，其中to accept是advice的定语，facing位于名词questions后，是其定语。

【译文】从哪里寻求专家的信息和如何决定采纳哪位专家的建议是现在许多人面临的问题。

三、状语从句

在阅读长句的时候，状语从句是树枝部分，是找到树干后，第二个层次要考虑的问题。判断从句是否为状语从句，主要看关系连词，比如since，when，if，lest等。由此可见，关系连词是状语从句的重点，状语从句的考点也是围绕它们展开的。状语从句的阅读重点主要有以下3点。

➢ 是否知道一些特殊的关系连词的意思，比如provided（如果）等。

➢ 是否知道哪些状语从句要详读，哪些要略读。

➢ 是否理解until，unless等引导的复杂状语从句的意思。

主要的关系连词总结如下。

序　号	连　词	考　点	阅 读 技 巧
1	when，if，after，before等	从句中无主语，连词后面接分词	当状语从句的主语和主句的主语一致时，为了避免重复，从句中可省略主语，把谓语动词变成分词。如果是主动语态，则为现在分词；如果是被动语态，则为过去分词。例如：When meeting you, I felt very happy.（时间状语从句的主语就是主句的主语）
2	while	"尽管"的意思	位于句首，和although同义，是可以略读的从句，因为主句才是作者真正的意思。
3	although	让步状语从句	可以略读的从句，因为主句才是作者真正的意思。
4	in that	"由于"的意思	因果状语从句，是考点所在，因此是详读部分。
5	provided	"如果"的意思	条件状语从句，是考点所在，因此是详读部分。
6	lest	"以防"的意思	考点所在，因此是详读部分，后面可以接虚拟语气。
7	in case	"以防"的意思	考点所在，因此是详读部分，后面可以接虚拟语气。
8	even if	"即使"的意思	考点所在，因此是详读部分。
9	as long as	"只要"的意思	考点所在，因此是详读部分。
10	only if	"只要"的意思	考点所在，因此是详读部分。
	if only	"（某事）该多好啊！"的意思	虚拟语气的标志词。例如：If only I could fly. 我要是能飞该多好啊！
11	until	动作的截止点	I will wait for you until 7.（是"等"这个动作的截止点）
	not until	动作的开始点	I didn't get up until 7.（是"起床"的开始点）
12	unless	if not	不要翻译为"除非"，把从句变成否定句即可。

下面举一些具体例子来解析这些考点。

1. while和although引导的状语从句要略读

例句：**Although** Fisher wrote before the mathematical theory of games had been developed, his theory contains the essential feature of a game that the best strategy to adopt depends on what others are doing.

【句式解析】although引导的让步状语从句，重点在句子的后半句话，而前半句的让步成分很少作为出题点，故读although引导的句子时可以略读前半句话，把重心放在后半句。本句话的主干为his theory contains the essential feature，that放在名词后，是递进修饰关系，修饰feature，是同位语从句。

【译文】虽然费希尔是在数学博弈理论建立起来之前发表其著作的，但他的理论已囊括了博弈的本质特征——所能采用的最佳策略取决于他人在做什么。

2. until和not until句子的区别

例句：You are not in Stage 3 until your iron reserves go to zero.

　　　　Until recently, it is not easy for college students to find a job.

【句式解析】until本身的含义是动作的截止点，而not until则是开始点。

【译文】第一句话的意思是："当你的铁储备接近0时，你才进入第三阶段。"而第二句话的意思是："大学生现在找工作不容易。"

3. unless句式

例句：Radiation can cause serious consequence at the lowest level unless the damaged cells can reproduce themselves.

【句式解析】我们首先把unless引导的从句变成否定句：the damaged cells can not reproduce themselves，然后把unless变成if，则此句的意思为：如果受损的细胞没有自我复制，那么最低量的辐射就会造成严重的后果。如果我们没有这样分析句子，而直接把unless翻译为"除非"，则该句变为：除非受损的细胞自我复制，那么最低量的辐射就会造成严重的后果。这和原来的句意正好相反，这也是考生经常出错的地方。

【译文】如果受损的细胞不能自我复制，那么最低量的辐射就会造成严重的后果。

4. 状语从句的省略

例句：While talking to you, your could-be employer is deciding whether your education, your experience, and other qualifications will pay him to employ you.

【句式解析】本句的主干为：your could-be employer is deciding whether...其中，whether引导decide的宾语从句。宾语从句的主语是your education, your experience, and other qualifications; 谓语动词是will pay，him为宾语，to employ you动词不定式为宾补。句子开头While引导状语从句，因为其主语就是主句的主语your could-be employer（招聘人），所以将从句的主语省略，把谓语动词变为现在分词。

【译文】当招聘人在和你谈话的时候，他在判断你的教育程度、经历和其他的资质是否值得他来雇用你。

四、同位结构

在长句中，同位结构是细节，是修饰名词的，应该是第二个层次要考虑的问题。在阅读考题中，同位结构是重点考点，每年都有涉及同位语的细节类题。其考查点主要有如下2个。

序 号	项 目	考 点	阅 读 技 巧
1	同位语从句	与定语从句的区别	定语从句先行词在从句中充当句子成分，而同位语从句的先行词在从句中不做任何成分。即同位语从句的主谓宾是齐全的，that只起连接作用；而定语从句的连接代词that在从句中做主语或宾语。
2	N1, +N2+后置定语（N2是N1的同位语，和其意思相同）	N2是N1的简单重复	例如：I like the girl, the girl who has the same opinion with me. 第二个the girl就是重复第一个the girl, who引导的定语从句做后置定语。
		N2代替N1	例如：I like your gift, a red scarf bought in France. 其中a red scarf就是指前面的gift。bought过去分词短语做后置定语。
		N2代替前面一句话的内容	例如：Every student should study hard, the important factor for a good school. 其中the important factor就是指前面的主句"每个学生都要努力学习"。

下面举一些具体例子来解析这两个考点。

1. 同位语从句充当后置定语

例句：In talking to some scientists, particularly younger ones, you might gather the **impression that** they find the "scientific method" — a substitute for imaginative thought.

【句式解析】本句的主干为：you might gather the impression（你可能得到如下印象），In talking...是介宾结构，放在句首做状语，that放在名词impression后，是后置定语。因为从句中they find the "scientific method" — a substitute...主谓宾都齐全，that没有充当任何成分，所以为同位语从句，解释impression的具体内容。

【译文】当谈及一些科学家时，特别是年轻的科学家们，你可能会有这样的印象：他们发现了科学的方法而不是虚幻的想象。

2．"N1，+N2+后置定语"的句型

例句：Rather, we have a certain conception of the **American citizen**, **a character** who is incomplete if he cannot assess how his livelihood and happiness are affected by things outside of himself.

【句式解析】本句的主干为：we have a certain conception（我们有一定的概念），of the American citizen是介宾短语做后置定语，修饰conception，概念是关于美国人的。a character是N2，是American citizen的同位语，who引导的定语从句修饰a character，if引导定语从句中的状语从句，how引导状语从句中assess的宾语从句。

【译文】我们对于美国市民有了一定的概念—— 如果他不能估算出身外之物在多大程度上影响他的生计和快乐，那他就不是纯粹的美国人。

五、并列结构

1．并列结构的实质

首先看下面三个句子：

➤ A long-held view of the history of the English colonies has been as following.（人们一直拥有如下几点关于英国殖民地历史的观点。）

➤ England's policy toward these colonies before 1763 was controlled by commercial interests.（1763年以前，英国对这些殖民地的政策主要是由商业利益决定的。）

➤ A change to a more imperial policy generated the tensions that ultimately led to the American Revolution.（进一步向着帝国主义政策的方向而改变，产生了紧张局势，最终导致了美国革命。）

以上三句话的意思表达已然完整清晰，但是为了增加阅读难度，出题人硬是把这三句话用and并列结构把两个that引导的表语从句糅合在一起。

A long-held view of the history of the English colonies that became the United States has been **that** England's policy toward these colonies before 1763 was controlled by commercial interests **and that** a change to a more imperial policy, dominated by expansionist militarist objectives, generated the tensions that ultimately led to the American Revolution.

从这个例子可以看出，并列结构是通过并列连词把形式相同的部分连接在一起的一种语言形式，是把句子写长的一种重要方法。它有几个特殊的要求。

（1）前后并列的部分，形式必须一致，即动词和动词并列、名词和名词并列、从句和从句并列、句子和句子并列。如果形式不一致，则是语法错误。

（2）如果是三者或三者以上并列，则中间要有逗号，在最后一个并列部分前加并列连词，而不必在每个并列部分的前面加上并列连词。例如：swimming, playing chess and dancing，而不能写成swimming, and playing chess and dancing。细心的考生可能会遇到如下情况：dancing and singing and swimming，这并不是语法错误，它是词组dancing and singing 和动名词swimming先并列，dancing和singing再并列，因为dancing and singing语义接近。

（3）并列连词并不只有and，还有一些其他的词或词组，分别代表不同的逻辑关系，请考生将此记牢。例如：

> but表示转折关系。

> or表示选择关系。

> for表示因果关系，是"由于"的意思，连接并列的两个句子。

> rather than表示否定关系，是"而不是"的意思。

> not... but...否定前者，肯定后者，是"不是……而是……"的意思。

> whether... or...表示选择关系。

> neither... nor...表示否定两者。

> both... and...，not only... but also...表示肯定两者。

2．如何找并列关系

根据并列前后的语法成分必须一致的原则，可以采用三个步骤来找到并列关系。

第一步，在并列连词and，but等处分割句子，然后定位到并列连词后面的内容。

第二步，根据并列连词后面内容的形式，向前找第一个与其形式一样的部分。

第三步，找到并列的内容后，把并列部分拆分为原始的分句结构。

下面举例说明如上三个步骤。

Over and over again, the Revolutionary generation asserted **that** the welfare of the Republic rested upon an educated citizenry **and that** schools would be the best means of educating the citizenry in civic values and the obligations.

第一步，在and处拆分，并定位到and后面的内容that。

第二步，由于that是从句的连词，我们也要向前寻找从句的连词，在asserted后找到第一个that，于是我们可以判定是asserted的两个并列宾语从句。

第三步，将句子拆分为：

➤ The Revolutionary generation asserted that the welfare of the Republic rested upon an educated citizenry.（革命一代宣称：共和国的安宁依赖于受教育的人民。）

➤ The Revolutionary generation asserted that schools would be the best means of educating the citizenry in civic values and the obligations.（革命一代宣称：上学受教育是培养市民价值观和责任感的最好方式。）

【译文】革命一代一遍又一遍地指出：共和国的安宁依赖于受教育的人民，上学受教育是培养市民价值观和责任感的最好方式。

可以看出，一旦把并列成分拆开，句意就变得比较容易理解。由此可见，并列结构是英文句式"大树"分叉的部分，如果能把枝杈分开来看，理解起来就容易得多。所以，写作是把语义相关的中文短句用并列的形式连成长句，而阅读则是把英文的长句拆成短句的过程。

3．并列结构的主要模式

在并列结构中，主要有以下几种模式是考生经常无法辨认出的，通常是考点所在，请看下面的表格。

序　号	项　目	模　式	阅读技巧
1	介词的并列	介词……＋and＋介词……	如果并列连词后是介词，到前面找与这个介词一样的介词，或者其他的介词，而不要定位到其他词性的词身上（见"介词的并列"）。
2	从句的并列	从句连词……＋and＋从句连词（that，what，which等）……	如果并列连词后出现that等，不是that这个代词和前面某个名词并列，更多的情况是从句的并列，找相同的连词，或类似的连词。写作中注意，写并列从句时，一般不能省略连词（见"从句的并列"）。
3	句子的并列	主谓宾＋and＋主谓宾	并列连词后出现he／she等，很大程度上是句子的并列，而不是he／she跟前面句子主语或宾语的名词并列。判断是否是句子的并列，关键还是要看并列连词后的名词后面有没有动词（见"句子的并列"）。
4	两个并列连词	both A and B nor A but B whether A or B neither A nor B not only A but also B	如果是两个并列连词组成的句子，则并列连词后的内容必然是并列的。在阅读句子的时候，连词只是表明肯定或否定的逻辑关系，我们可以把连词当成插入成分对待。之后，我们再拆分句子（见"两个并列连词的并列"）。

下面举例说明这四种并列模式。

（1）介词的并列

例句：It applies equally **to** traditional historians who view history as only external and internal criticism of sources **and to** social science historians who equate their activity with specific techniques.

【句式解析】本句的句子主干为：It applies **to** traditional historians，后面的who view history as only external and internal criticism of sources是historians的后置定语，属于"定语从句充当后置定语"的情况；and处分割，后面是介词to，我们就要找前面的to，出现在applies的后面，于是把句子拆分为：

➢ It applies equally **to** traditional historians.

➢ It applies equally **to** social science historians.

historians后面的who equate their activity with...是定语从句，修饰先行词social science historians。

【译文】传统的历史学家把历史仅看成对史料的内部和外部的批评，社会科学历史学家把科研看作具体的技巧，它适用于他们两者。

（2）从句的并列

例句：And it is imagined by many **that** the operations of the common mind can be by no means compared with these processes, **and that** they have to be acquired by a sort of special training.

【句式解析】本句的主干是：it is imagined by many。其中it是形式主语，而that引导的从句才是真正的主语。由于这个从句较长，为了避免头重脚轻，使用it来代替that引导的主语从句。主语从句的主干是the operations can be compared with these processes，by no means是状语，表示否定含义，是"绝不"的意思。然后，我们在and处拆分，因为后面出现了that，我们首先想到的是从句的并列，向前寻找另外一个that，它在many后面，所以可以判断出是两个主语从句并列，因此把句子拆分为：

➢ It is imagined by many that the operations of the common mind can be by no means compared with these processes.

➢ It is imagined by many that they have to be acquired by a sort of special training.

【译文】大家都能想象得到，普通大脑的思维是不能和这些方法进行比较的，而且这些思维方法必须通过特殊的培训才能掌握。

（3）句子的并列

例句：The manager was in more direct relation with the men and their demands, **but** he **had seldom had** that familiar personal knowledge of the workmen which the employer had often had in the old family firms.

【句式解析】逗号前是一个简单句，主语是The manager，系表结构为：was in more direct relation... 并列连词but后出现的he是第二个简单句的主语，因为后面出现谓语动词had seldom had，所以是两个简单句的并列。在第二个分句中，which引导定语从句，做knowledge的后置定语，属于递进修饰的形式。

【译文】经理直接和员工接触并处理他们的要求，但是却不了解职工的个人信息，而这通常是旧式家族企业中一个管理者应该知道的。

（4）两个并列连词的并列

例句：The casual friendliness of many Americans should be interpreted **neither** as superficial **nor** as artificial, **but** as the result of a historically developed cultural tradition.

【句式解析】本句话共有3个并列连词：neither，nor和but，其后面的as superficial，as artificial和as the result是并列的。我们可以忽略这些连词，直接连成句，因为它们只是表示肯定或否定的关系，于是句子可以拆分为：

> The casual friendliness...should be interpreted as superficial.（由于有neither，所以是否定）

> The casual friendliness...should be interpreted as artificial.（由于有nor，所以是否定）

> The casual friendliness...should be interpreted as the result of...tradition.（由于有but，所以是肯定）

【译文】这种很随意的美国式朋友关系并不意味着肤浅和做作，而是美国传统文化发展的结果。

六、比较结构

than句型是考生比较熟悉的内容，这里主要讲解一个经常在阅读理解中出现的复杂的比较结构，那就是as... as...句型。

为了理解该词组，需要注意以下几个位置：

| A | **as** | B | **as** | C |

可以分以下四步理解该词组。

第一步：从C位置入手，由于as是连词，我们首先要在第一个as前的句子中寻找C的并列成分，假设我们找到了A。这个并列既有可能是名词的并列，也有可能是句子的并列。

第二步：忽略第一个as，把A和B直接连成句子。

第三步：本词组的含义就是，A和C在"B位置中的形容词或副词"方面是一致的，据此，理解句意。

第四步：根据中文表达习惯，翻译句子。

下面用具体例子来说明这四步。

例1：There are almost **as** many definitions of history **as** there are historians.

【句式解析】首先从第二个as后入手，是一个句子there are historians，然后读主句，发现它和There are...这个句子并列；第二步，我们忽略第一个as，把主句连接成为There are almost many definitions of history；第三步，"有历史学家"和"有历史定义"在B位置中的形容词many上是一致的；第四步，这句话的意思是："有多少历史学家，就有多少对历史的定义。"

例2：I was **as** interested in the famous people advertising the service **as** I was in ordinary people talking about the life-transforming help they had received.

【句式解析】首先从第二个as后入手，这是一个句子：I was in ordinary people，再阅读主句就能发现它和I was...是并列的；第二步，忽略第一个as，把主句连接成为I was interested in the famous people advertising the service（我对做广告的名人很感兴趣）；第三步，"我对名人"和"我对普通人"在B位置中的形容词interested（感兴趣）方面是一致的；第四步，这句话的意思是："我对为此服务做广告的名人很感兴趣，同时，对于那些谈论自己接受了改变命运帮助的普通人，我也同样很感兴趣。"

七、分裂结构

分裂结构就是把紧密相连的语法成分分割开来，这些成分是英语句式"树干"中的蛀虫，因此要把它们去掉，以免影响主干。找到主干之后，可以再读一下分裂结构，这是第二层次的内容。

分裂结构的4个考点系统总结如下。

序 号	考 点	位 置	结构及范例	备 注
1	插入结构（详见P26）	主谓之间	后置定语的6种形式充当插入成分	因为主语是名词，所以较长的后置定语就自然而然地将主谓分割开。
			同位语表示职位、头衔、身份等，充当插入成分	
			状语充当插入成分	
		谓宾之间	状语结构充当插入成分	插入结构多出现在两个逗号或两个破折号之间，但通常都是两个逗号或破折号同时存在，缺一不可。否则可能是其他结构。
			"……说"的结构	
		词组之间	动词短语间多是状语结构插入	
			名词短语间多是后置定语插入	
2	谓语分割主语和其后置定语	名词和后置定语之间	主语+谓语（很短）+后置定语（详见P22"后置定语的使用"部分）	因为谓语比起后置定语来很短，所以为了避免头重脚轻而采取分裂结构。
3	宾补分割动词和宾语	动宾之间	动词+宾补+宾语（熟悉常见的动词词组）	动词词组的重要用法
4	紧密相连的词组被修饰成分分割	词组间	from A+后置定语+to B，如果后置定语很长，则看到to B时，就应知道和from相连（熟悉常见的动词词组）	要求对词组深刻把握

1. 谓语分割主语和其后置定语

例句：The **sense** is growing **that** Americans need to turn things round fast, militarily and politically, if they ensure that events are not out of control.

【句式解析】本句的主干为：The sense is growing（意识在增长），that引导sense的同位语从句。由于谓语is growing很短，同位语从句很长，所以中心词sense和其后置同位语被分割了。同位语从句的主语为Americans，谓语是need，不定式to turn things round fast充当need的宾语，militarily and politically在两个逗号间，是状语结构充当的插入语，可以忽略。后面的if引导条件状语从句，that引导状语从句中ensure的宾语从句。

【译文】美国人越来越意识到：要让局势不失控的话，就需要马上在政治上和军事上行动起来。

2. 宾补分割动词和宾语

例句：The goal of all will be to try to **explain** to a confused and often unenlightened citizenry **that** there are not two equally valid scientific theories for the origin and evolution of universe and life.

【句式解析】本句的主干为：The goal will be to try to explain that…to a citizenry. 其中，to try动词不定式做表语，to explain动词不定式做try的宾语。explain的宾语是后面that there are not…宾语从句，to a citizenry是宾补。explain词组的正常语序应该为：explain sth. to sb.（向某人解释某事），但由于宾语从句很长，则用宾补分割了动词和其宾语。

【译文】所有的目标就是向迷惘、懵懂的公民解释，没有两种同样合理的科学理论解释了宇宙和生命的起源。

3. 紧密相连的词组被分割

例句：Each of these characteristics sharply **distinguishes** the 21,000 people who left for New England in the 1630's **from** most of the approximately 377,000 English people who had immigrated to America by 1700.

【句式解析】本句的主干为：Each of these characteristics distinguishes the 21,000 people from most of the 377,000 English people。其中distinguishes A from B是固定词组，意思是"把A从B中区分出来"。who left for…为定语从句，做21,000 people的后置定语，分割了distinguishes和from，考生只有先忽略后置定语，才可以把词组连接在一起。who had immigrated to America也是定语从句，充当后置定语，修饰English people。

【译文】这些特点中的每一项，都使17世纪30年代移居新英格兰的21 000人与截至1700年移居美洲的约377 000个英国人中的绝大多数鲜明地区分开来。

八、倒装结构

倒装结构是一种特殊的句式，在阅读中出现的频率并不是很高，但是这种句式一旦出现，就有可能成为细节类题的考点。它主要有三个考点：一个是完全倒装；一个是部分倒装；还有一个就是as的特殊句式。请看下面的表格，特别是阅读技巧部分。

序　号	考　点	结构及范例	阅 读 技 巧
1	完全倒装	（状语＋）谓语＋主语 例：Here comes the bus. The bus comes here.（正常语序）	状语一般为副词短语，谓语没有任何助动词，不论是什么形式，就直接置于主语前。阅读时要把其语序变成"主语＋谓语＋状语"。

（续）

序　号	考　点	结构及范例	阅　读　技　巧
2	部分倒装	部分倒装标志词＋助动词＋主语＋谓语 例：Neither did I come to the party yesterday.	部分倒装的标志词主要有： ➤ 表示否定关系的副词，比如neither，nor 等。 ➤ so位于句首，表示"也"。 ➤ only位于句首，表示"只有"的意思。 ➤ not only位于句首，表示"不仅"的意思。 ➤ "hardly…when"和"no sooner…than…"句型需要部分倒装，且从句需要使用过去完成时。 阅读时把这种句型变成：主语＋谓语（陈述句语序）＋部分倒装标志词
3	as，though的倒装	名词/形容词/副词＋as/though＋主语＋谓语 例："Teacher as I am…（尽管我是一名老师……）"这句话相当于"Although I am a teacher…（让步状语从句）"。	➤ 如果表语是名词，则在使用倒装句的时候，名词前不能加不定冠词或定冠词。 ➤ 如果是主谓宾结构，则不能将宾语提到句首使用该倒装句式。例如下面的错误：you as I beat。 ➤ 如果是主谓宾结构，在使用倒装时，as的前面只能是状语，而把整个主谓宾置于后面。例如：severely as I beat you（尽管我打你打得很重）。

　　通过上面的表格可以看出，在阅读倒装句的时候，不熟练的考生应尽量把句子结构改为正常语序，这样就不会造成理解障碍了。当熟练掌握这种结构之后，就可以不用转变语序来理解句意了。下面举几个例子演示转变句式。

　　1．"状语+谓语+主语"的完全倒装结构

　　例句：**Out of** our emotional experiences with objects and events **comes** a social feeling of agreement that certain things and actions are "good" and others are "bad".

　　【句式解析】因为本句开头是一个副词短语Out of…，紧接着是动词comes，这时谓语动词已经出现，而没有出现名词主语，所以可以判断这个句子符合"状语＋谓语＋主语"的结构。由此分析可知句子的主语是a social feeling of agreement，谓语是comes，状语是Out of our emotional experiences，本句的正常语序为：a social feeling of agreement comes out of our emotional experiences。that引导的从句是同位语从句，修饰feeling，属于递进修饰的结构。

【译文】某些事物和行为是好的，而另外一些是不好的——这种社会认同感来自我们对物体和事件的情感体验。

2. "谓语＋主语"的完全倒装结构

例句：**Scattered** around the globe **are** more than 100 small regions of isolated volcanic activity known to geologists as hot spots.

【句式解析】掌握倒装结构的关键是找到主句，然后将它还原为正常语序："More than 100 small regions are scattered around the globe."通过这个办法，理解倒装句就变简单了。of isolated volcanic activity是介宾结构做后置定语，修饰名词regions；known to geologists as hot spots为过去分词短语做后置定语，也修饰regions，属于递进修饰的逻辑关系。

【译文】被地理学家认为是热点的孤立的火山活动区域，有100多个零零星星地分布于全球各处。

3. so位于句首，表示"也"的意思，部分倒装

例句：Nonstop waves of immigrants played a role, too — and **so did** bigger crops of babies as yesterday's "baby boom" generation reached its child-bearing years.

【句式解析】and引导了两个并列句，第二个分句中as引导状语从句，表示因果关系。其中，did就是前面played a role的意思。

【译文】绵延不断的移民潮，还有当年"婴儿潮"时期出生的孩子已经到了生育年龄，这些因素都在发挥作用。

4. 否定词位于句首，部分倒装

例句：**Nor**, if regularity and conformity to a standard pattern are as desirable to the scientist as the writing of his papers would appear to reflect, **is** management to be blamed.

【句式解析】本句的主干为："**Nor is** management to be blamed."if引导的状语从句在两个逗号之间，是插入成分，所以应当首先忽略。找到主干后，我们再阅读插入成分，它是as…as…句型。首先我们阅读第二个as后的内容，writing of his papers would appear to reflect（他的论文要反映的），再忽略第一个as，连成句为regularity and conformity to a standard pattern are desirable to the scientist（科学家想看到规律性和与某种标准模式相符的一致性）。第一个as前的内容和第二个as后的内容在desirable方面是一致的，本部分可以翻译为：如果像他的论文所反映的那样，科学家也想看到规律性和与某种标准模式相符的一致性。

【译文】如果像他的论文所反映的那样，科学家也想看到规律性和与某种标准模式相符的一致性，那么管理人员也是无可指责的。

九、强调结构

强调结构主要就是指"It is / was...that..."句式。理解这个句式需要考生注意以下3点：

（1）本结构只有两种时态，即is和was的形式，没有完成时。

（2）本结构不能强调谓语动词，也就是is或was后面不能出现谓语动词。

（3）It is / was...that...没有任何语法作用，只起到加强语气的作用，也就是说，把"It is / was...that..."去掉后剩下的内容应该是一个完整的句子。例如：It is you that help me. 把It is和that去掉，就剩下you help me，正好是一个句子，本句强调的是主语。再例如：It is you that we love. 把It is和that去掉，剩下you和we love，调整语序后，变为：we love you，强调的是宾语。所以，即使It is / was后出现复数名词，也不可以把is / was变为are / were。

在阅读强调句时，为了理解句意，可以把"It is / was...that..."去掉，然后把剩下的部分连接成句。请看下面的例句。

例1：Perhaps **it is** humankind's long suffering at the mercy of flood and drought **that** makes the idea of forcing the waters to do our bidding so fascinating.

【句式解析】把句中的it is和that去掉，剩下的部分是humankind's long suffering at the mercy of flood and drought和makes the idea of forcing the waters to do our bidding so fascinating，这两者之间是主谓关系。

【译文】也许因为人类长期饱受洪水和干旱之苦，所以我们想尽办法来协调水源的想法十分具有吸引力。

例2：Thus, in the American economic system **it is** the demand of individual consumers, coupled with the desire of businessmen to maximize profits and the desire of individuals to maximize their incomes, **that** together determines what shall be produced and how resources are used to produce it.

【句式解析】在本句中，coupled with the desire...这个过去分词短语在两个逗号之间，是插入成分，所以首先应当忽略。简缩出句子主干it is the demand of individual consumers that together determines...后，可以看出这是个强调句型，然后再把it is和that去掉，剩下的结构为"the demand of individual consumers determines what shall be produced and how resources are used to produce it"。其中，what shall be produced是determines的宾语从句，and后是连接副词how，所以how引导的从句和前面的what从句并列，也是determines

的宾语从句。在插入成分中，and后的the desire和前面的the desire of businessmen并列，都是with的宾语。

【译文】因此，在美国的经济体系中，正是客户的需求、商家实现利益最大化的愿望和个人希望工资最大化的愿望，一起决定了生产产品的种类和如何使用资源来生产这些产品。

十、双否结构

双否结构一共有两类：一类是两个否定词出现在一个简单句内；另一类是主从句双重否定结构，即两个否定词分别出现在主句和从句中。

在第一种情况下，双重否定句结构形式主要体现在：前面一个否定词，往往是not，后面直接连用另一个否定词，即两个否定词之间没有其他词出现；但是偶尔也会在它们之间出现一些隐含情感的程度副词，如so，very，too，much等。

例如：It is **not impossible** to pass the Band-Four examination next time if you work harder. （如果你更加努力学习的话，下次通过四级考试还是有可能的。）

在第二种情况下，主句否定时常借助一般否定词（即not）或绝对否定词（如no，nothing，nobody，never等）；从句否定同样也可借助一般否定词或绝对否定词，但也可以使用一些含有否定含义的连词，如unless等，或是含有否定含义的"关系代词+but"。

例如：In the neighborhood there is **nobody** who **does** not know me. （在这儿，我绝对是个名人。）

在阅读中出现如上两种双否结构时，要把两个否定词全部去掉，组织出新的句子，这样就可以理解句意了。请看下面的分析：

1. 句内双否

例句：No language is perfect, and if we admit this truth, we must also admit that it is **not unreasonable** to investigate the relative merits of different languages or of different details in languages.

【句式解析】and后出现if从句，由于前面没有同样的从句，可知and连接两个并列分句，if从句是第二个分句的状语从句。第二个句子的主干为：we must also admit that...，that引导admit的宾语从句。宾语从句的主干为：it is **not unreasonable** to investigate...，这是一个句内双否结构，直接把not unreasonable变成it is reasonable to investigate...。or是并列连词，后面是介词of，所以of different details与前面的of different languages并列，都是merits的后置定语。

【译文】没有任何语言是尽善尽美的，假如我们承认这一真理，我们同样也必须承认，对不同语言的相对优势或对语言中的不同细节进行分析，这并非不合情理。

2．主从句间的双否

例句：Perhaps he believed that he could **not** criticize American foreign policy if he **did not** endanger the support for civil rights that he had won from the federal government.

【句式解析】句子主干为 "he believed that..."，that引导的是believed的宾语从句。宾语从句中又套了if引导的状语从句，且宾语从句的谓语和状语从句的谓语均是否定形式，我们把它们全部去掉后，可以得到：he could criticize American foreign policy if he endanger the support for civil fights。that在fights后，引导定语从句做fights的后置定语。

【译文】或许他认为，如果他批评美国的外交政策，这必将危及他从联邦政府那里业已赢得的对民权运动的支持。

> **Tips**：
>
> 分析英语句式结构时，需注意以下几点：
>
> ➤ 阅读不是翻译，要提高速度就不能调整语序。
>
> ➤ 分析句子结构，找动词，看主语，简缩出句子主干。
>
> ➤ 一个句子至少有一个动词，如果有两个动词，它们之间就应该有连词。
>
> ➤ 如果是并列句，就应找连词；如果是复合句，就应有关联词。
>
> ➤ 逗号不能连接两个句子。
>
> ➤ 迅速对英语的长句进行分割。
>
> ➤ 熟练掌握"后置定语"的6种结构和2种形式。
>
> ➤ 熟练掌握"阅读十大惯用句式及其考点"。
>
> ➤ 背下"王牌句"。

第四节 阅读基础能力训练

Passage One

At all ages and at all stages of life, fear presents a problem to almost everyone. ① "We are largely the playthings of our fears," wrote the British author Horace Walpole many years ago. "To one, fear of the dark; to another, of physical pain; to a third, of public ridicule; to a fourth, of poverty; to a fifth, of loneliness — for all of us our particular creature waits in a hidden place."

Fear is often a useful emotion. When you become frightened, many physical changes occur within your body. Your heartbeat and responses quicken; your pupils expand to admit more light; large quantities of energy-producing adrenaline are poured into your bloodstream. Confronted with a fire or accident, fear can fuel life-saving flight. Similarly, when a danger is psychological rather than physical, fear can force you to take self-protective measures. ② It is only when fear is disproportional to the danger at hand that it becomes a problem.

Some people are simply more vulnerable to fear than others. ③ A visit to the newborn nursery of any large hospital will demonstrate that, from the moment of their births, a few fortunate infants respond calmly to sudden fear-producing situations such as a loudly slammed door. Yet a neighbor in the next bed may cry out with profound fright. ④ From birth, he or she is more prone to learn fearful responses because he or she has inherited a tendency to be more sensitive.

Further, psychologists know that our early experiences and relationships strongly shape and determine our later fears. ⑤ A young man named Bill, for example, grew up with a father who regarded each adversity as a temporary obstacle to be overcome with imagination and courage. Using his father as a model, Bill came to welcome adventure and to trust his own ability to solve problems.

Phil's dad, however, spent most of his time trying to protect himself and his family. Afraid to risk the insecurity of a job change, he remained unhappy in one position. He avoided long vacations because "the car might break down". Growing up in such a home, Phil naturally learned to become fearful and tense.

医学考博阅读理解高分全解

▶ 重点词汇：

present	现在；现在的；展示（n./adj./v.）
plaything	玩物（n.）
ridicule	愚弄（n./v.）
poverty	贫穷（n.）
emotion	情绪（n.）
adrenaline	肾上腺素（n.）
slam	（砰地）关上（v.）
confront	面临，遭遇（v.）
flight	逃离（n.）
disproportional	不匀称的（adj.）
vulnerable	脆弱的（adj.）
demonstrate	展示，显示；说明（v.）
adversity	逆境（n.）
temporary	暂时的（adj.）
obstacle	障碍（n.）
adventure	冒险（n.）
be prone to	倾向于
inherit	继承（v.）
tendency	倾向，趋势（n.）
vacation	节日，假期（n.）
tense	时态；紧张的（n./adj.）

🔍 难句解析：

① "We are largely the playthings of our fears," wrote the British author Horace Walpole many years ago. To one, fear of the dark; to another, of physical pain; to a third, of public ridicule; to a fourth, of poverty; to a fifth, of loneliness — for all of us our particular creature waits in a hidden place.

【结构分析】解析本句要注意前后照应。并列结构to one...to another...to a third...to a fourth... to a fifth... 后的of介宾结构，变成完整结构应该是：We are playthings of fear of the dark / physical pain / public ridicule / poverty / loneliness.

② It is only when fear is disproportional to the danger at hand that it becomes a problem.

【结构分析】本句为强调句，强调句型为"it is＋被强调的部分＋that＋句子的其他部分"。如果去掉it is和that，句子结构仍然是完整的，那么可以判断此句为强调句。本句强调的是时间状语从句。要注意本句中disproportional to...的意思是"与……不匀称"，暗含"超过"或者"小于"的意思。

③ A visit to the newborn nursery of any large hospital will demonstrate that, from the moment of their births, a few fortunate infants respond calmly to sudden fear-producing situations such as a loudly slammed door.

【结构分析】句子主干为：A visit will demonstrate that... that引导的宾语从句中主语为infants，谓语为respond，such as...是situation的后置定语。from the moment of their births是插入语。

④ From birth, he or she is more prone to learn fearful responses because he or she has inherited a tendency to be more sensitive.

【结构分析】he or she是主语，谓语动词用单数形式；如果主语为he and she，谓语动词则用复数形式。be prone to的意思是"更易于，倾向于"，与have a tendency to 的含义相近。sensitive的意思是"敏感的"，与sensible"理智的"要区分开。

⑤ A young man named Bill, for example, grew up with a father who regarded each adversity as a temporary obstacle to be overcome with imagination and courage.

【结构分析】A young man是主语，named Bill是过去分词做后置定语，for example为插入语。grew up为谓语，who引导定语从句充当father的后置定语。定语从句中的谓语部分为固定搭配regard...as，to be overcome是动词不定式充当obstacle的宾语补足语。

▶ 全文翻译：

在人生的各个年龄和每个阶段，恐惧几乎是人人都要面临的问题。"我们在很大程度上是自身恐惧的玩物，"英国作家霍勒斯·沃波尔许多年前曾写道，"有人恐惧黑暗，有人恐惧肉体的病痛，有人恐惧被嘲弄，有人恐惧贫困，有人则恐惧孤独——对所有人来说，我们对某种事物特殊的恐惧就隐藏在某个地方。"

通常情况下，恐惧是一种有用的情绪。当受到惊吓的时候，人的体内会产生很多生理变化。如心跳加速、反应加快；瞳孔放大去吸收更多的光线；大量有助于产生能量的肾上腺素涌入血液。在面对火灾或突发事件时，恐惧能够驱使人快速逃离自救。同样，当危险来自心理而非生理因素时，恐惧也能迫使人采取自我保护的措施。只有当恐惧与即将来临的危险不相称时，恐惧才会成为一个问题。

　　有些人就是会比其他人对恐惧更加敏感。参观任何大医院的新生儿保育室都能说明这个问题，从他们出生的那刻起，一些幸运的婴儿对突然产生的恐惧情境反应平静，比如关门的巨大声响。而邻床的婴儿可能会因为巨大的恐惧而大哭。从刚出生开始，他或她就比别人更倾向于（学习）对恐惧做出反应，因为他或她遗传了一种较为敏感的心理倾向。

　　此外，心理学家们确信，我们早期的经历和社会关系强有力地塑造并决定了我们日后的恐惧情绪。例如，一位名叫比尔的年轻人跟着父亲长大，他的父亲将每次挫折都看作是用想象力和勇气就可以克服的暂时的困难。比尔将父亲当作榜样，逐渐变得敢于冒险，并相信自己解决问题的能力。

　　然而，菲尔的父亲把自己绝大部分时间都用在努力保护自己和家庭上。由于害怕工作的改变而带来的不稳定因素，他始终坚守一个职位，却工作得不开心。他逃避长途旅行，因为"轿车可能会发生故障"。在这样的家庭环境里长大，菲尔自然变得易于恐惧和紧张。

Passage Two

Scientists are hoping to eliminate malaria（疟疾）by developing a genetically modified mosquito that cannot transmit the disease. Malaria has long troubled the populations of South America, Africa, and Asia, where mosquito bites infect up to 500 million people a year with this serious and sometimes fatal parasitic blood disease. For generations, scientists have been trying to eliminate malaria by developing new drugs and using pesticides（杀虫剂）to wipe out local mosquito populations. ①But these measures aren't working—and some scientists, like Greg Lanzaro, say that because of drug resistance and population changes, malaria is actually more prevalent now than it was 20 years ago. Lanzaro says he has a better way to stop the spread of malaria: genetically modify mosquitoes so they are unable to carry the disease.

Lanzaro and his colleagues are planning a multi-year project to produce malaria-resistant mosquitoes—and he thinks they can do it within five years. ②"We can get foreign genes into mosquitoes and they go where they're supposed to go," Lanzaro says, pointing out that scientists have already succeeded in genetically engineering mosquitoes that cannot transmit malaria to birds and mice. And, he says, scientists are quickly making progress on genes that block transmission of the disease to humans as well.

The most difficult part scientifically, Lanzaro says, is figuring out how to get the lab-engineered mosquitoes to spread their genes into natural populations. ③After all, he points out, it's useless to engineer mosquitoes in the lab that can't transmit malaria when there are millions out in the wild. To solve this problem, Lanzaro wants to load up a mobile piece of DNA with the malaria-resistant gene, and then insert it into a group of mosquito embryos. ④The malaria-resistant gene would be integrated directly into the mosquitoes' DNA, making it impossible for those mosquitoes to transmit the parasite that causes malaria. In this way a small group of lab-raised mosquitoes could be released into the wild, and by interbreeding with wild mosquitoes, eventually transmit the beneficial gene to the entire population.

▶ 重点词汇：

eliminate	消除（v.）
malaria	疟疾（n.）
genetically modified	转基因的
transmit	传播；传递（v.）
infect	感染，传染（v.）
fatal	致命的（adj.）
parasitic	寄生的（adj.）
pesticide	杀虫剂（n.）
resistance	抵抗（n.）
prevalent	流行的；普遍的（adj.）
embryo	胚胎（n.）
block	阻碍（v./n.）
release	发放；发行；释放（v./n.）

🔍 难句解析：

① But these measures aren't working — and some scientists, like Greg Lanzaro, say that because of drug resistance and population changes, malaria is actually more prevalent now than it was 20 years ago.

【结构分析】破折号连接了两个分句，第一个分句为these measures aren't working，此处work的意思是"起作用"。第二个分句中主语为scientists，谓语为say，宾语为that引导的从句。该从句中表语为比较级，是malaria流行程度now与20 years ago的比较，because of...是宾语从句中的原因状语。

② "We can get foreign genes into mosquitoes and they go where they're supposed to go," Lanzaro says, pointing out that scientists have already succeeded in genetically engineering mosquitoes that cannot transmit malaria to birds and mice.

【结构分析】本句的主干为Lanzaro says，pointing out是现在分词充当伴随状语，out后面是that引导的宾语从句，宾语从句的主干为scientists have succeeded in engineering mosquitoes, that cannot transmit malaria to birds and mice是mosquitoes的定语从句。

③ After all, he points out, it's useless to engineer mosquitoes in the lab that can't transmit malaria when there are millions out in the wild.

【结构分析】本句的主干是"it is+形容词+to do"结构。it为形式主语，动词不定式为真正的主语。在动词不定式中，that引导的定语从句修饰先行词mosquitoes。when引导从句充当定语从句中的时间状语。

④ The malaria-resistant gene would be integrated directly into the mosquitoes' DNA, making it impossible for those mosquitoes to transmit the parasite that causes malaria.

【结构分析】本句中的making it impossible结构是现在分词充当伴随状语。此处的it是形式宾语，后面的动词不定式为真正的宾语。for those mosquitoes to…中的mosquitoes为动词不定式中动作的逻辑主语。

▶ 全文翻译：

科学家们希望通过培育出一种不能传播疾病的转基因蚊子来根除疟疾。疟疾长期困扰着南美洲、非洲和亚洲的居民。在这些地方，每年有多达5亿的人口因蚊子叮咬而传染上这种严重的，有时甚至是致命的寄生虫性血液疾病。历代的科学家们一直试图通过研制新药或使用杀虫剂来消灭当地蚊子的方法来根除疟疾。但是这些方法都没有奏效——一些科学家，如格雷格·兰萨罗说，因为蚊子的抗药性以及其种群的演变，实际上疟疾现在的传播程度比20年前有过之而无不及。兰萨罗说他有一套更好的办法可以切断疟疾的传播：对蚊子进行基因改造，这样它们就无法携带疟疾的病原体。

兰萨罗和他的同事正在规划一个为期多年的项目，培育携带疟疾抗体的蚊子——他认为他们能够在五年内培育成功。兰萨罗说："我们可以把异体基因植入蚊子体内，然后让它们飞到指定的地方。"兰萨罗指出科学家已经成功地在蚊子身上进行了基因改造，使它们无法将疟疾传播给鸟类和老鼠。同时他还说，科学家们在研究基因方面正迅速取得进展，以杜绝蚊子将疟疾也传播给人类。

兰萨罗说，科技上最困难的部分是让在实验室内接受了疟疾基因改造工程的蚊子将抗疟疾基因传播到蚊子的自然种群中去。他指出，毕竟，当数百万的蚊子还能在野外传播疟疾时，在实验室中改造蚊子基因，使其不传播疟疾是没有用的。为了解决这个问题，兰萨罗打算将携带动态单体DNA的抗疟疾基因植入一组蚊子的胚胎中。抗疟疾基因将会直接和蚊子的DNA结合在一起，这就阻断了疟疾致病菌的传播。这样一来，一小群实验室培育的蚊子被释放到野外，然后通过与野生蚊子交配繁殖，最终将有益的基因传播到整个种群中。

Passage Three

All day long, you are affected by large forces. Genes influence your intelligence and willingness to take risks. Social dynamics unconsciously shape your choices. Instantaneous perceptions set off neural reactions in your head without you even being aware of them.

Over the past few years, scientists have made a series of exciting discoveries about how these deep patterns influence daily life. Nobody has done more to bring these discoveries to public attention than Malcolm Gladwell.

Gladwell's new book *Outliers* seems at first glance to be a description of exceptionally talented individuals. But in fact, it's another book about deep patterns. Exceptionally successful people are not lone pioneers who created their own success, he argues. They are the lucky beneficiaries of social arrangements.

Gladwell's non-controversial claim is that some people have more opportunities than others. Bill Gates was lucky to go to a great private school with its own computer at the dawn of the information revolution.

Gladwell's book is being received by reviewers as a call to action for the Obama Age. ①It could lead policy makers to finally reject policies built on the assumption that people are coldly rational profit-maximizing individuals. ②It could cause them to focus more on policies that foster relationships, social bonds and cultures of achievement.

Yet, I can't help but feel that Gladwell and others who share his emphasis are preoccupied with the coolness of the discoveries. ③They've lost sight of the point at which the influence of social forces ends and the influence of the self-initiating individual begins.

Most successful people begin with two beliefs: the future can be better than the present, and I have the power to make it so. They were often showered by good fortunes, but relied at crucial moments upon achievements of individual will. These people also have an extraordinary ability to consciously focus their attention. Control of attention is the ultimate individual power. People who can do that are not prisoners of the stimuli around them. They can choose from the patterns in the world and lengthen their time horizons.

Gladwell's social determinism overlooks the importance of individual character and individual creativity. And it doesn't fully explain the genuine greatness of humanity's talents. As the classical philosophers understood, examples of individual greatness inspire achievement more reliably than any other form of education.

▶ 重点词汇：

dynamics	动力（ *n.* ）
instantaneous	即时的（ *adj.* ）
perception	观点（ *n.* ）
neural	神经的（ *adj.* ）
pattern	模式（ *n.* ）
exceptionally	例外地；尤其（ *adv.* ）
talent	天才；天赋（ *n.* ）
beneficiary	受益者（ *n.* ）
non-controversial	没有争议的（ *adj.* ）
revolution	革命（ *n.* ）
assumption	假设（ *n.* ）
be preoccupied with	被占据
self-initiating	自我激发的（ *adj.* ）
crucial	关键的（ *adj.* ）

🔍 难句解析：

① It could lead policy makers to finally reject policies built on the assumption that people are coldly rational profit-maximizing individuals.

【结构分析】主语为It，谓语为could lead，宾语为policy makers。built on为过去分词短语充当policies的后置定语，that引导assumption的同位语从句。profit-maximizing的意思是"利益最大化"。

② It could cause them to focus more on policies that foster relationships, social bonds and cultures of achievement.

【结构分析】主语为It，谓语为could cause，宾语为them。that引导的定语从句修饰policies。foster的意思是"培育，培养"。relationships, social bonds and cultures of achievement为并列结构，充当定语从句中的宾语。

③ They've lost sight of the point at which the influence of social forces ends and the influence of the self-initiating individual begins.

【结构分析】主干为They've lost sight。at which引导介词前置的定语从句，从句为and引导的并列句。

▶ 全文翻译：

一天到晚你都在受到巨大力量的影响。基因会影响你的智商、倾向冒险的程度；社会动态潜移默化地决定了你的选择；瞬时的感知也在不知不觉中触发你头脑中的神经反应。

过去数年，在这些深层模式如何影响日常生活方面，科学家们有着一系列激动人心的发现。在将这些发现引起大众关注上，马尔科姆·格莱德威尔所做的工作超过了任何人。

格莱德威尔的新书《不凡者》乍看上去似乎是在描述那些拥有非凡才华的人。而事实上，它还是一本关于"深度模式"的书。作者认为异常成功的人们并不是创造出自己成功的孤独先锋，而是社会安排中的幸运受益者。

格莱德威尔的一个没有引起争议的主张是有些人比其他人拥有更多的机会。比尔·盖茨在信息化革命到来之时就读于一所拥有计算机的优秀私立学校，那是他的幸运。

格莱德威尔的书被评论家们看作奥巴马时代的行动呼吁，可能让决策者最终拒绝采纳那些建立在假设人们都是冷漠、理智、极端利益化的个体之上的政策，而更多地关注那些能巩固关系、加强社会关系以及创造文化成就的政策。

然而，我只是觉得格莱德威尔和那些认同他观点的人们被新发现的好处冲昏了头脑。他们已经看不见在社会影响力和个人主动影响力之间的"临界点"。

多数成功人士的出发点中有两个信念：未来会比现在更好，我能够让它实现。虽然他们经常是好运当头，但在关键时刻依靠的还是个体意志力的成功。这些人还具备有意识地集中注意力的超凡能力。控制注意力是最基本的个人力量。那些能做到这一点的人们不会成为周围刺激的囚徒。他们能从整个世界的各种模式中进行选取并延长它们的时间跨度。

格莱德威尔的社会决定论忽视了个体个性及个体创造力的重要性。而且它没有充分说明人类中那些不凡者的真正伟大之处。正如古典哲学家的观点，个体伟大的典范比任何形式的教育更能激发人们创造出成就。

Passage Four

Loneliness has been linked to depression and other health problems. Now, a study says it can also spread. A friend of a lonely person was 52% more likely to develop feelings of loneliness. And a friend of that friend was 25% more likely to do the same. ①Earlier findings showed that happiness, fatness and the ability to stop smoking can also grow like infections within social groups. The findings all come from a major health study in the American town of

Framingham, Massachusetts.

The study began in 1948 to investigate the causes of heart disease. Since then, more tests have been added, including measures of loneliness and depression.

The new findings involved more than 5,000 people in the second generation of the Framingham Heart Study. The researchers examined friendship histories and reports of loneliness. The results established a pattern that spread as people reported fewer close friends.

For example, loneliness can affect relationships between next-door neighbors. The loneliness spreads as neighbors who were close friends now spend less time together. The study also found that loneliness spreads more easily among women than men.

Researchers from the University of Chicago, Harvard and the University of California, San Diego, did the study. The findings appeared last month in the *Journal of Personality and Social Psychology*.

The average person is said to experience feelings of loneliness about 48 days a year. The study found that having a lonely friend can add about 17 days. But every additional friend can decrease loneliness by about 5%, or two and a half days.

Lonely people become less and less trusting of others. ②This makes it more and more difficult for them to make friends—and more likely that society will reject them.

John Cacioppo at the University of Chicago led the study. He says it is important to recognize and deal with loneliness. He says people who have been pushed to the edges of society should receive help to repair their social networks.

③The aim should be to aggressively create what he calls a "protective barrier" against loneliness. This barrier, he says, can keep the whole network from coming apart.

▶ 重点词汇：

loneliness	孤独（*n.*）
depression	压抑；萧条（*n.*）
infection	感染（*n.*）
investigate	调查（*v.*）
additional	额外的；富余的（*adj.*）
aggressively	强有力地；有敌意地（*adv.*）
barrier	障碍（*n.*）

难句解析:

① Earlier findings showed that happiness, fatness and the ability to stop smoking can also grow like infections within social groups.

【结构分析】主干为findings showed that, that引导宾语从句, 从句的主语为并列结构 happiness, fatness and the ability, ability后面的动词不定式做后置定语, 从句的谓语为can also grow。

② This makes it more and more difficult for them to make friends — and more likely that society will reject them.

【结构分析】本句中的it为形式宾语, to make friends为真正的宾语, for them中的them 是make friends的逻辑主语。and more likely是与more and more difficult并 列的成分。

③ The aim should be to aggressively create what he calls a "protective barrier" against loneliness.

【结构分析】句子主干为The aim should be to create, what引导的名词性从句做create 的宾语从句, he calls的意思是"他所谓的; 他所说的"。

全文翻译:

孤独感会引发抑郁症以及其他疾病。而现如今, 一项研究表明孤独感也会传染。孤独人士的朋友有52%的可能会产生孤独感。同时, 这个朋友的朋友有25%的可能会有相同感觉。早期的发现表明: 幸福感、肥胖症以及戒烟能力会像传染病一样在社会群体内传播。这些发现都出自一项在美国马萨诸塞州弗雷明汉镇开展的一项重要健康研究。

这项旨在调查心脏病起因的研究开始于1948年。从那时开始, 更多的试验被列入其中, 包括孤独感和抑郁症的测定。

这项新发现调查涉及5000多人, 这些人都是弗雷明汉镇心脏病研究受众的子女。研究人员调查了他们的友谊史以及关于孤独感的记录。研究结果建立了一个模式——孤独感在仅拥有较少朋友的人当中传播。

比如: 孤独感会影响邻里之间的关系。当曾经是亲密友人的邻居逐渐疏远时, 孤独感会蔓延。研究还表明, 比起男性, 孤独感更容易在女性中传播。

来自芝加哥大学、哈佛大学以及加州大学圣地亚哥分校的研究人员进行了这项研究。研究结果于上个月发表在《人格与社会心理》杂志上。

据说, 普通人一年有大约48天会产生孤独感。研究发现, 有一个孤独的朋友, 孤独感会增加17天。但是, 每多一个朋友, 可以消除约5%或者是两天半的孤独感。

孤独的人变得越来越不信任其他人。这让他们交朋友变得越来越困难——而社会也更有可能遗弃他们。

来自芝加哥大学的约翰·卡乔波是这项研究的领头人。他说，认识并处理好孤独感是很重要的。他认为曾被社会所孤立的人们应该接受帮助以修复他们的社会关系。

目标应该是积极创建他所称的用来抵制孤独的"防护栏"。他说，防护栏可以保护整个社会关系不会瓦解。

Passage Five

Doctors in Britain are warning of an obesity time bomb, when children who are already overweight grow up. So, what should we do? Exercise more? Eat less? Or both? The government feels it has to take responsibility for this expanding problem.

①The cheerful Mr. Pickwick, the hero of the novel by Charles Dickens, is seen in illustrations as someone who is plump and happy. In 18th century paintings beauty is equated with rounded bodies and soft curves. ②But nowadays being overweight is seen as indicating neither a cheerful character nor beauty but an increased risk of heart disease and stroke.

So what do you do? Diet? Not according to England's chief medical officer, Sir Liam Donaldson. He says that physical activity is the key for reducing the risks of obesity, cancer and heart disease. And the Health Secretary John Reid even said that being inactive is as serious a risk factor in heart disease as smoking.

So, having bought some cross trainers, how much exercise should you do? According to Sir Liam Donaldson, at least 30 minutes of moderate activity five days a week. Is going to the gym the answer? Luckily for those who find treadmills tedious, the Health Development Agency believes that physical activity that fits into people's lives may be more effective. ③They suggest taking the stairs rather than the lift, walking up escalators, playing active games with your children, dancing or gardening. And according to a sports psychologist, Professor Biddle, gyms "are not making the nation fit", and may even cause harm.

There's new scientific evidence that too much exercise may actually be bad for you. ④Scientists at the University of Ulster have found that unaccustomed exercise releases dangerous free radicals that can adversely affect normal function in unfit people. The only people who should push their bodies to that level of exercise on a regular basis are trained athletes.

So, should we forget about gyms and follow some experts' advice to increase exercise in our daily life? After all, getting off the bus a stop early and walking the rest of the way can't do any harm! One final thought. How come past generations lacked gym facilities but were leaner and fitter than people today?

▶ 重点词汇：

obesity	肥胖（ *n.* ）
cheerful	高兴的（ *adj.* ）
curve	曲线（ *n.* ）
illustration	例证（ *n.* ）
plump	胖乎乎的（ *adj.* ）
stroke	中风（ *n.* ）
treadmill	跑步机（ *n.* ）
radical	极端的；极端分子（ *adj. / n.* ）
adversely	不利地（ *adv.* ）
athlete	运动员（ *n.* ）

🔍 难句解析：

① The cheerful Mr. Pickwick, the hero of the novel by Charles Dickens, is seen in illustrations as someone who is plump and happy.

【结构分析】主语部分为 "N1，N2+后置定语" 结构，Mr. Pickwick与the hero为同位语，is seen as是谓语部分，someone是介词as的宾语，who引导定语从句修饰someone。

② But nowadays being overweight is seen as indicating neither a cheerful character nor beauty but an increased risk of heart disease and stroke.

【结构分析】主语为动名词结构being overweight，谓语部分为被动语态is seen as，介词as后面的宾语结构为neither...nor...but（既不是……也不是……而是）。

③ They suggest taking the stairs rather than the lift, walking up escalators, playing active games with your children, dancing or gardening.

【结构分析】本句是个简单句，主干为 "They suggest+宾语"，宾语由doing形式的短语充当。在宾语中有两个并列结构，第一个为大并列taking the stairs, walking up escalators, playing active games, dancing or gardening，这个并列结构的

一个成分中还有一个由rather than引导的并列结构，一定要注意区分。

④ Scientists at the University of Ulster have found that unaccustomed exercise releases dangerous free radicals that can adversely affect normal function in unfit people.

【结构分析】主语为Scientists，谓语为have found，that引导宾语从句。宾语从句中主语为exercise，谓语为releases，宾语为radicals，后面又有that引导的从句，做定语修饰radicals。定语从句中主语为that（radicals），谓语为can affect，宾语为function。因此这是个从句里含从句的句子。

▶ 全文翻译：

英国的医生提醒人们，那些体重已经超重的孩子长大以后，要警惕"肥胖"这一定时炸弹。那我们应该做些什么？多运动？少吃饭？抑或是两者兼顾？英国政府觉得应当为这一不断扩大的问题负起责任。

狄更斯小说当中的主人公—— 快乐的匹克威克先生被塑造成一个胖乎乎又很开心的角色。在18世纪，画中的美人都被赋予丰满的体态和柔美的曲线。而现如今，超重却不再被视为快乐或是美丽，而是罹患心脏病和中风的风险。

那么你该如何应对？节食吗？英国政府首席医疗官利亚姆·唐纳森先生并不这么认为。他说，体育锻炼才是减少肥胖、癌症以及心脏病风险的关键。卫生大臣约翰·里德甚至说，不活动就像吸烟一样，是引发心脏病的危险因素。

因此，如果已经购买了一些健身器材，你的运动量应该多大呢？亚姆·唐纳森先生说，每周至少五次三十分钟的中等强度的活动。得去健身房锻炼吗？那些发现跑步机很乏味的人们是很幸运的。英国卫生发展局认为，融入人们生活中的运动才更有效。他们建议以爬楼梯取代乘坐电梯；沿着扶梯向上走；和孩子们玩一些竞技类游戏；跳跳舞或者种种花。运动心理学家比德尔教授认为，健身房"不但不能让人们保持健康"，甚至会带来危害。

有新的科学证据表明，过多的运动其实是有害的。阿尔斯特大学的科学家们发现不寻常的运动会释放危险的自由基，对不健康人群的正常身体机能有不良影响。只有经过长期训练的运动员，才可以让他们的身体经受那种水平的运动。

那么，我们是不是应该忘记健身房，并按照专家们的建议在日常生活中进行锻炼呢？毕竟提前一站下车然后步行走完剩下的路不会有半点危害！最后再想想，为何过去的人们缺乏健身设施，但却比现在的人们苗条，比现在的人们健康呢？

Passage Six

People are living longer than ever, but for some reason, women are living longer than men. A baby boy born in the United States in 2003 can expect to live to be about 73; a baby girl, about 79. This is indeed a wide gap, and no one really knows why it exists. The greater longevity of women, however, has been known for centuries. It was, for example, described in the seventeenth century. However, the difference was smaller then — the gap is growing.

A number of reasons have been proposed to account for the differences. ①The gap is greatest in industrialized societies, so it has been suggested that women are less susceptible to work strains that may raise the risk of heart disease and alcoholism. ②Sociologists also tell us that women are encouraged to be less adventurous than men (and this may be why they are more careful drivers, involved in fewer accidents).

Even smoking has been implicated in the age discrepancy. ③It was once suggested that working women are more likely to smoke and as more women entered the work force, the age gap would begin to close, because smoking is related to earlier deaths. Now, however, we see more women smoking and they still tend to live longer although their lung cancer rate is climbing sharply.

One puzzling aspect of the problem is that women do not appear to be as healthy as men. That is, they report far more illnesses. But when a man reports an illness, it is more likely to be serious.

Some researchers have suggested that men may die earlier because their health is more strongly related to their emotions. For example, men tend to die sooner after losing a spouse than women do. Men even seem to be more weakened by loss of a job. (Both of these are linked with a marked decrease in the effectiveness of the immune system.) Among men, death follows retirement with an alarming promptness.

Perhaps we are searching for the answers too close to the surface of the problem. Perhaps the answers lie deeper in our biological heritage. After all, the phenomenon is not isolated to humans. Females have the edge among virtually all mammalian species, in that they generally live longer. Furthermore, in many of these species the differences begin at the moment of conception; there are more male miscarriages. In humans, after birth, more baby boys than baby girls die.

▶ 重点词汇：

gap	差距（ n. ）
longevity	长寿（ n. ）
account for	解释

strain	压力（n.）
susceptible	容易受影响的（adj.）
alcoholism	酗酒（n.）
adventurous	冒险的（adj.）
implicate	牵涉（v.）
discrepancy	差异；不符合（之处）（n.）
spouse	配偶（n.）
immune system	免疫系统
alarming	令人担忧的（adj.）
promptness	敏捷，迅速（n.）
biological heritage	生物遗传
virtually	几乎（adv.）
mammalian	哺乳动物的（adj.）
species	物种（n.）
miscarriage	流产（n.）

🔍 难句解析：

① The gap is greatest in industrialized societies, so it has been suggested that women are less susceptible to work strains that may raise the risk of heart disease and alcoholism.

【结构分析】这是一个主从复合句，so表示结果状况。it has been suggested翻译成"人们/有人建议……"，it是形式主语，真正的主语是that women are less susceptible to work strains，strains后又有一个that引导的定语从句。

② Sociologists also tell us that women are encouraged to be less adventurous than men (and this may be why they are more careful drivers, involved in fewer accidents).

【结构分析】这里需要注意的是括号中的内容。此处括号表示对主句内容的补充，this为主语，may be为谓语部分，why引导表语从句，involved in fewer accidents是drivers的后置定语。

③ It was once suggested that working women are more likely to smoke and as more women entered the work force, the age gap would begin to close, because smoking is related to earlier deaths.

【结构分析】这里It为形式主语，that 引导的是主语从句，是真正的主语。be more likely to意为"更有可能……"。要注意这个主语从句比较长，该主语从句包含两个并列分句，由and连接，and后面分句的主干为the age gap would begin to close，as引导时间状语从句，because则引导原因状语从句。

⏵ 全文翻译：

　　人们比以往任何时候活得都长，但是由于一些原因，女性比男性活得更长。2003年在美国出生的男婴，预期可能活到73岁，但是女婴大约会活到79岁。这的确是一个很大的差距，但是没有人知道它为什么会存在。女性的长寿几个世纪以来都被人们熟知。例如，17世纪它就已经被描述过了。然而，那时的差异较小，而现在的差距在不断加大。

　　许多原因都被提出来解释这种差异。在工业社会，差距更大了，所以有人提出女性不易被工作压力所影响，而这些压力会增加患心脏病和酗酒的风险。社会学家也说女性比男性更少受鼓励去冒险（这可能就是女性开车更小心、更少被卷入车祸中的原因）。

　　甚至吸烟也被牵扯到年龄差距上来。有人曾经提出随着更多的女性进入职场，职业女性更有可能吸烟，这使得年龄差距开始接近，因为吸烟与早逝有关。然而，现在我们看到更多的女性吸烟，但是女性仍然倾向于活得更长久，尽管她们得肺癌的概率在急剧上升。

　　令人百思不得其解的是女性看起来似乎不像男性那样健康。更确切地说，她们得病的次数更多。但是，男性一旦得病，就会很严重。

　　一些研究者认为，男性的过早死亡可能与他们的情绪有关。例如，在失去配偶后，男性比女性更早地死亡。男性在失去工作后也更为脆弱（这些都与明显的免疫系统功能下降有关）。在男性中，退休后的死亡率令人震惊。

　　也许我们追寻的答案与问题的表象很接近。也许更深层次的答案在于我们的生物遗传上。毕竟，这一现象并不孤立存在于人类当中。几乎所有哺乳动物中的雌性都拥有这一优势，这使它们通常活得更长久。因此，许多物种的差异开始于胚胎时期，流产掉的更多是雄性动物。人类在出生之后，男婴比女婴夭折的人数多。

Passage Seven

On how the world has changed over the last 50 years, not all of it has been good. ① As you are looking for organic food information, you have obviously become aware that a better alternative exists and you are taking a critical look at the source and production practices of the companies producing the world's food supplies.

The purpose of organic food information is to give you an understanding of what is going into your food. You will see that there are many benefits to organic food that you didn't know before. ②The basis behind knowing about organic food information is the fact that farmers are resorting to using artificial fertilizers and pesticides to control disease and insect attack in order to produce more crops to satisfy growing demand. ③These artificial fertilizers leave something poisonous in and on the fruit and vegetables we consume which in turn is absorbed and stored by our bodies.

Even the quality of food has gone down in recent years. Today's fruits have nowhere near the Vitamin C levels they did at one time. ④However, with organic food information you learn that organic food has fifty percent more nutrients, minerals and vitamins than any other form of produce that has been grown under intensive farming. If you are eating non-organic produce you will have to eat more fruit in order to make up for this deficiency. But then the dangerous cycle continues since you will be eating more chemicals that are worse for your health than they are good for you.

Another aspect of organic food information is the production of meat and poultry. ⑤Most only consider produce when it comes to organic food information disregarding the antibiotics and hormones that are given to both cattle and poultry that are being force-fed. Ask yourself what happens to all these antibiotics and hormones when the animal is killed, and the remaining of these antibiotics and growth hormones reside in the meat which are then consumed, digested and stored in human bodies. There is no way that an animal that isn't kept in healthy conditions can produce healthy food for humans to eat.

You have nothing to lose by trying organic product, not only will it be healthy for you but you will also be able to eat produce and meat the way they are supposed to be. You will likely be so impressed with the taste of organic fruit that you will never return to the mass-produced fruit again. While cost and availability can be a big issue for some, you can do a bit of research online and find a local store that stocks organic produce for a reasonable price.

▶ 重点词汇：

alternative	选择；二择其一的（n. / adj.）
critical	挑剔的（adj.）
resort to	借助于
artificial	人工的（adj.）
pesticide	杀虫剂（n.）
consume	食用；消费（v.）
deficiency	不足（n.）
disregard	不考虑（v.）
mass-produced	批量生产的（adj.）
availability	可获得（n.）
poultry	家禽（n.）

🔍 难句解析：

① As you are looking for organic food information, you have obviously become aware that a better alternative exists and you are taking a critical look at the source and production practices of the companies producing the world's food supplies.

【结构分析】本句的主干为you have become aware that...and you are taking a look at...，As引导时间状语从句。主干中第二个并列分句主干为you are taking a critical look at the source and practices，of结构是practices的后置定语，producing为现在分词充当companies的后置定语。

② The basis behind knowing about organic food information is the fact that farmers are resorting to using artificial fertilizers and pesticides to control disease and insect attack in order to produce more crops to satisfy growing demand.

【结构分析】本句主干为The basis is the fact，that...为fact的同位语从句。同位语从句中to control disease and insect attack为using artificial fertilizers and pesticides的目的状语，in order to produce...为control的目的状语。

③ These artificial fertilizers leave something poisonous in and on the fruit and vegetables we consume which in turn is absorbed and stored by our bodies.

【结构分析】本句主干为These fertilizers leave something，we consume为省略了that的定语从句，修饰fruit and vegetables，which引导第二个定语从句修饰something poisonous。

④ However, with organic food information you learn that organic food has fifty percent more nutrients, minerals and vitamins than any other form of produce that has been grown under intensive farming.

【结构分析】本句主干为you learn that...，that引导宾语从句。从句中有比较结构more...than，将有机食品（organic food）所含有的nutrients，minerals and vitamins与其他形式的农产品进行比较。produce在这里是名词，意为"农产品"，第二个that引导定语从句修饰produce。with organic food information为方式状语。

⑤ Most only consider produce when it comes to organic food information disregarding the antibiotics and hormones that are given to both cattle and poultry that are being force-fed.

【结构分析】本句主干为Most consider produce，when引导时间状语从句，come to的意思是"谈及，谈到"。disregarding为现在分词充当状语，该状语中第一个that引导定语从句修饰antibiotics and hormones，第二个that引导定语从句修饰cattle and poultry。

▶ 全文翻译：

对于世界在过去50年所发生的变化的问题，答案并非全是正面的。当你在寻找有机食品信息时，很明显你已经意识到还有更好的选择，因此会比较挑剔地审视生产世界食品供给的公司的原料和制造行为。

有机食品信息的目的是告知你食物里面有什么。你会看到前所未知的很多益处。了解有机食品信息之前要先明白这样一个事实：农民借助于人工肥料和杀虫剂，从而控制疫病、虫害，生产出更多的粮食以此满足越来越大的需求。这些人工肥料遗留了某些有毒物质在我们食用的蔬菜和水果的里里外外，反过来这些有毒物质会被我们的身体吸收并储存。

近年来甚至食品的质量都有所下降。如今的水果根本无法达到过去的维生素C的含量水平。然而，根据有机食品信息可知，有机食品所含的营养物、矿物质和维生素比其他精耕形式的农产品高出50%多。如果你食用非有机产品，你不得不多吃来弥补营养上的不足。但是这样一来危险的循环就会持续，你会吃更多的化学物质，对你的身体会造成更大的伤害。

有机食品信息的另一个方面是肉类和家禽的生产。提及有机食品信息，很多人只考虑到农作物，而没有考虑到强行喂养家畜和家禽时加入的抗生素和激素。问问自己，当动物被宰杀后，这些抗生素和激素去了哪儿？它们会留存在肉里，然后被我们食用、消化，并在身体里储存起来。在不健康的条件下喂养的动物是不可能为人类创造出健康食品的。

尝试有机产品，你不会损失什么，它不仅对你的健康有益，你还能以原本应该的方式来食用农产品和肉类。你可能会对有机水果的味道印象非常深刻，以至于不会再去食用批量生产的水果。尽管成本和获取渠道对某些人来讲是个比较大的问题，但你可以在网上找一找，在本地找到一家价格合理的出售有机食品的商店。

Passage Eight

Facelift followed by a week on a beach in Thailand? Hip surgery with a side of shopping in Singapore? Over the last 10 years, Asia's rise on the medical tourism scene has been quick. Eastern nations dominate the global scene. Now Bali wants a slice of the action.

The Indonesian island recently opened its first facility specifically targeting medical tourists with packages and services, Bali International Medical Centre (BIMC) Nusa Dua. BIMC already has an international hospital in Kuta, which opened in 1998.

The new internationally managed facility offers surgical and non-surgical cosmetic procedures and dental care.

Unlike most of the region's hospitals, BIMC is designed to feel more like a spa or resort than a medical facility.

①The 50-bed hospital has a 24-hour medical emergency entrance and hotel-like lobby at the front of the building servicing the hospital's medical, and dental centres.

If you're a celebrity who doesn't want everyone to know you're here for a bit of lipo（吸脂术）, no worries. There's a private entrance that leads to the CosMedic Centre, which offers views of a golf course.

②BIMC has even teamed up with the nearby Courtyard by Marriott Bali, which provides specific after-care services like tailor-made meals and wellness programs for patients.

③Latest technology and cool interiors are a start, but breaking into a regional industry that already has some of the world's top international hospitals will be tough, says Josef Woodman, CEO of U.S.-based medical travel consumer guide Patients Beyond Borders (PBB).

"As a newcomer, Bali faces stiff competition from nearby international healthcare providers. To compete, Bali will need to demonstrate a quality level of care and promote its services to the region and the world. On the positive side, Bali is blessed as one of the region's safest, most popular tourist destinations, with a built-in potential to attract medical travelers."

The Indonesian island couldn't have picked a better time to get into the game, says PBB. ④ "The world population is aging and becoming wealthier at rates that surpass the availability of quality healthcare resources," says the company's research.

▶ 重点词汇：

facelift	紧肤术（n.）
surgery	手术（n.）
tourism	旅游业（n.）
dominate	控制，主导（v.）
target	目标；瞄准（n./v.）
cosmetic	化妆的，美容的（adj.）
dental	牙齿的（adj.）
emergency	紧急（n.）
resort	度假村（n.）
celebrity	名人（n.）
specific	具体的（adj.）
tailor-made	定制的（adj.）
stiff	坚硬的（adj.）

| demonstrate | 显示（v.） |
| surpass | 超过（v.） |

🔍 难句解析：

① The 50-bed hospital has a 24-hour medical emergency entrance and hotel-like lobby at the front of the building servicing the hospital's medical, and dental centres.

【结构分析】主干为hospital has entrance and lobby, servicing the hospital's medical, and dental centres是现在分词充当后置定语，修饰emergency and lobby。这里的service为动词。

【理解难点】emergency entrance的中心词为entrance，当两个名词在一起时，中心名词为第二个名词。同时要注意本句中的并列结构entrance and lobby, medical and dental。

② BIMC has even teamed up with the nearby Courtyard by Marriott Bali, which provides specific after-care services like tailor-made meals and wellness programs for patients.

【结构分析】主干为BIMC has teamed…，which引导定语从句修饰先行词BIMC。定语从句中的主干为which provides services，此处的services为名词，like tailor-made meals and wellness programs为services的后置定语。

【理解难点】tailor-made meal的意思是"定制餐"，wellness的意思是"康健，康复"。

③ Latest technology and cool interiors are a start, but breaking into a regional industry that already has some of the world's top international hospitals will be tough, says Josef Woodman, CEO of U.S.-based medical travel consumer guide Patients Beyond Borders (PBB).

【结构分析】本句为宾语从句提前，主谓在最后says Josef Woodman…，CEO为同位语，of…为CEO的名词扩展。宾语从句为并列句，由but连接。第一个分句的主干为technology and interiors are a start,第二个分句的主干为breaking into a regional industry will be tough。第二个分句的主语由动名词充当，定语从句that already has some of the world's top international hospitals修饰先行词industry。

④ The world population is aging and becoming wealthier at rates that surpass the availability of quality healthcare resources.

【结构分析】本句的主干为population is aging and becoming wealthier，at rates为状语，that引导定语从句修饰rates。

▶ 全文翻译：

　　整容后在泰国海滩上享受一周？接受提臀术后在新加坡购物一周？在过去的10年间，亚洲医疗旅行的增长景象十分迅速。亚洲东部的国家控制着这种全球景象。现在巴厘岛想来分一杯羹。

　　印度尼西亚群岛最近开设了第一家机构——巴厘岛努沙杜瓦国际医疗中心（BIMC），专门针对"打包"享受医疗和服务的医疗旅行者。该中心已于1998年在库塔开设了一家国际医院。

　　这个新的国际化管理机构提供外科手术与非手术美容项目及牙齿护理。

　　与该地区多数医院不同，BIMC的设计更像是一个水疗吧或者度假村，而不是一家医疗机构。

　　这家拥有50个床位的医院有24小时急诊通道，大楼前的大厅就像酒店一样服务医院的医疗和牙科中心。

　　如果你不想公众知道你是在这里做吸脂术的名人，不用担心。有一条私人通道带你进入医学美容中心，还能让你看到高尔夫球场的全景。

　　BIMC甚至与附近的巴厘岛万怡庭院度假酒店合作，可以提供细致的后续服务，比如定制餐和病人康复服务项目。

　　以美国为基地的医疗旅游客服指导中心PBB首席执行官约瑟夫·乌德曼说："最新科技和酷炫的内饰只是开始，但要进入已经拥有世界顶级国际化医院的地区很艰难。"

　　"初来乍到，巴厘岛面临严酷的、来自附近国际化医疗保健服务供应商的竞争。要想赢得竞争，巴厘岛需要显示医疗保健服务的高质量水平，将服务提升到地区和世界领先水平。从积极的一面来看，巴厘岛被认为是该地区最安全、最受欢迎的旅游胜地之一。"

　　PBB说，印度尼西亚群岛挑了一个最佳时间参与竞争。"世界人口老龄化与财富增长速度，超过了可利用的优质医疗保健资源的增长速度，"该公司的调研声称。

Passage Nine

　　In a purely biological sense, fear begins with the body's system for reacting to things that can harm us — the so-called fight-or-flight response. "An animal that can't detect danger can't stay alive," says Joseph LeDoux. Like animals, humans evolved with an elaborate mechanism for processing information about potential threats. At its core is a cluster of neurons deep in the brain known as the amygdald.

LeDoux studies the way animals and humans respond to threats to understand how we form memories of significant events in our lives. The amygdala receives input from many parts of the brain, including regions responsible for retrieving memories. ①Using this information, the amygdala appraises a situation — I think this dog wants to bite me — and triggers a response by radiating nerve signals throughout the body. These signals produce the familiar signs of distress: trembling, perspiration and fast-moving feet, just to name three.

This fear mechanism is critical to the survival of all animals, but no one can say for sure whether beasts other than humans know they're afraid. That is, as LeDoux says, "if you put that system into a brain that has consciousness, then you get the feeling of fear."

Humans, says Edward M. Hallowell, have the ability to call up images of bad things that happened in the past and to anticipate future events. ②Combine these higher thought processes with our hardwired danger-detection systems, and you get a near-universal human phenomenon: worry.

That's not necessarily a bad thing, says Hallowell. "When used properly, worry is an incredible device," he says. After all, a little healthy worry is okay if it leads to constructive action like having a doctor look at that weird spot on your back.

Hallowell insists, though, that there's a right way to worry. "Never do it alone, get the facts and then make a plan," he says. Most of us have survived a recession, so we're familiar with the belt-tightening strategies needed to survive a slump.

Unfortunately, few of us have much experience dealing with the threat of terrorism, so it's been difficult to get facts about how we should respond. ③That's why Hallowell believes it was okay for people to indulge some extreme worries last fall by asking doctors for Cipro and buying gas masks.

重点词汇：

biological	生物的，生物学的（adj.）
react	反应，回应（v./n.）
elaborate	复杂的；精密的（adj.）
mechanism	机制（n.）
potential	潜在的；潜力（adj./n.）
neuron	神经元（n.）
amygdala	杏仁体（n.）

retrieve	搜索（ *v.* ）
trembling	颤抖（ *n.* ）
perspiration	出汗；汗水（ *n.* ）
anticipate	期待（ *v.* ）
incredible	难以置信的（ *adj.* ）
indulge	沉浸，沉溺（ *v.* ）

难句解析：

① Using this information, the amygdala appraises a situation — I think this dog wants to bite me — and triggers a response by radiating nerve signals throughout the body.

【结构分析】该句主干为the amygdala appraises a situation and triggers a response，Using this information是现在分词充当方式状语，破折号后的内容为对situation的解释。I think后的this dog wants to… 为宾语从句。

【理解难点】根据对并列结构的认知，triggers与appraises为并列谓语，and并列的前后成分一致，形式一致。

② Combine these higher thought processes with our hardwired danger-detection systems, and you get a near-universal human phenomenon: worry.

【结构分析】本句的结构是"祈使句+and+句子"，意思是"如果……那么……"，祈使句相当于一个if引导的条件状语从句。combine…with是固定搭配，意思是"……与……相结合"。

③ That's why Hallowell believes it was okay for people to indulge some extreme worries last fall by asking doctors for Cipro and buying gas masks.

【结构分析】本句的主干为主系表结构，表语为why引导的从句，表语从句中的主干为Hallowell believes。it was okay…为believes的宾语从句，从句为"it was+形容词+for sb.+to do sth."句型，by asking…and buying是方式状语。

全文翻译：

从纯粹的生物学意义上讲，恐惧始于身体系统对可能伤害我们的事物做出反应，也就是所谓的战斗或逃跑反应。"不能察觉到危险的动物无法生存下去，"勒杜说。像动物一样，人类进化出了精密的机制来处理关于潜在威胁的信息。其核心是位于大脑深处的一束神经元，称为杏仁体。

勒杜研究动物和人类应对威胁的方式，以理解我们对生活中的重要事件是如何形成记忆的。杏仁体从大脑中的很多部位接受输入的信息，包括负责提取记忆的区域。杏仁体利用这些信息评定一个现象：我认为狗想要咬我，通过向全身发射神经信号来做出响应。这些信号产生熟悉的痛苦的迹象，颤抖、出汗和快速移动脚，或者三个迹象同时发生。

所有动物的这种恐惧机制对生存都是很重要的，但是没有人能确定除了人类，野兽是否也知道害怕。正如勒杜说："如果你把这个系统变成一个大脑意识，那么你会感觉到恐惧。"

爱德华·哈洛威尔说，人类有能力调用过去发生的糟糕的事情图像和未来的预期事件。把这些高级思维过程与我们固有的危险探测系统相联系，你会获得一个几乎是人类所共有的现象：担心。

"这并不一定是坏事，"哈洛威尔说。"如果使用恰当，担忧是一个难以置信的策略。"毕竟，一些健康的担忧是正常的，如果它带来建设性的行动，比如你背上出现奇怪的斑点，那就得让医生检查一下。

然而，哈洛威尔坚持认为，可以以一种正确的方式去担心。"不能只是担心，要了解事实，然后制订一个计划。"他说。我们大多数人都在经济衰退中幸存了下来，所以我们熟悉度过低潮的节约攻略。

不幸的是，很少有人有很多处理恐怖主义威胁的经验，因此，很难得到关于应该如何回应的事实。这就是为什么哈洛威尔相信允许人们去年秋天沉溺于一些极端的担忧是可以的，比如要求医生开环丙沙星和买防毒面具。

Passage Ten

①Do you remember all those years when scientists argued that smoking would kill us but the doubters insisted that we didn't know for sure? That the evidence was inconclusive, the science uncertain? That the antismoking lobby was out to destroy our way of life and the government should stay out of the way? Lots of Americans bought that nonsense, and over three decades, some 10 million smokers went to early graves.

There are upsetting parallels today, as scientists in one wave after another try to awaken us to the growing threat of global warming. ②The latest was a panel from the National Academy of Sciences, enlisted by the White House, to tell us that the Earth's atmosphere is definitely warming and that the problem is largely man-made. The clear message is that we should get moving to protect ourselves. The president of the National Academy, Bruce Alberts, added this key point in the preface to the panel's report: "Science never has all the answers. ③But science does provide us with the best available guide to the future, and it is critical that our nation and the world base important policies on the best judgments that science can provide concerning the future consequences of present actions."

④Just as on smoking, voices now come from many quarters insisting that the science about global warming is incomplete, that it's OK to keep pouring fumes into the air until we know for sure. This is a dangerous game: by the time 100 percent of the evidence is in, it may be too late. With the risks obvious and growing, a prudent people would take out an insurance policy now.

Fortunately, the White House is starting to pay attention. But it's obvious that a majority of the president's advisers still don't take global warming seriously. ⑤Instead of a plan of action, they continue to press for more research—a classic case of "paralysis by analysis".

To serve as responsible stewards of the planet, we must press forward on deeper atmospheric and oceanic research but research alone is inadequate. If the Administration won't take the legislative initiative, Congress should help to begin fashioning conservation measures. A bill by Democratic Senator Robert Byrd of West Virginia, which would offer financial incentives for private industry, is a promising start. Many see that the country is getting ready to build lots of new power plants to meet our energy needs. If we are ever going to protect the atmosphere, it is crucial that those new plants be environmentally sound.

▶ 重点词汇：

inconclusive	非结论性的，不确定的（adj.）
lobby	门厅，接待室（n.）
antismoking	禁止吸烟（n.）
nonsense	胡说，废话（n.）
grave	墓穴，坟墓（n.）
panel	面板；座谈小组；全体陪审员（n.）
definitely	明确地；肯定地（adv.）
parallel	类似的事物；平行线（n.）
pour	倾泻，涌出；倒（v.）
fume	[浓烈或难闻的]烟，气味；愤怒，生气（n./v.）
prudent	审慎的，谨慎的（adj.）
paralysis	瘫痪（n.）
steward	管家，管事；服务员，乘务员（n.）

legislative	立法的（adj.）
initiative	主动的行动；首创精神（n.）
crucial	至关重要的，决定性的（adj.）
negligence	疏忽（n.）
aggravate	使恶化，加重（v.）

🔍 难句解析：

① Do you remember all those years when scientists argued that smoking would kill us but the doubters insisted that we didn't know for sure? That the evidence was inconclusive, the science uncertain? That the antismoking lobby was out to destroy our way of life and the government should stay out of the way?

【结构分析】这里有三个问句，第一个问句的主干是Do you remember all those years...，后面的when引导定语从句修饰前面的名词years，定语从句由but连接的两个句子组成；第二个问句和第三个问句句首的That都引导一个宾语从句，承接第一个问句，that前省略了主句Do you remember all those years when scientists argued that smoking would kill us but the doubters insisted；the science uncertain承前省略了was。

【理解难点】通过结构分析我们知道这几个句子都是围绕第一个问句的主干部分展开的并列疑问句，因此我们在阅读中应弄清楚句子的层次，逐一分析。

② The latest was a panel from the National Academy of Sciences, enlisted by the White House, to tell us that the Earth's atmosphere is definitely warming and that the problem is largely man-made.

【结构分析】主干部分是The latest was a panel，表语panel后接有两个定语成分：from介词短语和enlisted过去分词短语，意思为"白宫召集的、来自国家科学院的专家团"。不定式结构to tell us...表示目的，即"为了告诉我们……"。

③ But science does provide us with the best available guide to the future, and it is critical that our nation and the world base important policies on the best judgments that science can provide concerning the future consequences of present actions.

【结构分析】该句的主干是由and连接的两个并列句，前一个分句的主干是science does provide us with guide；后一个分句的主干是it is critical，其中it为形式主语，真正的主语是that引导的主语从句。从句的主干是our nation and the world base policies on judgments，judgments后接两个定语结构，一个是that引导的定语从句，另一个是concerning分词结构。

④ Just as on smoking, voices now come from many quarters insisting that the science about global warming is incomplete, that it's OK to keep pouring fumes into the air until we know for sure.

【结构分析】该句的主干是voices now come from many quarters，句首Just as结构做比较状语，意为"正如……一样"。insisting引导的分词结构做定语修饰主语voices，分词结构中含有两个并列的由that引导的宾语从句，第二个宾语从句的真正主语是不定式结构to keep...。

⑤ Instead of a plan of action, they continue to press for more research — a classic case of "paralysis by analysis".

【结构分析】instead of表示否定；破折号后面的部分不是修饰前面的名词research，而是说明前面的整个句子。paralysis by analysis的意思是"分析导致瘫痪"，就是无休止地研究一件事，致使最终没有任何行动。

▶ 全文翻译：

还记得那些年科学家们曾认为吸烟会致人死亡，而那些怀疑者们却坚持认为我们无法对此得出定论吗？还记得怀疑者们坚持认为缺乏决定性的证据，科学也不确定的时候吗？还记得怀疑者们坚持认为反对吸烟的游说是为了毁掉我们的生活方式，而政府应该置身事外的时候吗？许多美国人相信了这些胡言乱语，在三十多年里，差不多有一千万烟民早早地进了坟墓。

现在出现了与吸烟类似的令人感到难过的事情。科学家们前仆后继，试图使我们意识到全球气候变暖所带来的日益严重的威胁。最近的行动是由白宫召集了一批来自国家科学院的专家团，他们告诉我们，地球气候毫无疑问正在变暖，并且这个问题主要是人为造成的。明确的信息是我们应该立刻着手保护自己。国家科学院院长布鲁斯·艾伯茨在专家团报告的前言中加上了这一重要观点："科学解答不了所有问题。但是科学确实为我们的未来提供了最好的指导，关键是我们的国家和整个世界在做重要决策时，应该以科学能够提供的关于人类现在的行为对未来影响的最好判断为依据。"

就像吸烟问题一样，来自不同领域的声音坚持认为有关全球变暖的科学资料还不完整。在我们证实这件事之前可以继续向大气中不断地排放气体。这是一个危险的游戏：到了有百分之百的证据的时候，可能就太晚了。随着风险越来越明显，并且不断增加，一个谨慎的民族现在应该准备一份保单了。

幸运的是，白宫开始关注这件事了。但是显然大多数总统顾问并没有认真看待全球气候变暖这个问题。他们没有出台行动计划，相反只是继续迫切要求进行更多的研究——这是一个经典的"分析导致瘫痪"的案例。

为了成为地球上有责任心的一员，我们必须积极推进对于大气和海洋的深入研究。但仅有研究是不够的。如果政府不争取立法上的主动权，国会就应该帮助政府开始采取保护措施。西弗吉尼亚州民主党议员罗伯特·伯德提出一项议案，建议从经济上激励私企，就是一个良好的开端。许多人看到这个国家正准备修建许多新的发电厂，以满足我们的能源需求。如果我们准备保护大气，关键要让这些新发电厂对环境无害。

Passage Eleven

Of all the components of a good night's sleep, dreams seem to be least within our control. In dreams, a window opens into a world where logic is suspended and dead people speak. ① A century ago, Freud formulated his revolutionary theory that dreams were the disguised shadows of our unconscious desires and fears; by the late 1970s, neurologists had switched to thinking of them as just "mental noise"—the random byproducts of the neural-repair work that goes on during sleep. ② Now researchers suspect that dreams are part of the mind's emotional thermostat, regulating moods while the brain is "off-line". ③ And one leading authority says that these intensely powerful mental events can be not only harnessed but actually brought under conscious control, to help us sleep and feel better. "It's your dream," says Rosalind Cartwright, chair of psychology at Chicago's Medical Center. "If you don't like it, change it."

Evidence from brain imaging supports this view. ④ The brain is as active during REM (rapid eye movement) sleep—when most vivid dreams occur—as it is when fully awake, says Dr. Eric Nofzinger at the University of Pittsburgh. But not all parts of the brain are equally involved, the limbic system (the "emotional brain") is especially active, while the prefrontal cortex (the center of intellect and reasoning) is relatively quiet. "We wake up from dreams happy or depressed, and those feelings can stay with us all day," says Stanford sleep researcher Dr. William Dement.

The link between dreams and emotions shows up among the patients in Cartwright's clinic. ⑤ Most people seem to have more bad dreams early in the night, progressing toward happier ones before awakening, suggesting that they are working through negative feelings generated during the day. Because our conscious mind is occupied with daily life we don't always think about the emotional significance of the day's events—until, it appears, we begin to dream.

And this process need not be left to the unconscious. Cartwright believes one can exercise conscious control over recurring bad dreams. As soon as you awaken, identify what is upsetting about the dream. Visualize how you would like it to end instead, the next time it occurs, try to wake up just enough to control its course. With much practice people can learn to, literally, do it in their sleep.

⑥At the end of the day, there's probably little reason to pay attention to our dreams at all unless they keep us from sleeping or "we wake up in a panic", Cartwright says. Terrorism, economic uncertainties and general feelings of insecurity have increased people's anxiety. Those suffering from persistent nightmares should seek help from a therapist. For the rest of us, the brain has its ways of working through bad feelings. Sleep — or rather dream — on it and you'll feel better in the morning.

▶ 重点词汇:

neurologist	神经病学家,神经科医师(n.)
switch	转变,转向(n./v.)
random	随机的,任意的(adj.)
byproduct	副产品(n.)
thermostat	调温器(n.)
regulate	调节;管理,控制(v.)
harness	马具;治理,利用(n./v.)
occur	出现;发生(v.)
limbic system	[大脑]边缘系统
prefrontal cortex	[大脑]前额叶皮层
recur	反复出现,再发生(v.)
visualize	想象;使形象化(v.)
significance	重要性;重要的状态或性质(n.)
persistent	持续的;坚持不懈的(adj.)
nightmare	梦魇,噩梦(n.)
therapist	治疗学家(n.)

🔍 难句解析:

① A century ago, Freud formulated his revolutionary theory that dreams were the disguised shadows of our unconscious desires and rears; by the late 1970s, neurologists had switched to thinking of them as just "mental noise" — the random byproducts of the neural-repair work that goes on during sleep.

【结构分析】本句被分号分为两部分，其中第一部分的主干是Freud formulated his revolutionary theory…，宾语theory后面是一个以that引导的同位语从句，说明theory的内容；在第二部分中，代词them指代的是dreams，破折号后面的部分the random byproducts of the neural-repair work…进一步解释什么是mental noise，work后面的that引导一个定语从句，修饰work。

② Now researchers suspect that dreams are part of the mind's emotional thermostat, regulating moods while the brain is "off-line".

【结构分析】suspect后面是that引导的宾语从句；逗号之后的现在分词短语regulating moods…做定语，解释thermostat的意思，句末的while引导一个时间状语从句。

③ And one leading authority says that these intensely powerful mental events can be not only harnessed but actually brought under conscious control, to help us sleep and feel better.

【结构分析】该句的主干是one leading authority says，其宾语是that引导的宾语从句。宾语从句的主干是these events can be not only harnessed but actually brought…，其中并列连词结构not only…but（also）连接两个过去分词，表示"不仅被驾驭……而且被有意识地加以控制"。动词不定式to help…在宾语从句中做结果状语。

④ The brain is as active during REM (rapid eye movement) sleep — when most vivid dreams occur — as it is when fully awake, says Dr. Eric Nofzinger at the University of Pittsburgh.

【结构分析】该句是一个倒装句，句首是间接引语的宾语从句，主谓结构后置，即says Dr. Eric。宾语从句的主干是比较结构The brain is as active during REM as it is when fully awake。两个破折号之间是插入语，做定语从句，修饰REM sleep，即"出现清晰梦境的快速动眼睡眠"。

⑤ Most people seem to have more bad dreams early in the night, progressing toward happier ones before awakening, suggesting that they are working through negative feelings generated during the day.

【结构分析】该句的主句后跟有两个现在分词结构，第一个分词结构表伴随，其动作和主句中的动作几乎同时发生；第二个分词结构表结果，即"因此表明……"。

⑥ At the end of the day, there's probably little reason to pay attention to our dreams at all unless they keep us from sleeping or "we wake up in a panic", Cartwright says.

【结构分析】句首的At the end of the day是时间状语，there's probably little reason to pay attention to our dreams at all是主句，后面的unless引导条件状语从句，其中包含以or连接的两个并列分句。

【理解难点】在英语中，如果要表示一句话或一个观点是某个人说的，这个说话的人通常出现在句子中间或者末尾。

▶ 全文翻译：

　　在高质量睡眠的所有因素中，梦似乎是最无法控制的一个。在梦中，进入这样一个世界：逻辑暂时失去了效用，死人会开口说话。一个世纪前，弗洛伊德阐述了革命性的理论，即梦是人们潜意识中欲望和恐惧经伪装后的预示；到了20世纪70年代末期，神经病学家们转而认为梦是"精神噪声"，即睡眠时进行的神经修复活动的一种杂乱的副产品。目前，研究人员猜想梦是大脑情感自动调节系统的组成部分，会在大脑处于"掉线"状态时对情绪进行调整。一名重要的权威人士说，梦这种异常强烈的精神活动不仅能被驾驭，事实上还可以有意识地加以控制，以帮助我们得到更好的睡眠和感受。芝加哥医疗中心心理学系主任罗莎琳德·卡特赖特说："梦是你自己的，如果你不喜欢，就改变它。"

　　大脑造影的证据支持了以上观点。匹兹堡大学的埃里克博士说，在出现清晰梦境的快速动眼睡眠中大脑和完全清醒时一样活跃。但并非大脑的所有部分都一样，脑边缘系统（"情绪大脑"）异常活跃，而前额皮层（思维和推理的中心地带）则相对平静。斯坦福睡眠研究员威廉·德蒙特博士说："我们从梦中醒来，或者高兴或者沮丧，这些情绪会伴随我们一整天。"

　　梦和情绪之间的联系在卡特赖特诊所里的病人身上显露出来了。多数人似乎在晚上入睡的较早阶段做更多不好的梦，而在快睡醒前会逐渐做开心一些的梦，这说明人们在梦里渐渐克服了白天的不良情绪。因为清醒时我们的头脑被日常琐事占据着，所以并不会总是想着白天发生的事情对我们情绪的影响，直到我们开始做梦，这种影响才出现。

　　这一过程不一定是无意识的。卡特赖特认为人们可以练习有意识地控制噩梦的重现。你一醒来就立刻确定梦中有什么在困扰你，设想一下你所希望的梦的结局，下次再做同样的梦时，试图醒过来以控制它的进程。通过多次练习，人们完全可以学会在梦中这样做。

　　卡特赖特说，说到底，只要梦不使我们无法睡眠或"从梦中惊醒"，就没有理由太在意所做的梦。恐怖主义、经济不稳定及通常的不安全感都增加了人们的焦虑。那些长期受到噩梦折磨的人应该寻求专家帮助，而对其他人来说，大脑有自动消除不良情绪的方法。安心睡觉甚至做梦，早上醒来时你会感觉好多了。

Passage Twelve

Currently, the economic costs of pediatric obesity in the United States are relatively small. ①Without effective intervention, the costs of obesity might well become catastrophic, arising not only from escalating medical expenses but also from diminished worker productivity, caused by physical and psychological disabilities. Future economic losses would be incalculable.

Like global warming, the obesity epidemic is a looming crisis that requires action before all the scientific evidence is in. ②And as with climate change, some have questioned experts' forecasts, doubting the far-reaching impact of obesity, though skepticism is gradually being overcome by accumulating data. ③Others would delay concerted efforts to address the problem, placing hope in the development of new drugs or surgical procedures that might offer a painless technological fix. Or they argue that the costs of action are too great, not recognizing that our survival depends on solving the problem. But I believe that obesity differs in one important respect from global warming: simple solutions are available, and with a comprehensive national strategy, we may be able to implement them without great sacrifice.

Certainly, we have much to learn about the regulation of body weight. Low-fat diets have yielded disappointing results, and very-low-carbohydrate diets appear to be more effective only in the short term. Novel approaches that focus on the quality rather than the ratio of macronutrients appear promising, and other areas warrant study, including the effects of sleep deprivation, stress, and infectious agents on weight. Unfortunately, we lack a comprehensive strategy for encouraging children to eat a healthful diet and engage in physical activity. ④Such a strategy would include legislation that regulates junk-food advertising, provides adequate funding for decent lunches and regular physical activities at school, restructures the farm-subsidies program to favor nutrient-dense rather than calorie-dense produce, and mandates insurance coverage for preventing and treating pediatric obesity.

Parents must take responsibility for their children's welfare by providing high-quality food, limiting television viewing, and modeling a healthful lifestyle. Fortunately, with the exercise of both personal and social responsibility, we have the power to choose the shape of things to come.

▶ 重点词汇：

catastrophic	灾难性的（*adj.*）
escalate	增加；上升（*v.*）
incalculable	无法估算的（*adj.*）
skepticism	怀疑态度（*n.*）
concerted	同心协力的（*adj.*）
carbohydrate	碳水化合物（*n.*）
subsidy	补贴（*n.*）

🔍 难句解析：

① Without effective intervention, the costs of obesity might well become catastrophic, arising not only from escalating medical expenses but also from diminished worker productivity, caused by physical and psychological disabilities.

【结构分析】该句的框架为the costs might become catastrophic...arising not only from A but also from B，如果没有有效干预，肥胖的代价会变成灾难，这个代价不仅仅是医疗开销上的，而且还有劳动力的萎缩。caused引导的过去分词结构充当productivity的后置定语。

【理解难点】并列结构not only...but also的考点和and结构一致。比如本句可以对应这样一个句子：What can cause the escalating cost of obesity?

② And as with climate change, some have questioned experts' forecasts, doubting the far-reaching impact of obesity, though skepticism is gradually being overcome by accumulating data.

【结构分析】as with climate change充当状语，意思是"和……一样"。some have questioned forecasts是主干，doubting为现在分词结构充当伴随状语，though则引导让步状语从句。

【理解难点】这句话的结构并不复杂，句内语义的逻辑关系走向是重点。比如，阅读理解中可以这样命题：What does the author want to emphasize? 答案应该是"怀疑"或者"质疑"，而不是已经能克服怀疑的海量数据，转折后是重点。

③ Others would delay concerted efforts to address the problem, placing hope in the development of new drugs or surgical procedures that might offer a painless technological fix.

【结构分析】主干为Others would delay efforts，placing为现在分词结构充当伴随状语，that引导定语从句修饰new drugs or surgical procedures。

【理解难点】句内的语义关系是考点。new drugs，surgical procedures，concerted efforts，哪一个才是解决问题的希望？

④ Such a strategy would include legislation that regulates junk-food advertising, provides adequate funding for decent lunches and regular physical activities at school, restructures the farm-subsidies program to favor nutrient-dense rather than calorie-dense produce, and mandates insurance coverage for preventing and treating pediatric obesity.

【结构分析】这是个简单句：a strategy would include legislation。that引导的定语从句修饰legislation，其为并列结构that regulates...provides...restructures... and mandates...（that A，B，C，and D），其中C这个部分又因为使用了C1...rather than C2显得复杂了，rather than是一个二者择其一的并列结构。

【理解难点】要找准并列结构的成分，把握"形式一致、成分一致"的原则。

▶ 全文翻译：

目前，美国儿童肥胖的经济代价相对较小。但如果没有有效的干预措施，肥胖的代价很可能会成为灾难性的，这不仅会使医疗费用增加，而且身体和心理残疾会导致劳动者的生产力下降。未来的经济损失将无法估量。

与全球变暖一样，肥胖流行病也是一场迫在眉睫的危机，需要在所有科学证据都出现之前采取行动。与气候变化类似，一些人质疑专家的预测，怀疑肥胖的深远影响，尽管越来越多的数据已经逐渐消除了这种怀疑。其他人则会推迟解决这个问题的共同努力，寄希望于开发出可能提供无痛技术修复的新药或手术。或者他们认为行动的代价太大，没有意识到我们的生存取决于解决问题。但我认为，肥胖与全球变暖在一个重要方面有所不同：有简单的解决方案可用，这就是综合的国家战略，我们或许能够在不付出巨大牺牲的情况下实施这些方案。

当然，我们有很多关于体重调节的知识要学习。低脂饮食产生了令人失望的结果，而且极低碳水化合物饮食似乎只在短期内更有效。关注大量营养素的质量而非比例的新方法似乎很有前途，还有其他领域值得研究，包括睡眠不足、压力和传染性因素对体重的影响。不幸的是，我们缺乏一个全面的战略来鼓励孩子们健康饮食和参加体育活动。这样的战略要包括立法监管垃圾食品广告，为像样的午餐和学校的常规体育活动提供充足的资金，重组农场补贴计划以支持营养密集而非热量密集的农产品，并将预防和治疗儿童肥胖强制纳入保险范围。

父母必须通过提供高质量的食物、限制观看电视和塑造健康的生活方式来为孩子的幸福负责。幸运的是，通过履行个人和社会责任，我们有能力选择未来的事情。

Passage Thirteen

①Several weeks after Erica Taylor recovered from her COVID-19 symptoms of nausea and cough, she became confused and forgetful, failing to even recognize her own car, the only Toyota Prius in her apartment complex's parking lot; ②Lisa Mizelle, a veteran nurse practitioner at an urgent care clinic who contracted the virus in July, finds herself forgetting routine treatments and lab tests and has to ask colleagues about terminology she used to know automatically.

It's becoming known as COVID brain fog: troubling cognitive symptoms that can include memory loss, confusion, difficulty focusing, dizziness and grasping for everyday words. Increasingly, COVID survivors say brain fog is impairing their ability to work and function normally.

③Scientists aren't sure what causes brain fog, which varies widely and affects even people who became only mildly physically ill from COVID-19 and had no previous medical conditions. ④Leading theories are that it arises when the body's immune response to the virus doesn't shut down or from inflammation in blood vessels leading to the brain. "The simplest answer is: people still have persistent immune activation after the initial infection subsided," said Dr. Avindra Nath, chief of infections of the nervous system at the National Institute of Neurological Disorders and Stroke.

⑤Inflammation in blood vessels, or cells lining the vessels, may be involved and inflammatory molecules, released in effective immune responses can also be sort of toxins, particularly to the brain, said Dr. Serena Spudich, chief of neurological infections and global neurology at Yale School of Medicine.

⑥Tiny strokes may cause some symptoms, said Dr. Dona Kim Murphey, a neurologist and neuroscientist, who herself has experienced post-COVID neurological issues, including "alien hand syndrome", in which she felt a "superbizarre sense of my left hand, like I didn't understand why it was positioned the way it was". Other possible causes are autoimmune reactions "when antibodies mistakenly attack nerve cells," Dr. Spudich said.

So far, MRI scans haven't indicated damaged brain areas, neurologists say.

▶ 重点词汇：

nausea	恶心（n.）
veteran	熟练的（adj.）
practitioner	从业人员（n.）
dizziness	头晕眼花（n.）
impair	破坏（v.）
inflammation	发炎，炎症（n.）
persistent	持续的（adj.）
subside	下降，减退（v.）
molecule	分子（n.）
neurological	神经的（adj.）
alien	不相容的；陌生的；外来的（adj.）
syndrome	综合征（n.）
superbizarre	超级怪异的（adj.）

🔍 难句解析：

① Several weeks after Erica Taylor recovered from her COVID-19 symptoms of nausea and cough, she became confused and forgetful, failing to even recognize her own car, the only Toyota Prius in her apartment complex's parking lot.

【结构分析】本句主干为she became confused and forgetful，主干前为时间状语，该状语成分包含一个after引导的时间状语从句，主干后现在分词结构failing to do做伴随状语，解释主干的状态（也可认为是结果状语），该状语中又包含一个同位语结构，即"名词1，名词2（同位语）+后置定语"。

【理解难点】要注意句子结构隐含的时间关系，感染COVID-19在先，症状为nausea和cough，康复几周后才confused和forgetful，症状为failing to recognize her own car。这可能会成为阅读理解中的命题点。

② Lisa Mizelle, a veteran nurse practitioner at an urgent care clinic who contracted the virus in July, finds herself forgetting routine treatments and lab tests and has to ask colleagues about terminology she used to know automatically.

【结构分析】该句的主干为Lisa Mizelle finds herself...and has to ask，主语后有同位语的复合结构，即"名词1，名词2（同位语）+后置定语"，该后置定语有两个并列结构at an urgent care clinic和who引导的定语从句，都是直接修饰名词

practitioner。谓语动词中finds sb. doing往往表达意料之外的结果，要注意并列结构and前后的并列成分为finds和has。

【理解难点】要注意同位语的复合结构成为考点的可能性，Mizelle有不止一个信息，veteran nurse、在急护门诊工作、7月份感染病毒，命题时是可以出排除题的。同时要注意并列结构前后的"三个一致"要求：形式一致、成分一致、语义走向一致。

③ Scientists aren't sure about what causes brain fog, which varies widely and affects even people who became only mildly physically ill from COVID-19 and had no previous medical conditions.

【结构分析】该句主干为Scientists aren't sure，what为about的宾语从句，which引导定语从句修饰brain fog，该定语从句中又嵌套了一个who引导的定语从句修饰people。每个定语从句中都有and并列结构。第一个and前后的并列成分为varies and affects，第二个and前后的并列成分为became and had。

【理解难点】要非常小心定语从句的指向对象。扩大来看，要注意多个后置定语并置时的修饰对象，有的是并列指向同一个对象，有的则是嵌套。同时要注意并列结构的并列成分，这会引发传递效应。比如，阅读理解可以这样命题：What do we know about brain fog?

④ Leading theories are that it arises when the body's immune response to the virus doesn't shut down or from inflammation in blood vessels leading to the brain.

【结构分析】该句主干为theories are that...，that引导表语从句，该表语从句中有一个时间状语从句。该时间状语从句很长，主干为immune response doesn't shut down。要特别注意并列结构or前后的并列成分。这里的or from其实是or arises from，表示原因。即arises when or arises from，用来说明脑雾产生原因的主流观点。同时，本句出现了两个leading，第一个是形容词，意思是"主流的，领先的"，第二个是词组leading to现在分词，表示"通向，导致"。

【理解难点】这是个特别容易命题的句子，比如一种命题方式为：When does the brain fog occur? 这就需要通过句子的结构精确定位leading theories的内容。

⑤ Inflammation in blood vessels, or cells lining the vessels, may be involved and inflammatory molecules, released in effective immune responses can also be sort of toxins, particularly to the brain.

【结构分析】该句是由and引导的两个并列分句：Inflammation may be involved and

molecules can also be sort of toxins。第一个分句中的inflammation存在于两个地方，即blood vessels或者cells，cells是在血管里。第二个分句中的molecules也是有炎症的（inflammatory），是由有效的免疫反应释放的（released为过去分词，充当molecules的后置定语）。

【理解难点】该句出现两个主句的并列，容易混淆。对and和or引导的并列结构的精确分析，仍然是阅读理解和解题的重要内容，怎么强调都不为过。

⑥ Tiny strokes may cause some symptoms, said Dr. Dona Kim Murphey, a neurologist and neuroscientist, who herself has experienced post-COVID neurological issues, including "alien hand syndrome", in which she felt a "superbizarre sense of my left hand, like I didn't understand why it was positioned the way it was".

【结构分析】这个句子很长，但并不一定难，阅读时不要被长度吓倒。先去掉插入语said Dr. Dona Kim Murphey, a neurologist and neuroscientist, who herself has experienced post-COVID neurological issues，这是典型的"名词1，名词2+后置定语"的同位语复合结构。主干为strokes may cause symptoms，后面用including做后置定语，症状包含异手综合征，in which为修饰syndrome的定语从句。定语从句描述异手综合征的详细情况：she（医生）felt a sense, like为并列句，解释什么样的感觉。

【理解难点】插入语往往干扰阅读的流畅性，通常会出现对人物身份的解释和扩展，但有时也会成为命题的重点，我们需要根据题干进行精确定位。

▶ 全文翻译：

从新冠肺炎恶心和咳嗽的症状中恢复过来几周后，埃里卡·泰勒变得糊涂和健忘，甚至认不出自己的车，这可是她公寓停车场里唯一的丰田普锐斯。丽莎·米泽尔是一家急诊诊所的资深护士，今年7月感染了病毒，她发现自己忘记了常规治疗和实验室检查，不得不向同事询问她过去不加思索就知道的术语。

这种症状被称为COVID脑雾：令人困扰的认知症状，包括记忆力减退、困惑、注意力难以集中、头晕和难以掌握日常用语。越来越多的新冠肺炎幸存者表示，脑雾正在削弱他们正常工作的能力和日常生活的功能。

科学家们尚不确定是什么原因导致了脑雾，影响对象范围很大，连那些原本身体健康、在感染新冠病毒后仅出现轻微症状的患者也会患上脑雾。主流观点认为，当人体对病毒的免疫反应没有停止，或者是通向大脑的血管有炎症时，脑雾就会出现。"最简单的答案是，在最初的感染消退后，人们仍有持续的免疫激活，"美国国家神经疾病和中风研究所神经系统感染科主任阿维德拉·纳特博士说。

耶鲁大学医学院神经感染和全球神经学主任塞雷娜·斯普迪奇博士表示，原因可能还涉及血管或血管壁的炎症，因为有效的免疫反应释放的消炎物质有时可能反而是一种毒素，尤其对大脑而言。

神经病学家兼神经科学家唐纳·金·穆尔菲博士表示，轻微的中风可能会导致一些症状。她自己也经历过新冠肺炎后的神经问题，包括"异手综合征"，在这种情况下，她感觉到"我的左手有一种超级奇怪的感觉，就像我不明白它为什么是在这个位置"。斯普迪奇说："其他可能的原因是抗体错误地攻击神经细胞时的自身免疫反应。"

神经学家说，到目前为止，核磁共振扫描还没有显示大脑有受损区域。

Passage Fourteen

It was 3:45 in the morning when the vote was finally taken. ① After six months of arguing and final 16 hours of hot parliamentary debates, Australia's Northern Territory became the first legal authority in the world to allow doctors to take the lives of incurably ill patients who wish to die. The measure passed by the convincing vote of 15 to 10. Almost immediately word flashed on the Internet and was picked up, half a world away, by John Hofsess, executive director of the Right to Die Society of Canada. He sent it on via the group's on-line service, Death NET. Says Hofsess: "We posted bulletins all day long, because of course this isn't just something that happened in Australia. It's world history."

The full import may take a while to sink in. *The NT Rights of the Terminally Ill Law* has left physicians and citizens alike trying to deal with its moral and practical implications. ② Some have breathed sighs of relief, others, including churches, right-to-life groups and the Australian Medical Association, bitterly attacked the bill and the haste of its passage. But the tide is unlikely to turn back. ③ In Australia — where an aging population, life-extending technology and changing community attitudes have all played their part — other states are going to consider making a similar law to deal with euthanasia. In the US and Canada, where the right-to-die movement is gathering strength, observers are waiting for the dominoes to start falling.

Under the new Northern Territory law, an adult patient can request death — probably by a deadly injection or pill — to put an end to suffering. The patient must be diagnosed as terminally ill by two doctors. ④ After a "cooling off" period of seven days, the patient can sign a certificate of request. After 48 hours the wish for death can be met. For Lloyd Nickson, a 54-year-old Darwin resident suffering from lung cancer, the NT Rights of

Terminally Ill law means he can get on with living without the haunting fear of his suffering: a terrifying death from his breathing condition. "I'm not afraid of dying from a spiritual point of view, but what I was afraid of was how I'd go, because I've watched people die in the hospital fighting for oxygen and clawing at their masks," he says.

▶ 重点词汇：

parliamentary	议会的，国会的（*adj.*）
incurably	不可治愈地（*adv.*）
turn back	逆转；往回走
euthanasia	安乐死（*n.*）
domino	多米诺骨牌（*n.*）
diagnose	诊断（*v.*）
certificate	证书；证明（*n.*）
objection	反对（*n.*）
sink in	被理解
cool off	使冷静

难句解析：

① After six months of arguing and final 16 hours of hot parliamentary debates, Australia's Northern Territory became the first legal authority in the world to allow doctors to take the lives of incurably ill patients who wish to die.

【结构分析】句子的主体结构是Australia's Northern Territory became the first legal authority...。句首是表示时间的介词词组做状语：After six months of arguing and final 16 hours of hot parliamentary debates，后面的动词不定式to allow doctors to take the lives of incurably ill patients who wish to die相当于定语从句which allows doctors to...，修饰legal authority，who引导定语从句who wish to die修饰前面的patients。

【理解难点】理解句子的关键在于剔除庞杂的修饰成分，抓住句子的主干。

② Some have breathed sighs of relief, others, including churches, right-to-life groups and the Australian Medical Association, bitterly attacked the bill and the haste of its passage. But the tide is unlikely to turn back.

【结构分析】第一句话中，逗号松散地连接两个表示对比的句子：Some have breathed...

others...bitterly attacked...others之后是介词词组including churches, right-to-life groups and the Australian Medical Association对others做进一步的解释。its passage中的its指代前面提到的the bill。第二句与第一句是转折关系。

【理解难点】tide的本意是"潮水，潮汐"，这里的引申含义是"趋势，趋向"；turn the tide是"使形式转变，改变局面"的意思。bill在这里是"法案"的意思。另外还要理解some和others的对比关系。

③ In Australia — where an aging population, life-extending technology and changing community attitudes have all played their part — other states are going to consider making a similar law to deal with euthanasia.

【结构分析】这个句子的主体结构是：...other states are going to consider...句首的In Australia是介词词组做地点状语，后面的where引导定语从句where an aging population, life-extending technology and changing community attitudes have all played their part，进一步解释Australia的具体情况。

【理解难点】注意两个破折号之间的句子说各种因素都发挥了作用，是针对其他州考虑制定关于安乐死法律这件事而言的。另外注意consider的用法，consider后面一般接v.-ing形式或that引导的宾语从句。

④ After a "cooling off" period of seven days, the patient can sign a certificate of request. After 48 hours the wish for death can be met.

【结构分析】两个句子都是简单句。第一句话中前面是介词词组做时间状语：After a "cooling off" period of seven days。第二句使用了被动语态。

【理解难点】"cooling off"在这里是指"给病人充足的考虑时间以做出冷静的决定"。meet在这里是"满足"的意思，可以和wish, demand, need, requirement等词连用。

▶ 全文翻译：

凌晨3:45进行了最终表决。经过6个月的争论和最后16个小时国会的激烈辩论，澳大利亚北部地区（澳北州）成为世界上第一个允许医生根据绝症病人的个人意愿来结束其生命的合法当局。这一法案以令人信服的15票对10票通过。几乎同时，该消息就出现在互联网上。身处地球另一端的加拿大死亡权利协会执行主席约翰·霍夫塞斯在收到该消息后便通过协会的在线服务"死亡之网"发了公告。他说："我们一整天都在发布公告，因为这件事的意义不在于它是在澳大利亚发生的事情，而是因为这是世界历史上的一件大事。"

要充分理解这一法案的深刻意义可能需要一段时间。澳北州晚期病人权利法使得无论是内科医生还是普通市民都同样地力图从道义和实际意义两方面来对待这一问题。一些人如释重负，另外一些人，包括教会、生命权利组织以及澳大利亚医学会成员都对这一决议及其仓促的通过进行了猛烈的抨击。但这一潮流已无法逆转。在澳大利亚，人口老龄化、延长寿命技术和公众态度的变化都发挥着各自的作用。其他州也将考虑制定类似的法律来处理安乐死问题。在美国和加拿大，死亡权利运动正在积蓄力量。观察家们正在等待多米诺骨牌产生的效应。

根据澳北州所通过的这项新法案，成年病人可以要求安乐死——可能是通过注射致死药剂或服用致死药片——来结束痛苦。但此前病人必须由两名医生诊断其确实已病入膏肓，然后再经过7天的冷静思考期，方可签署一份申请证明。48小时后，才可以满足其安乐死的愿望。对于居住在达尔文市的现年54岁的肺癌患者利奥德·尼克森来说，这一法案意味着他可以平静地生活下去而无须整天惧怕即将来临的苦难：因呼吸困难而在煎熬中痛苦地死去。"从思想上说，我并不害怕死，但我怕的是怎样死，因为我在医院看到过病人在缺氧时苦苦挣扎，用手抓他们的面罩时的情景，"他说。

Passage Fifteen

Technically, any substance other than food that alters our bodily or mental functioning is a drug. Many people mistakenly believe the term drug refers only to some sort of medicine or an illegal chemical taken by drug addicts. They don't realize that familiar substances such as alcohol and tobacco are also drugs. This is why the more neutral term substance is now used by many physicians and psychologists. ① The phrase "substance abuse" is often used instead of "drug abuse" to make clear that substances such as alcohol and tobacco can be just as harmfully misused as heroin and cocaine.

② We live in a society in which the medicinal and social use of substances (drugs) is pervasive: an aspirin to quiet a headache, some wine to be sociable, coffee to get going in the morning, a cigarette for the nerves. When do these socially acceptable and apparently constructive uses of a substance become misuses? First of all, most substances taken in excess will produce negative effects such as poisoning or intense perceptual distortions. Repeated use of a substance can also lead to physical addiction or substance dependence. ③ Dependence is marked first by an increased tolerance, with more and more of the substance required to produce the desired effect, and then by the appearance of unpleasant withdrawal symptoms when the substance is discontinued.

Drugs (substances) that affect the central nervous system and alter perception, mood, and behavior are known as psychoactive substances. ④ Psychoactive substances are commonly grouped according to whether they are stimulants, depressants, or hallucinogens. Stimulants initially speed up or activate the central nervous system, whereas depressants slow it down. Hallucinogens have their primary effect on perception, distorting and altering it in a variety of ways including producing hallucinations. These are the substances often called psychedelic (from the Greek word meaning "mind-manifestation") because they seemed to radically alter one's state of consciousness.

▶ 重点词汇：

substance	物质；实质；财产（n.）
addict	使成瘾；成瘾者（v./n.）
psychologist	心理学家（n.）
cocaine	可卡因（n.）
pervasive	普遍的（adj.）
sociable	社交的（adj.）
negative	否定的；消极的（adj.）
poisoning	中毒；毒害（n.）
distortion	扭曲；曲解（n.）
tolerance	宽容；忍受（n.）
symptom	症状（n.）
psychoactive	药物等对心理起作用的（adj.）
depressant	抑制剂；镇静剂（n.）
hallucinogen	致幻剂（n.）
psychedelic	迷幻剂（n.）

🔍 难句解析：

① The phrase "substance abuse" is often used instead of "drug abuse" to make clear that substances such as alcohol and tobacco can be just as harmfully misused as heroin and cocaine.

【结构分析】句子的主干是句子的前半部分The phrase "substance abuse" is often used... to make clear..., to make clear that...是动词不定式做状语，表示目的。that后面接的是宾语从句，做动词make clear的宾语。

【理解难点】注意 "make＋sth.＋adj." 结构，make clear that...，因为sth.是一个that引导

的从句，所以放在了形容词clear的后面。另外注意as...as的用法。

② We live in a society in which the medicinal and social use of substances (drugs) is pervasive: an aspirin to quiet a headache, some wine to be sociable, coffee to get going in the morning, a cigarette for the nerves.

【结构分析】句子的主干是We live in a society...，后面的which引导定语从句in which the medicinal and social use of substances (drugs) is pervasive，修饰 society。冒号后面的部分是表示并列关系的名词词组，用于举例说明前面提出的观点，开始可以忽略不看。

【理解难点】注意冒号后面列举的前三个名词词组中的动词不定式都相当于定语成分，修饰前面的中心名词，表示其功效。

③ Dependence is marked first by an increased tolerance, with more and more of the substance required to produce the desired effect, and then by the appearance of unpleasant withdrawal symptoms when the substance is discontinued.

【结构分析】句子的主干结构是Dependence is marked first by..., and then by...，中间逗号隔开的成分是"with+*n.*+过去分词"结构：with more and more of the substance required to produce the desired effect，做状语，用于进一步解释药物依赖的第一种表现。when the substance is discontinued是表示时间的状语从句。

【理解难点】注意and连接的两个by介词词组是并列关系，这样就能抓住句子的主干了。另外注意名词在这里的特殊意义：dependence指"对药物的依赖"，withdrawal的意思是"停止用药"。

④ Psychoactive substances are commonly grouped according to whether they are stimulants, depressants, or hallucinogens.

【结构分析】句子的主干部分是Psychoactive substances are... grouped according to...，使用了被动语态。其中whether引导宾语从句whether they are stimulants, depressants, or hallucinogens，做介词according to的宾语。

【理解难点】group在句中用作动词，是"分类"的意思。

▶ 全文翻译：

从专业角度来说，除食品外，任何能改变我们生理和心理机能的物质都是药物。很多人错误地认为"药物"这个词仅仅指某些药品或是吸毒者服用的违禁化学品。他们没有意识到诸如酒精、烟草这些我们熟悉的物质也是药物。这也是现在许多内科医生和心理学家使用"物质"这个更加中性的词的原因。他们常用"物质滥用"而不用"药物滥用"来清楚地表明滥用酒精、烟草这样的物质如同滥用海洛因和可卡因一样有害。

我们生活在一个医疗和社交方面都广泛使用物质（药物）的社会里：用来缓解头痛的阿司匹林、用来应酬的酒、早晨用来提神的咖啡，还有定神用的香烟。使用这些物质得到了社会认可，且显然具有积极的作用，但什么时候就变成滥用了呢？首先，大多数物质的过量使用都会产生负面影响，如中毒或感知严重错乱。反复使用一种物质可以导致成瘾或对该物质的依赖。依赖的最初表现是不断增长的耐药量，要产生预期的效果需要的药剂量越来越大，而一旦中断使用就会出现难受的停药症状。

影响中枢神经系统、改变感知、情绪和行为的药物（物质）属于对神经起显著作用的物质，它们通常分为兴奋剂、镇静剂和致幻剂。兴奋剂主要起到加速或激活中枢神经系统的作用，而镇静剂则相反：减缓它的活动。致幻剂主要影响人的感知，通过多种方式对感知加以扭曲或改变，其中包括产生幻觉。这些物质常被认为能"引起幻觉"（psychedelic一词源于希腊语，意为"心灵显现"），因为它们似乎能彻底改变人的意识状态。

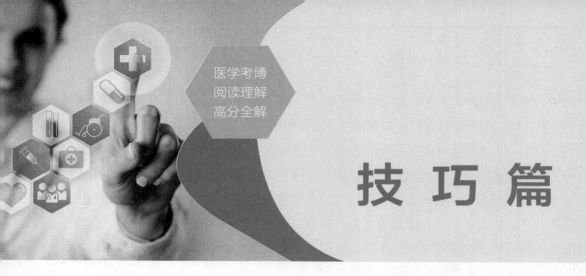

技 巧 篇

第一节 解题流程与技巧总结

在做过了一定量的阅读理解题目之后，我们再为大家梳理一下解题流程和技巧，以便考生在实际考试中快速解题。

本书所提到的解答各种题目的方法，主要强调答题时思维方式的客观性，即找到正确答案的客观依据一定是原文，而不是常理，更不是我们的主观臆断和想象。整个方法的讲述主要是为了培养考生客观思考问题的思维习惯，重点讲"怎样（how）"的问题，即怎样去读题干，怎样找题干与原文的对应关系，怎样对比选项并答题，而不是讲"为什么（why）"要选此选项。

为了实现上述目标，本书采用"三步法"来解答阅读题，同时强调"比"的概念，即选择答案时要抛开对与不对的观念，即答案是通过对比选项"比"出来的，而不是推理原文得出来的。

 一、"三步法"具体步骤

1. 读题干

考生在考场上首先应读问题的题干，这样做主要是为了下一步有针对性地阅读原文，因为每读一个题干，对文章重点内容的了解就会加深一步，从而避免眉毛胡子一把抓，读到最后却什么也没记住这一"千古难题"。在读题干的时候，我们要求大家做如下的工作。

（1）题干分类

为了方便对问题的阅读和记忆，我们首先应对题干进行分类，根据题干中是否出现了原文的具体内容和信息，把题目分为两种，从而把复杂的问题简单化。

　　第一种：题干主要由原文中的关键词或其他有实际意义的词语构成，即题干反映了文章的某些重要信息。（关键词指有助于我们在阅读原文时迅速找到应该画线的地方的词或词组）。

　　例1：The growth of specialization in the 19th century might be more clearly seen in sciences such as _____.

　　【译文】19世纪的专业化发展可能在 _____ 学科里看得更清楚。

　　【分析】在这个题干中，关键词是growth of specialization（专业化发展）和19th century（19世纪）。

　　例2：The author writes the development of geology to demonstrate _____.

　　【译文】作者写到地质学的发展，用来说明 _____。

　　【分析】在这个题干中，关键词是 development of geology（地质学的发展）。

　　例3：The direct reason for specialization is _____.

　　【译文】专业化的直接原因是 _____。

　　【分析】在这个题干中，关键词是direct reason（直接原因）和specialization（专业化）。

　　第二种：题干中没有出现原文的关键词或其他有实际意义的词语，也没有出现这些词的变形，即题干没有反映文章的具体信息。

　　例如：We can infer from the passage that _____.

　　【译文】根据这篇文章我们可以推断出 _____。

　　【分析】这一题干的问法是宽泛而笼统的，没有出现原文中的关键词或其他有实际意义的词语。

　　（2）应对办法

　　第一种：如果题干反映了文章的某些重要信息，则不仅要求考生读懂题干问的是什么，而且要记住题干中的关键词，尤其是名词，因为名词在原文中不易发生变动。这些关键词在很大程度上"透露"了文章的某些重要信息。对于那些基础很差、实在读不懂题干的同学，也请务必记住题干中表示时间、地点、人物等的名词。对于地点、人物等大写的名词，考生只需记住这些词的第一个大写字母就可以了，如Alan Greenspan，考生只需要记住A和G即可。之所以要记住这些关键词的"长相"，就是为了在阅读文章时能够"按图索骥"。这里需要提醒考生的是，如果两个题干中出现了同一个关键词，那么这个关键词就无须记忆了。

　　第二种：如果题干没有反映文章的具体信息，考生也就无须记忆，了解其内容即可，以便在阅读原文时大致圈定答案在原文中对应的位置。

（3）阅读题干的目的

总而言之，之所以要求大家先读题干并对题干进行分类，同时要求大家记住其中的关键信息，就是为了使考生在下一步阅读文章时能够抓住重点，即根据问题有针对性地去读原文并画出有用的信息。这样不仅可以使考生在现有水平的基础上迅速提高阅读速度，放弃对与题干无关的生词及信息的理解和记忆，而且可以使考生在答题时知其然，从根本上提高选择答案时的信心和准确率。

2. 读原文

第二步就是阅读原文，读文章时首先涉及的一个问题就是边读文章边答题，还是文章全部读完再答题。我们的要求是通篇读完文章再答题。因为这种阅读方法有助于抓住文章的主题和整篇文章的思路方向，从而为下一步选择答案提供宏观指导。但水平稍低的同学会说，当读完原文后，早就不知道讲什么了，就像没读一样。如果这样，也可以边读文章边答会做的题。但这样做的缺点就是会时常停顿，不利于从整体上把握文章的主题和结构模式。在阅读原文时，需要注意如下几点。

（1）考生在按顺序阅读原文时，一定要对重点内容与非重点内容有所区分，并用线画出重点内容。

1）重点内容如下：

➢ 涉及文章中心和段落主题的句子。这类句子出现的位置主要是文章的开头以及每段的段首，也有少量出现在段落末尾。如果最后一段很短，就全部画下来；如果很长就只画后面几句。这一点需要考生在阅读的过程中做出相应的判断。

➢ 与题干所反映的信息相关的句子。我们这里强调的是"相关"，即只要文章内容与你所记的题干（关键词）意思沾边时就可以画出，而不是完全一样时才画，画多了不要紧，但不能少画。这样在答题时不仅可以找到答案在原文中对应的位置，而且可以避免以偏概全。

➢ 表示转折关系的连词。对于文章中出现的but，however，nevertheless等表示转折关系的连词，也一定要画出来，因为由这些词连接起来的句子是一种转折关系，往往是出题的关键点所在。

➢ 表示"绝对化"意义和"第一"的词。文章中出现的none，all，never，nobody，only，absolute，utterly等有绝对化意义的词语以及the first（第一）等词，也是容易出题的地方，因此在阅读的过程中也要画出来。

2）非重点内容如下：

➢ 例子。文章所举的例子是用来进一步论证作者所提出的论点的，相当于论据，因此属于非重点内容，在阅读的过程中可以采取"略读"法，扫一眼了解其大概意思，看有没有与题干相关的信息，以防例子就是考点。无须将例子画出来，也不用记忆其内容。如果在题干中直接提到具体某个例子，这样你看一眼一定能记住；如果题干中根本没提到例子，而只是在选项中提到了，或者答题时要用到，那么可以到答题时再回去看。所以读原文时例子不需要细看。

➤ 生词。考生在按照上述要求阅读的过程中，如果遇到不认识的单词，千万不要纠缠于这一细节，更不必为此而"深深自责"，跳过去或权当没看见就是了。

（2）阅读原文的目的

之所以要求考生按顺序阅读并用线画出与题干相关的重点内容，是因为在阅读的过程中应尽可能多地找出题干与原文内容的对应关系。这样不仅加快了阅读速度，而且记住或找到了答题所需要的相关信息，同时对生词的恰当处理也减轻了考生的心理负担，以便考生下一步把精力集中在如何做对题目上。

3. 读选项，做题

在读选项和做题的时候，请考生注意如下三个大问题。

（1）答题方法

第一步，先做在原文中画出了信息的题。

1）原因

➤ 画有信息的题比没画信息的题做起来轻松、踏实。

➤ 做完这些题目后会对原文的信息有更多的了解，能帮助考生做剩下的题目。

2）方法

不管题目怎么变，但原文一定不会变，所以答题时要从原文中得出哪个选项更准确。当一个问题画了不止一处时，要弄清该题干答题点的真正来源。如果水平偏低判断不出来，那么只能全看。当问题涉及的信息多，不知道应先看原文做出判断，还是先看选项做出判断时，那就要看原文短还是选项短，哪边内容短就先看哪边。当先看选项时，要把四个全看完，但记忆的方法是不一样的，水平高的考生就把内容都记下来；水平不高的考生，就要按照前面说的方法，记住其中的名词。当不能准确判断选项时，我们的主张是："认为合适的"好于"不知道的"，但"不知道的"好于"似懂非懂的"。

第二步，对于没画线的题，对选项进行对比。

根据你对文章方向的把握及在做题时对文章信息的了解，排除你认为肯定不适合的选项，这样可以提高做题的速度。根据题干确定原文的信息点，千万不要在还没做排除时去研究问题，把该扔的都扔完后再研究。因为考试时人比较急躁，在一个人的心态不好时，出错率就较高。我们主张只读一遍原文，尽量通过选项之间的对比将选项区分开来。你脑中现有的信息是：

> 在做画线的题时留下的信息。

> 读原文时对整篇文章方向的把握。

到目前为止，可用的只有这两个信息，就用这两个信息帮助区别对比选项，把肯定不正确的去掉。所谓肯定不正确的选项，是指这个选项与留在你脑中的某些信息产生了冲突。但如果你自己觉得选项中的内容没见过，那就先留着，因为不能断定是文章中的确没有这个内容，还是你没看到。

（2）答题时需要注意的问题

1）在看任何问题的时候，一定要看懂问的是什么。

2）在读原文时，当百分之百确定没有问题，题干与所读的原文内容对应时，就马上放弃这句话；当不确定是否对应时，就将这句话先保留在脑子里，再看下面的内容；如果非常确定是对应的，那就看选项。

3）第一遍看选项时，不需要很仔细；遇到两个相似选项时，再仔细读并进行对比。

4）读文章时，只要求内容上的沾边，比如读了四个选项后，只有A项沾边时，那就选A，无须推理它为什么正确。（这里说的沾边就是与原文内容有关联。）

5）把握答题的出发点，区别以下两个问题：

> 主题干是"根据文章可以推断……（According to the passage, we can infer...）"时，一定要根据对文章主题、方向等的整体把握来答题。

> 主题干是"下面哪个是正确的？（Which of the following is TRUE?）"时，根据原文的某个细节来答题。

（3）对比选项时的技巧

1）AB原则：当已经把四个选项中的两个选项排除时，比如就剩A选项与B选项了，而且A与B又很像、很难对比，这时，如果假设A正确能推断出B也正确，那就应该选B。

2）褒贬原则：比如说一个事物在改进之前不好，但经过改进后就比较好了。选项中有三个说它在改进之前好，有一个选项说它不好，如果题干问的是改进之前的状况，那就选这个说它不好的选项。

3）虚实原则：在没有违背原文的情况下，选项越虚越好。"虚"就是我们所说的比较笼统的说法，"实"就是比较绝对化的说法。如：说法一描述了一个观点；说法二解释了女权运动。说法一是笼统的描述，我们称之为"虚"；说法二比较具体，我们称之为"实"。

二、"三步法"解题中的细微技巧

（1）单词量少不要紧，重要的是对认识的单词特别是动词的意思理解深刻。单词可以读不懂，但千万不要读错了。因为意思的偏差会对文章大概方向的把握产生影响，对解题不利。因此，读文章时对拿不准意思的内容权当不认识，不要乱猜。

（2）对于还没读完全文就已经画出全部题干在原文中对应的信息这种情况，如果能够确定你画的那些信息一定正确就可以不用再往下读了。但我们建议最好还是读下去，因为文章的重点一般是在后面，不过读的速度可以更快一点。

（3）当画线的内容不是答案所在的位置时，如果想要往下一段找的话，那么下一段的第一句话一定要提到有关上面的内容，才可以往下找。

（4）当看了选项后没什么概念时，要马上想到文章的方向。

（5）在平时练习的过程中，可以减少对同一段中例子的关注，增加对例子之外的句子的重视，同时要把转折关系精确地画出来。水平偏低、做不到这一点的同学，也至少要判断出所说内容的褒贬意思。

（6）关于局部问题的选项不能选，因为它只是问题的一个方面，不全面。

（7）在做根据原文具体信息得出答案的考题时，除了依据在原文中得到的信息外，对其他任何信息都应视其不存在，千万不要受到其他信息的干扰。

（8）阅读水平低的人，万一考试时读完文章没找到有什么要标记的，别再通读原文，就按题目直接回到原文中去找。

第二节　阅读方法总结

医学博士考试阅读理解文章具有以下三个特征：一是所选择的文章逻辑性强，结构紧密；二是用于解释说明细节的句子往往较长，理解起来有一定的难度；三是有一些位于段首或段末的句子，通常在文章中发挥承上启下的作用。

针对这些特点和做题的流程，我们要采用不同的阅读方法，现将这些方法总结如下。

1. 记忆阅读法

目的是通过快速阅读记住重要信息。大家可以采用句式分割的办法，重要的是记住主语和宾语的名词信息。这种阅读方法在最开始读题干时使用。

2．详略阅读法

不是逐字地读原文，而是抓住文章的梗概和作者的思路，对原文的内容进行有选择的阅读。这种方法适用于读原文找题目回现的阶段。

（1）详读的内容如下：

➢ 关键是阅读首段或各段首末句，迅速确定文章的主要内容、核心概念和作者态度等信息。

➢ 句子和句子之间衔接处的结构性句子。虽然句子是相对独立的表意单位，但各个句子之间并不是孤立的，上下文赋予了句子在整个文章中的完整含义。句子之间的关系在字里行间会有各种提示线索，如指代关系：it, this, that, these, those, here, he, she；因果关系：as a result, hence, therefore, consequently, thus；转折关系：though, but, however, in spite of, despite；承接关系：then, in addition, besides, in other words, moreover；列举关系：for instance, for example；类比关系：by comparison, likewise, compared to等。

（2）略读的内容如下：

➢ 重复与进一步解释说明的内容，如that is引导的句子、冒号后面的句子等。

➢ "反之亦然"的观点。

➢ 作者将要或者已经摒弃的论据、论证。

➢ 具体的过程、原理、证据、试验、数据等内容。

➢ 已知的例子、引用的内容。

➢ 一句话的重心如果在后面，则前面的内容可以略读。

3．跳读法

如果题干中有专有名词，考生可以不用细读文章，直接回原文找到这些专有名词的位置即可。

4．精读法

精读法就是前面提到的句式分析法，把句子拆分为主干和从句。此方法适用于回原文定位细节类题。

5．对比阅读法

精读的一种，要通过阅读分析出所读内容的相同点和不同点，适用于读答案中的四个选项。

总之，大比重分值使阅读理解成为测试的重心所在，是决定考试成败的关键。最后阶段的阅读复习主要是一个知识系统化和准确化的过程。本章的内容为全书的精华，是对所有考点系统的总结以及对所有解题方法和技巧的提炼。

第三节　分题型攻克阅读理解

一、文章结构类考题

➢ 文章结构类题的分类

所谓文章结构类考题，是指只有在通读原文的基础上才可以解答的题目。这种题目主要有两种类型：一种是主题类题，另一种是态度类题。这两种类型的题目都考查考生对篇章结构的整体把握，在逻辑上区分哪些语言范围广泛，引领主题；哪些语言细致入微地进行了解释说明；哪些是作者的观点；哪些又体现了作者的写作意图。这取决于考生能否把握文章的写作结构和脉络层次，只有了解了这一点，才能比较准确地确定应该选择哪个答案。

在阅读文章时应有意识地加强对文章写作思路和结构组织安排的理解，掌握英语文章常见的几种写作结构，这对迅速增强考试的应对能力是非常有帮助的。

通过对考试中出现的众多文章结构特点进行分析后不难发现，如果结构完整的话，不论这些文章的话题是什么，说明文和议论文体裁的文章都遵循着这样一个共同的模式：引入话题（即引子部分）—— 中心议题（即主题句）—— 分论点（说明扩展句）—— 得出结论（即主题句）。请考生以下表为模板，并详读表格说明，结合例题来熟悉文章的结构。

文章结构分类表

序　号	结构类型	逻辑关系	做题技巧
1	引子	列举例子	属于略读部分，例子说明的论点为详读部分。
		转折	重点考点，寻找后面的转折连词。
		递进式论述	难点，它的逻辑特点是前一句是后一句的基础，而非后一句是对前一句的解释。逻辑结构为"A→B→C"，中心在段落末尾。
		现象	可以预测，后面可能论述现象产生的原因。
		问题	可以预测，后面可能论述问题产生的原因和解决办法。
2	中心议题	中心句	如果是中心句，那么后面的句子是对其进行解释说明的。逻辑结构为"A←B"。

（续）

序　号	结构类型	逻辑关系	做题技巧
3	分论点	因果	解释中心句的原因。
		方法	提供解决问题的方法。
		作用意义	说明主题句内容的地位。
		例证	举例论证。
		解释说明	比如主题句说A很好，分论点就解释A如何好。
		列举	比如主题句说A有问题，分论点就罗列A有哪些问题。
4	总结	作者观点	态度类题语言回现处。
		中心议题的改写	与中心句意思相同，只是句式不同。
5	无主题句	并列关系	需要自己总结中心句。

表格说明：

（1）除了分论点部分，其余各项都可以不存在。比如，如果没有引子，那么这篇文章就是"总—分—总"结构；如果没有开头的主题句，那么这篇文章就是"分—总"结构；如果没有最后的中心句，那么这篇文章就是"总—分"结构；如果没有主题句而只有分论点，那么这篇文章采取的就是并列结构。对文章结构特点的把握有助于考生更加自觉地关注文章的开头和结尾，分清观点和事例，从而在阅读理解的考试中准确定位，快速答题。

（2）中心句也就是中心议题句，可能是第一句，也可能是最后一句，甚至可能是段中的某句（如表格中的引子结构出现的时候）。那么该如何判断主题句呢？它又有哪些特点呢？

1）判断首句是否是主题句，要看后面的句子是否围绕其展开。如果能够按照"文章结构分类表"看出分论点和首句的逻辑关系，那么就可以基本确定首句是主题句了。而如果首句是后面内容的铺垫，则可以判定它为引子。

2）具有归纳性、概括性、抽象性等特点。

3）多次在原文中重复。

（3）根据分论点和主题句的逻辑关系，可以把文章分成如下几种结构类型。只要考生能够把文章与如下类型的模板相对应，就说明考生已经基本掌握文章的主题。

1）描述性结构：主要介绍事物、问题或倾向的特点，对人物的描述如传记类文章，包括人物的身体特征、家庭背景、成长过程、个性爱好、成就贡献等，因此遇到此类文章时，时间、地点往往是出题重点。

2）释义性结构：解释某一理论、学科、事物，主要用例子进行比喻、类比、阐述。

3）比较性结构：把两个人或事物的功能、特点、优缺点进行对比。

4）原因性结构：这种结构主要分析事物的成因，是客观的还是主观的，直接的还是间接的。

5）问题解决性结构：文章开头提出存在的问题，然后论述如何解决该问题。

6）驳斥性结构：这种结构主要是先介绍一种观点，然后对其进行评论或驳斥，再分析其优点、缺点和危害性，最后阐明自己的观点。

➤ 文章结构类题的例题解析

为了让考生对前面的"文章结构分类表"的内容有更细致的了解，请看下面的具体解析。

1. How型文章

例文：Let us consider how voice training may contribute to personality development and an improved social adjustment. In the first place it has been fairly well established that individuals tend to become what they believe other people think them to be. When people react more favorably toward us because our voices convey the impression that we are friendly, competent, and interesting, there is a strong tendency for us to develop those qualities in our personality. If we are treated with respect by others, we soon come to have more respect for ourselves. Then, too, one's own consciousness of having a pleasant, effective voice of which he does not need to be ashamed contributes materially to a feeling of poise（泰然自若）, self-confidence, and a just pride in himself. A good voice, like good clothes can do much for an ego（自我）that otherwise might be inclined to droop（萎靡）.

The title that best expresses the ideas of this passage is "_____".

A. Our Ego

B. The Reflection of Our Personality

C. How to Acquire a Pleasant Voice

D. Voice Training in Personality Development

【解析】作者一开始就说明发声训练对个性发展和人的社会化可能产生的作用。基本可以判定这是"How型文章"，即作者马上就要论述它的作用如何大。接着，分别由in the first place及then并列了两个具体的方面，并展开讨论。第一个要点下，又分别由when和if引出两个细节加以论证。结尾一句总括全段，与首句呼应。不难看出，主题句是第一句，正确答案应选D。

另外，考生要特别注意此例中提到的in the first place，then，if等连接语，这些连接语能帮助我们把握文章内容的编排方式，领会文章的要点，准确而全面地理解文章。

2. 转折结构型文章

例文：If you were planning to buy a television set, the following advertisement would certainly attract your attention: "Color TV, only $79. Two-day sale. Hurry." However, when you go to the store ready to buy, you may discover that the advertised sets are sold out. But the salesman is quick to reassure you that he has another model, a more reliable set which is "just right for you". It costs $359. This sales tactic is called "bait and switch". Buyers are baited with a sales offer, and then they are switched to another more costly item. Buying items on sale requires careful consideration of the merchandise（商品）and the reasons for the sale.

（1）Which sentence best expresses the main idea?

A. The customer must be on his guard when purchasing items on sale.

B. Color television sets which sell for $79 are sold out quickly.

C. Many stores use the "bait and switch" technique to attract customers.

D. Anyone planning to buy a television set should look for a sale.

（2）The paragraph could be entitled "_____".

A. Buyer Beware   B. Closeout Sale

C. Crime Pays   D. Buying a TV Set

【解析】作者从一则电视机的广告入手，引入主题，然后用However进行转折，介绍了降价推销的惯用手段，称为bait and switch（廉价出售某种不打算出卖的商品，意在诱人购买昂贵的物品），属于我们模板中的转折结构。最后作者总结出自己的真正意图，即本段的主题句，告诫人们在购买降价商品时要警惕其中的圈套。因此正确答案为（1）A；（2）A。

转折法会将段落的主题句安排在段落的中间。例如：For adults a cold is not that serious. However, this is not the case for children. Cold symptoms in children may be signs of more serious diseases and should be given prompt medical attention.

本段主题句为第二句，因为However后面的内容才是作者真正的看法，并在下文中进一步做了说明。当主题句被安排在段中时，作者往往从具体的事例谈起，随之归纳出主题，然后再围绕这一主题展开讨论，使立论更加清楚，具有很强的说服力，即以"立"为主，对正面观点进行阐述。

3. 递进式文章

例文：Ever since humans have inhabited the earth, they have made use of various forms of communication. Generally, this expression of thoughts and feelings has been in the form of oral speech. When there is a language barrier, communication is accomplished through sign language in which motions stand for letters, words and ideas. Tourists, the deaf, and the mute have had to resort to this form of expression. Many of these symbols of whole words are very picturesque and exact and can be used intentionally. Spelling, however, cannot.

Body language transmits ideas or thoughts by certain actions, either intentionally or unintentionally. A wink（眨眼）can be a way of flirting（调情）or indicating that the party is only joking. A nod signifies approval, while shaking the head indicates a negative reaction.

Other forms of nonlinguistic language can be found in Braille (a system of raised dots read with the fingertips), signal flags, Morse code, and smoke signals. Road maps and picture signs also instruct people.

While verbalization（用语言表达）is the most common form of language, other systems and techniques also express human thoughts and feelings.

Which of the following statements best summarizes this passage?

A. When language is a barrier, people will find other forms of communication.

B. Everybody uses only one form of communication.

C. Nonlinguistic language is invaluable to foreigners.

D. Although other forms of communication exist, verbalization is the fastest.

【解析】这篇文章共有4段，谈的是肢体语言。第一段是递进式段落，第一句和第二句是引子，从肢体语言引入其作用，然后举例具体论述这些作用。第二段、第三段的首句从两个不同的方面引出了肢体语言的功能与分类。最后一段予以总结，强调肢体语言在表达人类思想和感情方面的作用，与第一段的中心句相呼应。因此正确答案应是A项。

4．例证型文章

例文：And yet, the myth of controlling the waters persists. This week, in the heart of civilized Europe, Slovaks and Hungarians stopped just short of sending in the troops in their contention over a dam on the Danube. The huge complex will probably have all the usual problems of big dams. But Slovakia is bidding for independence from the Czechs, and now needs a dam to prove itself.

What is the myth concerning giant dams?

A. They bring in more fertile soil.　　B. They help defend the country.

C. They strengthen international ties.　　D. They have universal control of the waters.

【解析】主题句为"And yet, the myth of controlling the waters persists.（控制该河段水域的神话依然继续着。）"下面的句子是两个具体例子说明主题句。属于例证型文章。所以D项"它们有对河流水域的完全控制权"正确。

从这些例题可以看出，绝大部分的文章都遵循前面所讲到的"文章结构分类表"中的模板，考生的任务无非是通过看懂英文的一些语义，把这个表格套在实际的文章中，找到主题句，理解分论点和主题句之间的逻辑关系，判断是问题解决型文章，还是例证型文章，或是因果型文章等。只要把握这些就可以掌握文章的结构。

（一）主题类考题

1. 主题类题的解题流程

主题类题是阅读考试中必然会出现的一类重点题目，它所考查的是考生能否看懂文章的结构脉络，也就是第一节讲到的文章结构分类表。建议考生在完成细节类题时，顺便查找各段的中心句，然后把所有的细节信息忘掉，对比在阅读时找到的各段的中心句，确定全文的中心句，最后解答主题类的题目。这样既可以节约时间，又可以保证正确率。

具体的解题流程如下：

步　骤	项　目	内　容	做 题 技 巧
第一步	阅读题目	判断题型	不要看选项，因为这对大家会有一定的心理暗示作用。有的考生根据答案回推文章，在语言能力不够的情况下，十分容易做错题。
		主题类题的常见提问方式有： The best title for this passage is _____. The topic/main idea of this article is _____. The author mainly discusses _____.	此类题是考查原文的主要内容。
		确定阅读方法	重视中心句和结构性的句子，而忽略细节。
第二步	寻找各段的中心句	根据文章结构模板寻找。	注意找到中心句，也可以帮助考生找到段落内相关的细节。
第三步	寻找全文的中心句	比较各段中心句，再根据文章模板，确定哪一句是全文的中心句。	细节类题解答完毕后，再进行该步骤。
第四步	画出全文的中心句	确定中心句是从原文中寻找出来的，而不是凭感觉杜撰出来的。	要特别关注段落的首尾。
第五步	选择答案	把全文的中心句和答案进行比较。	正确答案是对中心句的改写。

这五步当中最重要的是第二步、第三步和第五步。对于刚刚开始练习主题类题的考生来说，不可凭自己对一篇文章的感觉和对细节类题的印象来做题，这些都是选错答案的主

要原因。考生应该大量练习。在一定的练习后，思维会逐渐形成固定模式，对文章结构分类表了然于胸，对整个做题过程形成条件反射，那样做题速度自然会提高。

2. 主题类题的考点及例题解析

在了解了主题类题的做题步骤和文章篇章结构的准备知识后，考生就可以把自己想象成出题人，考虑一下可以设置哪些障碍，这些障碍也就是主题类题的考点所在。现将这些考点总结在下面的表格中，再用例题一一讲解。

序 号	步 骤	考 点	应 对 措 施
1	找主题句的过程	转折结构，把主题句置于段中或文章的中间。	注意寻找表示转折关系的连接词。
2		递进结构，把主题句置于段中或文章的中间。	开篇的例子或引言多为引子，考生可注意这之后的内容。
3		判断到底是"总—分"还是"分—总"结构——即主题句到底是首段的中心句，还是末段的中心句。	判断首段中心句和末段中心句的范围。如果末段中心句隶属于首段中心句的内容，则为"总—分"结构；反之则为"分—总"结构。
4		各段是并列关系，无法从原文中找到中心句。	这样的文章如果出主题类题，则要求考生自己进行引申、总结。
5	和答案进行对比	概括和具体之间	比主题句范围小的答案包括原文的细节、分论点。
			考生同样要注意，比主题句范围更加广泛的答案，也为错误答案。
6		对中心句进行偷换	可能出现偷换谓语、定语、状语等情况。

表格说明：

➢ 障碍的设置出现在两个环节：一个是找中心句的环节，另一个是和答案进行对比的环节。在找中心句的过程中，转折结构和"总—分、分—总"命题是重点，大约占到80%左右，而递进结构和无主题句的情况较少。

➢ 要注意95%的考题都是要求考生寻找主题句，而不是自己总结主要内容。只有在记叙文和无主题句的情况下，考生才可以引入自己的想法，进行提炼概括。

下面用具体的例题分析上面讲解的知识点。

（1）转折结构命题

例文：Nowadays, we hear a lot about the growing threat of globalization, accompanied by those warnings that the rich pattern of local life is being undermined, and many dialects and traditions are becoming extinct. But stop and think for a moment about the many positive aspects that globalization is bringing. Read on and you are bound to feel comforted, ready to face the global future, which is surely inevitable now.

Consider the Internet, that prime example of our shrinking world. Leaving aside the all-to-familiar worries about pornography and political extremism, even the most narrow-minded must admit that the net offers immeasurable benefits, not just in terms of education, the sector for which it was originally designed, but more importantly on a global level, the spread of news and comment. It will be increasingly difficult for politicians to maintain their regimes of misinformation, as the oppressed will not only find support and comfort, but also be able to organize themselves more effectively.

MTV is another global provider that is often criticized for imposing popular culture on the unsuspecting millions around the world. Yet the viewers' judgment on MTV is undoubtedly positive; it is regarded as indispensable by most of the global teenage generation who watch it, a vital part of growing up. And in the final analysis, what harm can a few songs and videos cause?

Is the world dominance of brands like Nike and Coca-Cola so bad for us, when all is said and done? Sportswear and soft drinks are harmless products when compared to the many other things that have been globally available for a longer period of time — heroin and cocaine, for example. In any case, just because Nike shoes and Coke cans are for sale, it doesn't mean you have to buy them — even globalization cannot deprive the individual of his free will.

Critics of globalization can stop issuing their doom and gloom statements. Life goes on, and has more to offer for many citizens of the world than it did for their parents' generation.

Which of the following could be the best title of the passage?

A. Globalization Is Standardization

B. Globalization: Like It or Lump It

C. Globalization: Don't Worry, Be Happy

D. Globalization Brings Equality

【解析】在分析这篇文章的时候，请结合第一节中的文章结构分类表。在这篇文章的首段中出现了明显的转折词，这说明第一句和第二句提出了两种对立的观点，but连接了两个明显的转折关系的句子，意思是 "当今我们听到了很多关于全球化带来的负面影响，但是我们冷静片刻就会发现全球化也有许多积极的因素"。

分论点部分是第二段、第三段和第四段，作者运用例证法来论证全球化与Internet，MTV，Nike一样利弊共存，但从总体上说是利大于弊。而且从文章的整体来看，作者支持后者的观点，也就是说全球化更多带来的是积极的影响。所以C为正确答案。

A选项指出"全球化是标准化"，与全文不符合，因此是错误的。B是"喜欢全球化，或是忍受它"，这个选项很具有迷惑性，因为它明显是从正反两个方面论证的。可是它与全文的中心议题不相符，因为全文虽然谈到了全球化利弊的两面性，但它们不是并列的关系，作者明显偏向转折后的论点，即对于全球化应该以乐观的态度去接受。

结合前面讲到的首段提出中心议题，再注意转折词，就可以很快地找到答案。请考生密切关注下面提到的一些表示转折的词汇，它们后面引导的句子往往是作者真正的意图。例如：however, nevertheless, on the other hand, still, unfortunately等。

（2）递进和"分—总"结构命题

例文：Next week, as millions of families gather for their Thanksgiving（感恩节）feasts, many other Americans will go without. According to the United States Department of Agriculture, more than 12 million households lack enough food for everyone in their family at some time during the year — including holidays.

Hunger is surprisingly widespread in our country — one of the world's wealthiest — yet the government estimates that we waste almost 100 billion pounds of food each year, more than one-quarter of our total supply.

Reducing this improper distribution of resources is a goal of America's Second Harvest, the nation's largest domestic hunger-relief organization. Last year, it distributed nearly 2 billion pounds of food to more than 23 million people in need.

America's Second Harvest is a network of 214 inter-connected food banks and other organizations that gather food from growers, processors, grocery stores and restaurants. In turn, the network distributes food to some 50,000 soup kitchens，homeless shelters and old people's centers in every county of every state.

A great deal of work is involved in distributing tons of food from thousands of donors（捐赠者）to hundreds of small, nonprofit organizations. Until a few years ago, America's Second Harvest lacked any effective way to manage their inventory. Without accurate and timely information, soup kitchens were sometimes empty while food was left to spoil in loading places.

In 2000, America's Second Harvest began to use a new inventory and financial-management system — Ceres. It is software designed specifically for hunger-relief operations. It is used by more than 100 America's Second Harvest organizations to track food from donation to distribution.

Ceres has helped reduce the spoiling of food and improve distribution. An evaluation found that the software streamlined food banks' operations by 23 percent in the first year alone. With more accurate and timely reports, Ceres saves time, flees staff members to focus on finding new donors, and promises more efficient use of donations.

Hunger in America remains a troubling social problem. Technology alone cannot solve it. But in the hands of organizations such as America's Second Harvest, it is a powerful tool that is helping to make a difference — and helping more Americans to join in the feast.

The main idea of the passage is that _____.

A. technology can help in the fight against hunger

B. America's Second Harvest has found more donors

C. America's Second Harvest promotes the development of technology

D. hunger is a problem even in the wealthiest country in the world

【解析】这篇文章既体现了递进式结构，又体现了"总—分、分—总"的命题思路。文章第一段描述了一个具体事例，more than 12 million households lack enough food for everyone；第二段的中心句提出了这个例子要说明的论点，即"饥饿仍然是美国存在的问题"，然后解释了出现这个问题的原因，即we waste almost 100 billion pounds of food each year（浪费太多）。如果考生十分熟悉文章结构表，就可知后面将要论述如何解决这个问题。所以第一段和第二段是一个引子，本文是"问题解决型"文章。

第三段果然提出了美国的Second Harvest这个组织试图解决这个问题；第四段是对Second Harvest的简介；第五段提出他们分发捐赠物的方法；第六段简单介绍Ceres；第七段指出Ceres的重要作用，围绕第六段展开；最后一段利用转折关系进行全文的总结。所以全文的中心句是But it is a powerful tool that is helping to make a difference，it就是前文的technology，故正确答案应该选择A。选项B和C从内容上看，都是细节型答案；而选项D是文章的引子，而非主题。

考生可以从这篇文章中体会出递进式论述和"分—总"的逻辑关系。由于第一段是例子，那它就不应该是主题。作者提出饥饿问题是为了引出解决的办法，即科技。这篇文章层层铺垫进行论述，因此，与其相关的主题类题有一定的难度。

（3）"总—分"结构命题

例文：The science of meteorology is concerned with the study of the structure state, and behavior of the atmosphere. The subject may be approached from several directions, but the scene cannot be fully appreciated from any point.

One may consider the condition of the atmosphere at a given moment and attempt to predict changes from that condition over a period of a few hours to a few days ahead. This approach is covered by the branch of the science called synoptic（天气图的）meteorology.

Synoptic meteorology is the scientific basis of the technique of weather forecasting by means of preparation and analysis of weather maps, which cannot be overestimated. In serving the needs of shipping, aviation, agriculture, industry, and many other interests and fields of human activity with accurate weather warnings and professional forecast advice, great benefits are reaped in terms of the saving of human life and property and in economic advantages of various kinds. One important purpose of the science of meteorology is constantly to strive, through advanced study and research, to increase our knowledge of the atmosphere with the aim of improving the accuracy of weather forecasts.

The tools needed to advance our knowledge in this way are the disciplines of mathematics and physics applied to solve meteorological problems. The use of these tools forms that branch of the science called dynamic meteorology.

Which of the following is the best title for the passage?

A. The Limitation of Meteorological Forecasting

B. New Advances in Synoptic Meteorology

C. Approaches to the Science of Meteorology

D. The Basics of Dynamic Meteorology

【解析】本文是一个典型的"总—分"结构文章。文章第一句The science of meteorology is concerned with...提出了一种"m科学"的定义。考生根本就不需要理解meteorology到底是什么意思，只要知道它是个专有名词即可。然后文章指出The subject may be approached from several directions...，意思是："它可以通过很多途径进行研究"。接下来的各段就在论述这些途径到底有哪些，和主题句是什么关系。第二段提出synoptic meteorology；第三段解释说明这种途径；第四段提出dynamic meteorology。

掌握了一定技巧的同学可以从线索词中发现正确答案。根据文章中多次提到的approach，science of meteorology可以很容易发现答案。A "气象预报的局限性"，这是文章分论点的一部分，不可以成为主旨。B"气象科学的进展"，这个选项是干扰项，仔细查看首尾段，我们就会发现，文章讨论的主题是气象学的研究途径。D出现在文章的最后，是文章的分论点。因此正确答案是C。

（4）全文没有中心句的文章概括题

例文：Americans usually consider themselves a friendly people. Their friendships, however, tend to be shorter and more casual than friendships among people from other cultures. It is not uncommon for Americans to have only one close friend during their life-time, and consider other "friends" to be just social acquaintances. This attitude probably has something to do with American mobility and the fact that Americans do not like to be dependent on other people. They tend to "compartmentalize（划分）" friendships, having "friends at work" "friends on the softball team" "family friends", etc.

Because the United States is a highly active society, full of movement and change, people always seem to be on the go. In this highly charged atmosphere, Americans can sometimes seem brusque or impatient. They want to get to know you as quickly as possible and then move on to something else. Sometimes, early on, they will ask you questions that you may feel are very personal. No insult is intended; the questions usually grow out of their genuine interest or curiosity, and their impatience to get to the heart of the matter. And the same goes for you. If you do not understand certain American behavior or you want to know more about them, do not hesitate to ask them questions about themselves. Americans are usually more eager to explain all about their country or anything "American" in which you may be interested. So much so in fact that you may become tired of listening. It doesn't matter because Americans tend to be uncomfortable with silence during a conversation. They would rather talk about the weather or the latest sports scores, for example, than deal with silence.

On the other hand, don't expect Americans to be knowledgeable about international geography or world affairs, unless those subjects directly involve the United States. Because the United States is not surrounded by many other nations, some Americans tend to ignore the rest of the world.

The general topic of the passage is _____.

A. American culture
B. American society
C. Americans' activities
D. Americans' personality

【解析】这篇文章各段落是并列的关系，没有全文的主题句。首段提到了friendships，指明了美国式友谊的特点是随意、短暂，并对友谊进行了分类；引子部分属于结构表中的转折关系，注意线索词however后面的一句话指出与其他国家文化不同的是美国式友谊趋向于短暂和随意。分论点部分为因果关系。第二段揭示了这种美国式行为的特点是节奏快、缺乏耐心、喜欢谈论而不是沉默，以及这些特点形成的原因。最后一段指出美国人的另外一个特性：一些美国人会漠视其他国家的存在。不难发现这三段的中心句是并列关系，再经过总结提炼就可以找出答案。

可以首先排除B"美国社会"和C"美国人的行为"，这两个答案缩小了外延，均属于文章的细节。在A"美国文化"和D"美国人的个性"中，通过对比发现D的范围比A要小。而综观全文，一直论述的是美国人，而不是美国，所以D是正确答案，而A扩大了外延。

应当特别注意的是：考生在总结和概括的时候切忌按自己的主观意愿扩大或缩小文章主旨的外延。同时，这道例题也为下面讨论"范围外延"的混淆项做了一个铺垫。

（5）概括和具体之间的区别

在这组例题当中，希望考生能够从逻辑上了解"范围"的意思，培养识别主题和细节的能力。同时，又不能随意扩大主题句的范畴。

中心句是文章中最基本、最具概括性的信息。这种信息应能归纳和概括文中其他信息所具有的共性。

例1：Choose the most general word.

A. Chemist.　　　　B. Physicist.　　　　C. Scientist.　　　　D. Biologist.

【解析】该问题要求找出最具概括性的词。C项Scientist符合题意，因为它包括了Chemist，Physicist和Biologist，而A，B和D都指某一具体学科的科学家，不能概括其他词。因此，Scientist最具概括性。

例2：Choose the most general sentence.

A. The hotel offers complimentary coffee from 7 to 10 a.m. daily.

B. There are many reasons why guests feel at home at the Glorietta Bay Inn.

C. The coin-operated laundry room has an ironing board.

D. There are a number of extra services at the Glorietta Bay Inn including baby-sitting.

【解析】A，C和D都是从不同的侧面说明旅馆的服务情况，相互间并无联系。而B却概括了A，C，D共性的东西，即：为什么旅客在这家旅馆里有宾至如归的感觉。因此，B符合题意。同样，如果在一段文章中，作者分几段来叙述几方面的内容，那么这些段落所要说明的问题就是本文的中心思想。

例3：Read the following passage and choose the best central thought.

Sugar history in the Hawaiian Islands is filled with pioneering. In sailing-ship days, Hawaiian sugar growers were many months away from sources of supplies and from markets. This isolation built up among the Hawaiian growers an enduring spirit of cooperation. Growers shared with one another improvements in production. Without government aid of any sort, they built great irrigation projects. Without government help, they set up their own research and experiment organization. Pioneering together over the years, they have provided Hawaii with its largest industry.

A.　In sailing-ship days, Hawaiian sugar growers were many months away from supplies and markets.

B.　Hawaiian sugar growers built their great industry without government help.

C.　Hawaiian sugar growers have set up their own research organization and have shared improvements.

D.　By pioneering together, sugar growers have provided Hawaii with its largest industry.

【解析】A，B，C只是文章中的具体内容，如果作为主题，其范围就太窄了。只有D才能概括全文要说明的问题，因此D是本文的主要思想。

例4：Read the following passage and choose the title that best expresses the ideas of the passage.

There is a simple economic principle used to determine prices. It is called the law of supply and demand. Supply means the amount of, or access to, certain goods. Demand represents the number of people who want those goods. If there are more goods than wanted, the price of them falls. On the other hand, if the demand for those goods is much greater than the supply, then price rises. Of course manufacturers prefer to sell more goods at increased prices.

A.　Economic Principles　　　　　B.　Law of Supply and Demand

C.　More Goods, Lower Prices　　　D.　Fewer Goods, Higher Prices

【解析】该问题中，A泛指经济规律，范围过宽；C和D只是供需规则的两个单独方面，不能包含全部，范围太窄。正确答案是B，因为这正是短文自始至终讨论的主题。

例5：Read the following passage and select the most appropriate title.

According to legend, the gods of the ancient Greeks lived in the clouds on the top of Mount Olympus. Zeus, the father of the gods, carried a bolt of lightning in his hand and ruled like an earthly king. Apollo was the sun god and his beams were golden arrows; he shielded the flocks of sheep and the fields of grain. Athena was the warrior goddess, standing in shining armor ready to protect the Greek cities. There were other gods as well, all with familiar human characteristics, but these were the leading gods.

A. The Gods of the Ancient Greeks
B. The Legend of the Sky God Zeus
C. Beliefs of the Ancient Greeks
D. Religions of the Past

【解析】该问题中，B只是文中提到的一项具体内容，作为主题思想面太窄了。C和D是泛指，面太宽。只有A才概括了全文要说明的问题，是全文的主题。

（6）答案对全文中心句偷换概念

例文：If you intend using humor in your talk to make people smile, you must know how to identify shared experiences and problems. Your humor must be relevant to the audience and should help to show them that you are one of them or that you understand their situation and are in sympathy with their point of view. Depending on whom you are addressing, the problems will be different. If you are talking to a group of managers, you may refer to the disorganized methods of their secretaries; alternatively if you are addressing secretaries, you may want to comment on their disorganized bosses. Here is an example, which I heard at a nurses' convention, of a story which works well because the audience all shared the same view of doctors. A man arrives in heaven and is being shown around by St. Peter. He sees wonderful accommodations, beautiful gardens, sunny weather, and so on. Everyone is very peaceful, polite and friendly until, waiting in a line for lunch, the new arrival is suddenly pushed aside by a man in a white coat, who rushes to the head of the line, grabs his food and stomps over to a table by himself. "Who is that? " the new arrival asked St. Peter. "Oh, that's God, " came the reply, "but sometimes he thinks he's a doctor. "

The best title for the text may be "_____".

A. Use Humor Effectively
B. Various Kinds of Humor
C. Add Humor to Speech
D. Different Humor Strategies

【解析】本文的中心句在第一句，"If you intend using humor in your talk to make people smile, you must know how to identify shared experiences and problems.（如果你想在谈话中使用幽默，令人发笑，那么你就要识别出你们共同的经历和问题。）"第二句话解释了为什么要这样做，和中心论点是因果关系。由此，我们首先排除了B项"不同种类的幽默"和D项"不同的幽默策略"，因为它们和中心句没有关系。而C项"谈话中增加幽默"偷换了中心句里面的动词，原文是using humor in your talk而不是add humor，所以正确答案是A"有效使用幽默"。如何有效使用幽默，就是要识别共同的经历和问题。

在将全文中心句和答案进行比较时，考生要十分仔细，看看哪个答案和原文最接近。通常这样的答案中包含几个原文中的原词，或者原词的近义词，这样的答案就叫作原文的正确改写型答案。

（二）态度类考题

1. 态度类题的解题流程及考点

态度就是评价。态度之中，作者的态度尤为值得关注，因为它反映了作者对事物的评价是肯定的还是否定的。这些评价决定了这些事物存在的价值和意义。

态度类题在考试中的数量并不是很多，大约出现2～3道。而且态度类题的考点也比较系统，现将解题流程和考点合并在下列表格中。

步　骤	项　目	考点	解题技巧
第一步	从题目入手根据关键词，即"对什么的态度"，回到原文定位	常用的提问方式如下： Which of the following is the author most likely to agree with? The author seems to be in favor of the idea of… What's the author's opinion/attitude? How does the author feel about…? What does the author think of…?	询问作者观点的题，才是态度类题。如果询问篇章中某人的观点，则为细节类题。
第二步	回归原文，寻找做题的语言回现	在转折处命题：文章如果是转折结构，考生既可以读到否定的论述，也可以读到肯定的论述，转折后才是作者真正的态度，即态度句在转折后。	寻找上下文的转折连词，在做题中十分重要。
		在两方观点的文章中（即驳斥型文章），要看有无作者的观点，判断是主观还是客观。	有作者的观点，则为主观性文章；无作者的观点，则为客观性文章，作者的态度是objective（客观的）或neutral（中立的）。
		优点句或缺点句	作者常常使用隐晦的暗示语言来表达其评价。
		注意混合态度I like it, but…	最精确的改写应是混合型，但是若无这样的答案，则转折后为作者真正的评价。
第三步	画出态度句	证明解题具有原文的证据	识别与理解态度句。
第四步	选择答案	别人的观点与作者的观点相混	区分别人的观点与作者的观点。
		中性词（如neutral, objective, unbiased, balanced）一般均为干扰项	识别词性。

表格说明：

（1）转折结构处命题是态度类题最常见的形式，大约占60%。所以当考生看到态度类题时，第一反应就是转折，找上下文的转折连词，切不可由于大意而错过真正的态度句。

（2）第二大类的题就是原文有优缺点句的类型，大约占30%。在说明文和议论文中，尽管作者没有直接说I think...，I believe...等，但如果有一些隐晦的说法，也可以判断其态度。作者通常通过副词状语或者形容词定语来表述态度，由于这些表述一般都比较隐蔽，不经过反复练习和强化很难形成挖掘它们的习惯。因此，在初期进行阅读练习时，读者可以试着圈出那些能表达作者褒贬态度的词汇，时间久了，就能形成关注它们的习惯。

1）能表明态度的特征词通常如下：

➤ 有感情色彩的形容词：accessible, accurate, approval, popular, novel, unrealistic等。

➤ 一些副词：fortunately, unfortunately, merely, only, unhappily, falsely等。

➤ 有感情色彩的动词和词组：mislead, overestimate, fail to, oversimplify, be blind to, advocate等。

➤ 一些固定名词：limitation, misconception, omission, shortcoming等。

2）下面通过两个例句来论述这个问题：

➤ After careful examination of the constitutional issues involved, the mayor, responding to the people's wishes, has announced that he will take immediate action.

➤ After hesitating for as long as he dared to, and taking refuge in the ambiguities of the constitution, the mayor has at long last yielded to pressure and grudgingly agreed to try to do something.

第一句和第二句内容基本相同，但第一句对市长的态度是肯定的，因为careful examination表示认真负责的态度，responding to the people's wishes, take immediate action表示积极的态度。而第二句对市长的态度是否定的，因为hesitating for as long as表示犹豫不决、尽量拖延的态度，taking refuge in反映逃避、回避矛盾的态度，has at long last yielded to pressure和grudgingly agreed表示采取行动是被迫的。

（3）双方观点型文章和混合态度命题较少，大约占5%。

2．态度类题的例题解析

下面结合例文的具体语境，分析态度类题的命题点之所在。

（1）转折结构处命题

例文：Taking charge of yourself involves putting to rest some very prevalent myths. At the top of the list is the notion that intelligence is measured by your ability to solve complex problems: to read, write and compute at certain levels, and to resolve abstract equations quickly. This vision of intelligence asserts formal education and bookish excellence as the true measures of self-fulfillment. It encourages a kind of intellectual prejudice that has brought with it some discouraging results. We have come to believe that someone who has more educational merit badges, who is very good at some form of school discipline is "intelligent". Yet mental hospitals are filled with patients who have all of the properly lettered certificates. A truer indicator of intelligence is an effective, happy life lived each day and each present moment of every day.

According to the author, the conventional notion of intelligence measured in terms of one's ability to write and compute _____.

    A. is a widely held but wrong concept

    B. will help eliminate intellectual prejudice

    C. is the root of all mental distress

    D. will contribute to one's self-fulfillment

【解析】根据题干中的关键信息notion of intelligence measured in terms of one's ability to write and compute（用读写能力衡量智商的观点），可以在段落的第二句定位到相关信息。如果能够读懂第一句话，就可以直接判断出这是一个转折结构："Taking charge of yourself involves putting to rest some very prevalent myths.（能够管理好自己就意味着放弃流行的观点。）"下面紧接着写出，最流行的观点就是At the top of the list...这正是题干中的内容，所以应该选择A"广泛接受却是错误的"。

而考生多半并不认识put...to rest这个词组，也无法辨认出分词词组的分裂结构，正常的语序是put myths to rest。如果这样就要继续读下去。后面几句话都是具体解释这种观点的内容，直到本段倒数第二句话，作者用yet进行转折，又列举出精神病医院的例子，从而引入其真正的观点：A truer indicator of intelligence is an effective, happy life（对智力更加准确的衡量是看一个人能否快乐而有意义地生活着），由此我们可以得出正确答案是A。C选项"精神疾病的根源"是一个比较大的迷惑项。选择该选项的人进行了自我引申，原文根本没有提到精神病的根源是什么，是考生自己在这两个现象上建立了因果关系。自我引申是我们在阅读理解中做错题的原因之一。

（2）识别优缺点句

例文：Nursing at Beth Israel Hospital produces the best patient care possible. If we are to solve the nursing shortage（不足）, hospital administration and doctors everywhere would do well to follow Beth Israel's example.

At Beth Israel each patient is assigned to a primary nurse who visits at length with the patient and constructs a full-scale health account that covers everything from his medical history to his emotional state. Then she writes a care plan centered on the patient's illness but which also includes everything else that is necessary.

The primary nurse stays with the patient through his hospitalization, keeping track with his progress and seeking further advice from his doctor. If a patient at Beth Israel is not responding to treatment, it is not uncommon for his nurse to propose another approach to his doctor. What the doctor at Beth Israel has in the primary nurse is a true colleague.

Nursing at Beth Israel also involves a decentralized（分散的）nursing administration; every floor, every unit is a self-contained organization. There are nurse-managers instead of head nurses; in addition to their medical duties they do all their own hiring and dismissing, employee advising, and they make salary recommendations. Each unit's nurses decide among themselves who will work what shifts and when.

Beth Israel's nurse-in-chief ranks as an equal with other vice presidents of the hospital. She also is a member of the Medical Executive Committee, which in most hospitals includes only doctors.

The author's attitude towards the nursing system at Beth Israel Hospital is _____.

A. negative   B. neutral   C. critical   D. positive

【解析】从文章的首段就可以看出作者的观点是正面的，在前面已经介绍过说明文中对优点的判断为正面态度。第二段和第三段具体介绍了护士对于病人全程接诊的过程，指出了这种护理方式给病人带来的好处；第四段和第五段介绍了护士的管理方式和在医院中的地位及作用。从文章的整体来判断作者的态度是积极的，所以D是正确答案。

（3）双方观点型文章——主客观命题

例文：In ancient Greek, the term euthanatos meant "easy death". Today euthanasia（安乐死）generally refers to mercy killing, the voluntary（自愿）ending of the life of someone who is terminally ill. Like abortion，euthanasia has become a legal, medical and moral issue over which opinion is divided.

Euthanasia can be either active or passive. Active euthanasia means that a physician or other medical personnel takes an action that will result in death, such as giving an overdose of deadly medicine. Passive euthanasia means letting a patient die for lack of treatment, or stopping the treatment that has begun. Examples of passive euthanasia include taking patients off a breathing machine or removing other life-support systems. Stopping the food supply is also considered passive.

A good deal of the debate about mercy killing originates from the decision-making process. Who decides whether a patient is to die? This issue has not been solved legally in the United States. The matter is left to state law, which usually allows the physician in charge to suggest the option of death to a patient's relatives，especially if the patient is brain dead. In an attempt to make decisions about when their own lives should end, several terminally ill patients in the early 1990s used a controversial suicide device, developed by Dr. Jack Kevorkian, to end their lives.

In parts of Europe, the decision-making process has become very flexible. Even in cases where the patients are not brain dead, patients have been put to death without their approval at the request of relatives or at the suggestion of physicians. Many cases of passive euthanasia involve old people or newborn infants. The principle justifying this practice is that such individuals have a "life not worthy of life".

In countries where passive euthanasia is not legal, the court systems have proved very tolerant in dealing with medical personnel who practice it. In Japan, for example, if physicians follow certain guidelines they may actively carry out mercy killings on hopelessly ill people. Courts have also been somewhat tolerant of friends or relatives who have assisted terminally ill patients to die.

The attitude of the writer toward euthanasia is _____.

A. negative   B. positive   C. objective   D. casual

【解析】从文章的首段很难看出作者对于安乐死的态度，因为作者只是十分客观地给出了安乐死的定义；第二段介绍安乐死的方法；第三段以美国和欧洲国家为例说明由谁来决定采取安乐死的方法。通读全文可以发现，这篇文章属于双方观点型文章。前面提到：在双方观点型文章中，要看有无作者的观点，判断是主观的还是客观的。阅读之后，也没有找到作者对于安乐死的肯定或否定的态度，所以我们可以推断出作者的态度是客观的。故C是正确答案。

（4）混合态度命题

例文：Computers manipulate information, but information is invisible. There's nothing to see or touch. The programmer decides what you see on the screen. Computers don't have knobs like old radios. They don't have buttons, not real buttons. Instead, more and more programs display pictures of buttons, moving even further into abstraction and arbitrariness. I like computers, but I hope they will disappear, that they will seem as strange to our descendants as the technologies of our grandparents appear to us. Today's computers are indeed getting easier to us, but look where they started: so difficult that almost any improvement was welcome.

Concerning the author's attitude towards computers, which of the following is most suitable?

A. He doubts the convenience of computers.

B. He loves them, but proposes to change them.

C. He doesn't like them at all, but has to rely on it for his job.

D. He is dissatisfied with nowadays technological development.

【解析】本题的态度句是：I like computers，but I hope they will disappear… 是明显的混合态度。A项没有错误，作者的确十分怀疑计算机的方便性，这点我们可以从字里行间里体会出来，比如 "moving even further into abstraction and arbitrariness（进一步走向抽象和随意）"。但是B项更加符合原文的混合态度，既喜欢又讨厌，因此是most suitable的答案。正是考虑到此，出题人才问："Which of the following is most suitable？"

Tips：

较高境界的阅读是把注意力集中在作者的思想上，而非个别零碎的单词上。比如读到but的时候，就应当能够预见下一句的意思与上一句的不同，意思相反。如果能够抓住作者的思路及文章的脉络，就会越读越明白，而不会只见树木，不见森林。为了做到这一点，需要熟练掌握如下知识点：

➤ 考试文章的常见脉络

● 时间顺序：按时间的先后说明某一理论的发展或某一研究成果由过去至现在的情况。

● 一般→具体：首段作总的说明，其他段落分别说明或具体论述首段观点。

● 具体→一般：前面几段分别说明，末段总结。

● 对比：以进行对比的两个事物之间的基本共同点或差异为主题展开。

➤ 根据分论点和主题句之间的逻辑关系，文章又可以分为：

● 问题解决型文章（见主题类题例2——科技解决美国饥饿）。

- 因果型文章（见主题类题例2的第二段——解释饥饿的原因）。
- 转折型文章（见主题类题例1——全球化的好处）。
- 例证型文章（见主题类题例6——段落最后进行举例）。
- 双方观点型文章（见态度类题例3—— 对安乐死的支持/反对观点）。

➤ 注意根据文章中的结构词把握文章的脉络。
➤ 熟悉主题类题的6大考点。
➤ 熟悉态度类题的4大考点。
➤ 请再仔细阅读本书选编的例题，最好能把它们背下来，这样就形成思维模式在实际考试中使用了。

二、局部细节类考题

局部细节类题在总题量中占相当大的比例，大约80%，而主旨题占大约20%。有的同学可能会问：难道没有别的题型了吗？其实很多题型之间的关系是重叠的，不能划分得十分清楚，很多时候是对同一问题不同角度的描述。比如说，某推断类题针对文章的细节进行推断，我们既可以说它是细节类题也可以说它是推断类题。如果是对全文的态度，那态度类题就很可能又属于主旨大意题；如果是针对文中某一具体事实的态度，就很可能属于细节类题。细节类题最主要的特征是针对文章中一句或几句的局部细节提问。这种题不需要考生了解文章的结构线索和主要内容，只需要知道局部的具体信息就可以了。主题类题和细节类题的关系就好比"中医"和"西医"的关系，主题类题就相当于"中医"，讲究"整体"；而细节类题就相当于"西医"，体现"头痛医头，脚痛医脚"的特征。所以在解答这两种题的时候，整体的思路完全不同。

局部细节类题主要有三种：事实细节类题、猜测词义类题和推断类题。

（一）事实细节类题

1. 事实细节类题的解题流程

解题的信息来自原文，且只能来自原文，而不能靠自己的主观臆断或其他的背景知识来选择答案。为了实现上述目标并且能够快速、客观、准确地解题，科学的做题流程就显得十分重要。根据多年的教学和实践经验，我们总结出如下四步解题流程，请大家熟记下面的表格。

步　骤	项　目	要　点	阅读或解题技巧
第一步	阅读题干	标注关键词，即可能在原文中出现的原词。	1．题干中的主语和宾语部分为重点词，可能在原文中出现。 2．题干中的专有名词，如人名、地名、数字等，肯定会在原文中出现。 3．如果多道细节类题提到同一个专有名词，则以此定位不科学，因为这个名词可能在文章中出现很多次。 4．题干中的谓语在原文中出现的概率不高，通常是出题人改写的内容，不要以此定位。
		标注修饰词，为精确定位奠定基础。	如果原文两次提到题干的内容，这就要靠限定的形容词或副词来精确判断到底是哪个位置才能解答题干的问题。
	阅读选项	属于"阅读题干"的要点。	这些逻辑词有：who, what, when, where, how和why。比如：标注出how，则可以判断原文是关于方法手段的关系，原句可能出现by（通过）或use等。
		如果题干中无关键信息，则可以直接阅读选项，再去原文中定位。	1．比如：题干为：Which of the following is TRUE? 2．当关键词少于或等于3个时，考生也可以直接看选项定位。
第二步	定位，寻找原文信息，解答题目	利用题干中的关键词，寻找其在原文中出现的地方。	此时可以采用浏览的方式，而不要细细地读。我们阅读原文的目的就是要找到和题目对应的相关信息，而不是精读文章。特别是有专有名词出现时，更要加快浏览的速度。
		有时无法找到题干中的原词，这是由于出题人常常不是采用文章中的原句，而是使用同义的词语来进行提问。	1．如果出现该情况，请考生不要再读题干，应该读选项，通过选项中的词来帮助你找到原文的回现。 2．找到各选项在原文中出现的位置，发现原文中有题干关键词的近义词时，一般就是解题点。
		找到原文回现，在下面画线，特别是在和题干重合的词或题干的近义词下面。	这是避免主观臆断的最好方式。
第三步	读选项，将选项进行比较	2-2型选项	两个选项是对比答案，或两个选项有重合的词，而另外两个选项与这两个选项相差较远。正确答案很有可能出现在相近选项当中。
		3-1型选项	3个选项相似，1个与其不同。这可能是最难的题，因为要从3个中比较出1个正确选项。也有可能是最简单的题，1个不同选项为正确答案。
		4-4型选项	4个选项无联系，这可能是简单题，也可能是出题人在定位处给考生设置了障碍。

（续）

步 骤	项 目	要 点	阅读或解题技巧
第四步	根据原文和选项比较出正确答案	混淆项的写法	1. 原文没有提到的答案——迷惑不会定位的学生。 2. 所答非所问的答案——迷惑定位不准确的学生。 3. 与原文相反的答案。 4. 偷换概念的答案——偷换主语、谓语、宾语等。
		正确项的写法	原文的同义改写

2. 事实细节类题的原文特征及考点

在熟悉了事实细节类题的解题流程后，我们还应关注细节类题的原文特征。因为，只有熟知出题人的出题规律，才能做到胸有成竹，把握阅读重点。其实考生自己也知道，并不是每个细节都能出题。那么命题的考点经常在哪里呢？主要有两个地方：一个是细节列举的逻辑关系处，另外一个就是我们在"基础篇"为大家讲解的十大惯用句式的长难句处。现将7个考点总结如下。

（1）列举处常考

列举处是指用first(ly)，second(ly)，third(ly)，finally；not only...but also；then；in addition；furthermore；moreover；above all；on the one hand...on the other hand等表示顺承关系的词语列举出的事实。要求考生从列举出的内容中，选出符合题干要求的答案项。

例文：Among the many shaping factors, I would single out the country's excellent elementary schools; a labor force that welcomed the new technology; the practice of giving premiums to inventors; and **above all** the American genius for nonverbal, spatial thinking about things technological.

According to the author, the great outburst of major inventions in early America was in a large part due to _____.

A. elementary schools

B. enthusiastic workers

C. the attractive premium system

D. a special way of thinking

【答案】D

【解析】文章列举了几个事实，分别用"；"分开，问题是："依据作者的观点，美国早期的发明大爆炸主要是因为什么？"首先回原文定位，题目中的中心词in a large part对应文章中的above all，所以答案为D项，意思是"特别的思维方式"。文章中提到了基础教育、热情的工人、奖金激励机制，它们都是shaping factors。但是题目问的是最主要的，所以其他三个选项不正确。考生在做此类题的时候需要特别注意上面提到的表示顺承关系的词语，它们可以帮助我们在考试中迅速地找到答案。

（2）例证处常考

为了使自己的观点更有说服力、更加明确，作者经常用具体的例子打比方，句中常由as，such as，for example，for instance，take...as an example等引导的短语或句子作为例证，这些例句或比喻就成了命题者提问的焦点。

例文：In talking to some scientists, **particularly younger ones**, you might gather the impression that they find the "scientific method" — a substitute for imaginative thought. I've attended research conferences where a scientist has been asked what he thinks about the advisability of continuing a certain experiment. The scientist has frowned, looked at the graphs, and said "the data are still inconclusive." "We know that," the men from the budget office have said, "but what do you think? Is it worthwhile going on? What do you think we might expect? " The scientist has been shocked at having even been asked to speculate.

It seems that some young scientists _____.

A. have a keen interest in prediction

B. often speculate on the future

C. think highly of creative thinking

D. stick to the "scientific method"

【答案】D

【解析】从"I've attended research conferences..."可知，文章明显是在通过阐述具体事例来说明第一句话的内容，所以，我们要详读第一句，而不读例子。第一句话 you might gather the impression that they find the "scientific method" — a substitute for imaginative thought中，that引导的是一个同位语从句，其中，substitute是核心词汇，在这里用作名词，是"代替"的意思。所以D是正确答案。

同时，本题也是一个3－1型选项模式，A，B，C三个选项都是一个意思，由此也可推出D项为正确答案。

（3）转折对比处常考

一般而言，转折后的内容常常是语义的重点，命题者常对转折处的内容进行提问。转折一般通过however，but，yet，in fact等词语来引导，强对比常由like，unlike，until，not so much...as等词语引导。

例文：Two key figures in American command arrangements in World War II were President Franklin D. Roosevelt and General George C. Marshall, Chief of Staff of the army who enjoyed Roosevelt's almost complete confidence. Even now **historians** are **not agreed** on the extent of Roosevelt's role as commander-in-chief, **nor** on the nature of his relations with Marshall and the other staff heads comprising the Joint Chiefs of Staff. **According to**

one view, Roosevelt was a somewhat passive war director, concerned only with winning the war quickly and largely reliant on the advice of his top military assistants. Professor Samuel P. Huntington, in *The Soldier and the State* (1957), states flatly that "the military ran the war". **Nevertheless**, says Professor William Emerson in military affairs the picture of the passive Roosevelt is deceiving. When the President wanted to, he could intervene in military affairs powerfully and decisively.

1）Professor Huntington and Emerson _____.

    A.　agree that Roosevelt was a somewhat passive war director

    B.　agree that the military ran the war

    C.　disagree as to the extent of Roosevelt's role as commander-in-chief

    D.　believe that the President could, and often did intervene in military affairs powerfully and decisively

【答案】C

【解析】通过原文第二句中的historians are not agreed可知他们二人肯定是对一个问题持有不同的态度，所以A，B，D三项排除；C项为historians的意见，所以是正确答案。

通过后文的nevertheless也可以推断出他们持有不同的态度。

2）According to Professor Emerson, Roosevelt _____.

    A.　sometimes took an active role in making military decisions

    B.　had a passive role in military affairs

    C.　was closely supervised by the Joint Chiefs of Staff

    D.　had little control of the war machine

【答案】A

【解析】问题中此人的意见就是文章最后一句话，罗斯福可以在任何他愿意的时候干预军队，所以答案为A项。

（4）比较处常考

含有比较级的选项应该说是应用更为广泛的选项，因为它不仅用于定位，也用于排除选项，因为无端的比较、相反的比较、偷换对象的比较经常出现在干扰选项中。只有我们标记并且关注到了原文中的比较，才能够较为顺利地排除这样的干扰。

例文：The victory of the welfare state is almost complete in northern Europe. In Sweden, Norway, Finland, Denmark and the Netherlands, government intervention in almost all aspects of economic and social life is considered normal. **In Great Britain, this is only somewhat less true.** Government traditionally has played a very active role in economic life in France and continued to do so. Only West Germany dares to go against the tide towards excessive interventionism in Western Europe. It also happens to be the most successful Western European economy.

Which of the following inferences is true, according to this passage?

A. The economy developed faster in welfare states than in non-welfare states.

B. French government is more active in regulating its economy.

C. The new protectionism is so called mainly because it is the latest.

D. Government plays a more active role in economic life in Northern Europe than in Great Britain.

【答案】D

【解析】A项是比较错误的选项，原文最后一句指出："没有过多干预经济的联邦德国是西欧最成功的经济体"，正好与A项的内容相反。B项是一个无端比较的选项，因为原文只拿英国和北欧进行了比较，而没有和法国进行比较。C项在原文中没有提到；原文的第三句中somewhat less true是明显的比较，所以D项为正确答案。

（5）因果句常考

命题者常依据文中的因果句，出一些考查文中两个事件内在因果关系的试题，或出一些概括文意、段意的试题。

例文：Kruger and co-author David Dunning found that when it came to a variety of skills — logical reasoning, grammar, even sense of humor — people who essentially were inept（无能的；笨拙的）never realized it, while those who had some ability were self-critical.

It **had little to do with** innate modesty, Kruger said, but rather with a central paradox: Incompetents lack the basic skills to evaluate their performance realistically. Once they get those skills, they know where they stand, even if that is at the bottom.

Why do incompetent people rarely know they are inept?

A. They are too inept to know what competence is.

B. They are not skillful at logical reasoning, grammar, and sense of humor.

C. They lack the basic skills to evaluate their performance realistically.

D. They have some ability to over-criticize themselves.

【答案】C

【解析】先根据题干中的关键词inept，定位到第一段的宾语从句中，可见这里讲的是结果，而题干问的是这种现象的原因，所以我们得再往下读。第二段第一句It had little to do with…（和……没关系）中，出现了因果关系连词，于是我们可以把答案定位到：Incompetents lack the basic skills to evaluate their performance realistically.（无能的人缺乏现实地评价自己表现的能力。）与C项内容正好一致，所以C项为正确答案。

A项在文章中没有提到，B项中提到的三种skills在文中只是作为例子来说明人们经常会在这些地方意识不到自己的无能，D项明显与题目的意思相反。

（6）复杂句常考

复杂句常是命题者的出题之处，包括同位语、插入语、定语、从句、动词不定式等，其考点就是我们在"基础篇"为大家讲解的十大惯用结构和长难句分析。

例文1：Although America has obviously not fulfilled the visionary hope entertained for it in the romantic heyday, Americans have, until recently, thought of themselves as an idea, a "proposition" (in Lincoln's word) **set up for** the enlightenment and the improvement of mankind.

The writer states that, until recently, Americans have thought of their country as a _____.

A.　source of enlightenment
B.　leader in technological progress
C.　recipient of European heritage
D.　peacemaker

【答案】A

【解析】原文画线部分属于（N1，+N2+名词扩展）句型。N1是"an idea"，N2是"proposition"，名词扩展是set up for the enlightenment，由此可推出"idea=proposition=being set up for the enlightenment"，所以A项为正确答案。而B，C和D三项的内容在原文中没有出现。

例文2：By having a right to everything, men want everything. Government is a contrivance（发明）of human wisdom to provide for human wants. Men have a right that these wants should be provided for by this wisdom. Among these wants is to be reckoned the want, out of civil society, of a sufficient restraint upon their passions.

According to the author, government _____.

A.　is made by men
B.　is made in virtue of natural rights
C.　has a right to everything
D.　wants everything

【答案】A

【解析】答案应是对这句话的改写："Government is a contrivance（发明）of human wisdom…（政府是人类智慧的发明）"，因此A项为正确答案。D项为最大的混淆项，第一句中"By having a right to everything, men want everything"，动名词having的逻辑主语为men，而不是题干中的government，所以D项为错误答案。

（7）指代处常考

我们做阅读理解题目时常碰到这样的问题：

➢ The word "it" in Line 3 most probably refers to _____.

➢ In Line 3, the word "one" could best be replaced by _____.

➢ What does the word "they" in Line 3 refer to?

这种指代性的题目有一定的难度。从历年考试中这种题目的得分来看，答对比率只有33%左右。因为它要求考生对代词所在句以及紧邻几个句子的结构和意思都要有准确的理解。指代通常有两种情况：指代单个词或词组；指代句子意思。

在具体解答这类问题时，我们应注意以下几点：

➢ 注意指代条件：每个代词都有自己的指代条件，如单数、复数、可数、不可数、先行词的远近等要求。

● it指代单数可数名词或不可数名词；指物不指人；可以指代前面一句话的意思。

● they指代复数可数名词；指物指人都可以；一般不能指代前面一句话的意思。

● one指代单数可数名词；可以指前面的人；一般不能指代前面一句话的意思。

● that指代单数可数名词或不可数名词；可以指代前面一句话的意思。

● this指代单数可数名词或不可数名词；可以指代前面一句话的意思。

● which在非限制性定语从句中，既可以指代名词，也可以指代句子。

➢ 如果代词周围有好几个名词或词组，而且都符合指代条件，就要分析哪一个选项符合文章的意思。

➢ 将四个选项试着代入，看哪一项符合搭配，包括句子的语法意义和逻辑意义。

（1）复数指代人的题目

例句：The basketball team never lacked vociferous supporters, but **they** rarely responded to this show of enthusiasm.

【解析】文中的黑体字they若是指高声呼叫的支持者，则与后面的意思（对这种热情很少做出回应）不符。因此，they只能指代球队球员。

（2）宾格指代型题目

例句：Scott Fitzgerald, who first introduced **him** to a publisher, was one of the few contemporary writers that Hemingway did not turn against.

【解析】文中黑体字him若指的是主语Scott Fitzgerald，则应该用反身代词himself，而不能用him，因此，这里的him指代后文中的Hemingway。

以上7点为事实细节类题经常考查的重要考点，为了让大家更为系统地掌握这些考点，我们用下方的这个表对它们进行了详细的总结。

序 号	项 目	要 点	阅读或解题技巧
1	列举处	哪一项与其他各项不同	注意各项的修饰成分，即定语和状语
		哪一项不在作者列举的范围内	注意选项中可能出现原文的近义词
		题干关键词如果不到3个	通过选项回原文定位
2	例证处	考查例子说明的论点	不要定位到例子，要定位到前后的论点
		考查例证的作用	"虚"的答案为正确答案的可能性大
3	转折对比处	通过转折前的内容推测转折后的意思	注意转折连词前后会出现反义词
		考查转折前后的细节	注意选项的修饰词
		转折后的内容为作者真正的意思	态度类题的解题点
4	比较处	无端比较	原文要出现比较级或最高级，否则为无端比较
		偷换比较双方	比较级句式分析
		和原文比较结果相反	
5	因果句	因果不要倒置	仔细阅读前后的因果关系连词
		定位到出现题干关键词的前后	阅读不要关注于"果"，要前后找因
6	复杂句	找出句子主干	详见"基础篇"
		十大惯用结构	详见"基础篇"
7	指代处	各代词的语法要求	先判断是指代"人"还是指代"物"；再判断"单数"和"复数"
		指代句子的意思	注意非限制性定语从句中which和it的区别

阅读时注意细节的安排方式，跳过那些与题目无关的细节，就可以迅速在相应的位置找到题目的原文回现，最后与选项一一对比，找出正确答案。

（二）猜测词义类题

猜词技巧是阅读中一项非常重要和常用的技巧，是应对生词、确定词汇在具体语言环境中确切含义的手段。阅读中的生词不是孤立的，而是与其上下文中的词、句乃至整个篇章，在意义、结构和逻辑上存在联系，这些联系便是我们推测词义的依据，通常简称为词的上下文线索（context clues）。所以，从根本上说，猜测词义题就是通过原文的已知线索，猜测出一些未知信息，而不是考查考生到底背了多少词汇。我们将从如下几方面来论述如何解答猜测词义题。

1. 猜测词义类题的解题流程

考生要坚信：猜测词义类题是根据原文的信息来猜，而绝非靠自己的主观臆断，所以找到原文的线索词就是解题的关键。同时，需要注意的是，一个单词通常有好几个意思，我们要解决的是这些词在文中所表达的意思。因此，不可脱离上下文的"线索词"而仅仅根据自己以前了解的词义来确定其意义。在下面的专题中，我们将介绍如何才能找到这些"线索词"。

2. 如何寻找上下文的"线索词"

猜测词义通常可采用以下几种方法。

（1）利用生词上下文中的解释线索猜测词义

例：Our earth is very old. It holds many secrets about life in the past. **Archaeologists** dig in the ground and bring out these secrets. They discover objects thousands of years old that inform us about how people lived long ago.

【解析】如果不熟悉Archaeologists的意思，可以根据上下文中的in the past（过去）、dig in the ground（挖掘土地）、objects thousands of years old（数千年前的物件）等推测，该词与"挖掘历史和过去"有关，该词词缀为-ist，即"做……的人"，综合来看，该词的意思为"考古工作者"。

（2）利用文中的举例猜测词义

例：Some artists plan their paintings around **geometric forms** like squares, circles and triangles.

【解析】如果不知道geometric forms的意思，可从文中所列举的三角形、正方形、圆形来猜出其意义为"几何图形"。

（3）利用后置的名词扩展结构猜测词义

例：The invention of **snorkel**, a long air tube that reaches up to the surface, has made it possible for submarines to use their diesel engine even when they are submerged.

【解析】句中snorkel一词的意思，可通过其同位语a long air tube that reaches up to the surface来猜，由此我们可以确定该词的意思为"通气管"。

（4）利用文中的反义词猜测词义

表示转折或对比的词有but, while, however, otherwise 等。

例：Unlike her **gregarious** sister, Jane is a shy person, who does not like to go to parties, or to make new friends.

【解析】根据句中的Unlike，可知"shy person, who does not like to go to parties, or to make new friends"应该表达了与gregarious相反的意思，所以gregarious的意思为"好交际的"。

（5）利用同义、近义词或词组猜测词义

例：One of the **predominant** concerns today is the future of our natural resources. This issue is **of greatest importance** because it is becoming clear to many people that our present resources will not last forever.

【解析】可猜测句中predominant的词义与of greatest importance的意思相近，因为第一句话中的concerns和第二句话中的issue所指相同，所以predominant是"十分重要的；压倒一切的"的意思。

（6）利用下文中下定义的句子猜测词义

例：An **expedition** is a long, organized trip or journey, which is made into an unfamiliar area for a particular purpose by a group of people.

【解析】句中"long, organized trip or journey（长期有组织的远行）"和后面which引导的定语从句which is made into an unfamiliar area（去不熟悉的地方）进一步解释了expedition之意为"远征"。

（7）利用构词法猜测词义

这种方法可以使考生知道所要猜测词的大概意思，至少知道这个词是肯定还是否定的含义。但是具体这个词是什么意思，考生还是要回归到原文的线索词中，切不可凭背景知识主观臆断。

构词法主要有两种,一种是前缀、后缀构词法;另一种是合成构词法。下面我们就为大家一一讲解。

1)英语中的前缀、后缀构词颇多,且特定的"缀"往往表示特定的含义,把握这一点,可做到"以不变应万变"。

例如:He had been **overworking** and fell ill at last.

overwork是由前缀over-加动词构成,over有"超过,过于"之意,overwork的意思就是"工作过多,劳累过度"。再如:overburden"负担过重";overcharge"要价过高";overdo"做得过分"。

英语中常用的前缀还有:

➤ mis-错、误:misfortune"不幸";mislead"误导";mismanage"处理不当"

➤ mid-中央:midnight"半夜";midway"半路"

➤ under-低于:underdone"半生不熟的";underestimate"低估"

➤ anti-反对:antibody"抗体";anticyclone"反气旋";antifreeze"防冻剂"

2)合成构词法指的是把英语中的两个单词连接在一起。

例如:Family members take turns choosing a special activity for the evening, and everyone **partakes** in for fun.

根据短语构成及上下文意思看,句中的partakes in相当于takes part in。

再如:break out→outbreak(名词"爆发");set out→outset(名词"起始");come in→income(名词"收入")。

3. 经典例题解析

在熟悉如何找到原文中的线索词后,我们通过几道例题,为大家讲解一下以上技巧在考试中的应用。

例文:In nations where workers can produce a large quantity of goods and services per unit of time, most people enjoy a high standard of living; in nations where workers are less productive, most people must endure a more meager existence.

The word "meager" in this paragraph is closest in meaning to "_____".

A. modest   B. poor   C. meaningless   D. plentiful

【答案】B

【解析】本段落中,前后两个分句是对比关系,并构成对仗,因为开头部分都是in nations where…。前半部分的谓语是can produce a large quantity of goods(能生产大量的货物）；后半部分因为有否定词less productive，所以应该是"生产量低"的意思。由此可知，meager应该和a high standard of living构成相反含义。a high standard of living是"高生活质量"的意思，正好与B项poor（贫穷）意义相反，所以B为正确答案。A项modest（谦虚的）和原文无关；C项meaningless（毫无意义的）和原文无关；D项plentiful（大量的，许多的）和原文语义相反。

例文：Moreover, demographers see the continuing shift South and West as joined by a related but newer phenomenon: more and more, Americans apparently are looking not just for places with more jobs but with fewer people, too. For some instances, regionally, the Rocky Mountain States reported the most rapid growth rate 37.1 percent since 1940 in a vast area with only 5 percent of the U.S. population.

The word "demographers" most probably means _____.

A. people in favor of the trend of democracy

B. advocates of migration between states

C. scientists engaged in the study of population

D. conservatives clinging to old patterns of life

【答案】C

【解析】根据题干中的关键词demographers，我们可以定位到第一句话。该词是此句的主语，所以后面的谓语动词和宾语为解题的解释线索。解释线索的意思是："不断向南方和西方移民又出现了一个相关的新现象。"冒号后为例证，解释这个新现象是什么，即美国人不仅在寻找工作机会多的地方，也在寻找人口更少的地方。由此分析可知：C项"研究人口的科学家"与这种现象的行为最相符，所以为正确答案。

A项中的democracy与题干中的demographers拼写相近，但语义却相距甚远，是"民主"的意思，为拼写上的混淆项；B项"倡导移民"是最大的混淆项，仔细阅读解释线索，它不是号召移民，而是解释了移民的方向，所以B项与原文不符；D项"坚守旧的生活方式的保守主义者"，与解释线索无关。

（三）推断类题

推断类题是阅读理解部分各种类型问题中最难解答的问题，因为它的答案没有直接通过一个明确的句子在文章中陈述出来，而是需要考生以作者表面的论述为基础，利用文章提供的暗示（如用词的选择、论述的详略等）体会作者的言外之意，层层剖析、推导，最后得出正确的判断。在阅读中，人们首先理解的是语言的字面意义。然而，语言所表达的内容常常超过其字面意义，这就需要我们掌握逻辑判断和推理的方法，根据事物发展的自然规律以及语言本身的内在联系，从一定的文字符号中获得尽可能多的信息。

例文1：A wise man once said that the only thing necessary for the triumph of evil is for good men to do nothing. So, as a police officer, I have some urgent things to say to good people.

Day after day my men and I struggle to hold back a tidal wave of crime. Something has gone terribly wrong with our once proud American way of life. It has happened in the area of values. A key ingredient is disappearing, and I think I know what it is: accountability.

We can learn from the first paragraph that it is _____.

A. unnecessary for good people to do anything in face of evil

B. certain that evil will prevail if good men do nothing about it

C. only natural for virtue to defeat evil

D. desirable for good men to keep away from evil

【答案】B

【解析】题目要求考生推断出智者的话的引申意思。智者的话"the only thing necessary for the triumph of evil is for good men to do nothing"的字面含义为"邪恶获得胜利的必要之处是好人什么都不做"，引申后，正好符合B项的说法"如果好人什么都不做，那么邪恶就会流行"。

例文2：Of course, we have no statistics on crimes that go undetected. But it's disturbing to note how many of the crimes we do know about were detected by accident, not by systematic inspections or other security procedures. The computer criminals who have been caught may have been the victims of uncommonly bad luck.

It is implied in this paragraph that _____.

A. many more computer crimes go undetected than are discovered

B. the rapid increase of computer crimes is a troublesome problem

C. most computer criminals are smart enough to cover up their crimes

D. most computer criminals who are caught blame their bad luck

【答案】A

【解析】A项的意思是："许多计算机犯罪并没有被发现。"文中提到：The computer

criminals who have been caught may have been the victims of uncommonly bad luck.（被抓到的实施计算机犯罪的罪犯是极其不幸的。）由此可以推知这句话实际的意思是很多实施计算机犯罪的罪犯都可以逍遥法外，因而A项最合适。

B项"计算机犯罪的增加是一个令人头痛的问题"，这个选项与文章意思不符，文中谈到的是计算机犯罪已经很多，而不是增加的问题；C项"计算机罪犯足够聪明能够掩盖其罪行"，原文说的是"我们偶尔查看，而不是通过具体的安全措施，就可以查出这么多罪犯"，可见罪犯没有被抓获，不是由于他们聪明，而是由于太多了，没办法查；D项"被逮捕的计算机罪犯要归于他们的坏运气"，是对原文错误的理解，文意是"由于太多了，无法全部查出，所以真的被抓获，是自己运气不好"，所以D项为错误答案。

例文3：There are some good arguments for a technical education given the right kind of students. Many European schools introduce the concept of professional training early in order to make sure children are properly equipped for the professions they want to join. It is, however, presumptuous to insist that there will only be so many jobs for so many scientists, so many businessmen, so many accountants. Besides, this is unlikely to produce the needed number of every kind of professionals in a country as large as ours and where the economy is spread over so many states and involves so many international corporations.

It could be inferred from the passage that in the author's country the European model of professional training is _____.

A. dependent upon the starting age of candidates

B. worth trying in various social sections

C. of little practical value

D. attractive to every kind of professionals

【答案】C

【解析】本段开头提到There are some good arguments for a technical education（对于职业教育，有一些好的方面），紧接着作者介绍了欧洲的职业教育是什么样的。第三句用however开始转折，由此可见，作者对于欧洲的职业教育持负面态度，是不支持的。A项"取决于入学者开始的年龄"，是原文提到的内容，不用推断。B项"值得在各种社会场合尝试"，为褒义答案，所以错误。C项

"没有什么实用价值"，为否定含义，所以正确。D项"吸引各行各业的专家"，是一个褒义答案，所以错误。

例文4：However, very few of us have actually been interviewed personally by the mass media, particularly by television. And yet, we have a vivid acquaintance with the journalistic interview by virtue of our roles as readers, listeners and viewers. Even so, true understanding of the journalistic interview, especially television interviews, requires thoughtful analyses and even study, as this book indicates.

The passage is most likely a part of _____.

A. a news article

B. a journalistic interview

C. a research report

D. a preface

【答案】D

【解析】这是一道推理题。我们通过as this book indicates做出判断，这段话属于前言（preface）的一部分。考生很容易会选B项 a journalistic interview，因为在原文中多处找到了对应，但是我们需要知道细节类题与推理题最大的不同就在于，后者需要透过现象看本质。直接找到文字对应的往往是陷阱，要特别小心。

第四节　阅读理解经典文章详解

为了能够让考生在阅读实践中巩固单词、句型等基础知识，同时练习本书提到的解题技巧，我们特地选编了若干难度适中、符合考点、有启发性的文章。这些文章都是医学专业的文章，但从考试角度讲，却是攻克考点的经典例文和例题。我们把这些文章按照文体分类，点明文章的主题句。同时罗列出文章的逻辑关系，配备了长句、难句的分析和讲解。考生可以先按照本书所讲的流程和技巧做题，争取10分钟完成一篇文章，在核查答案后，再阅读讲解部分。这样，考生既锻炼了解题技巧，又掌握了语言知识，两全其美。

Passage One

Breast cancer patients who take a multivitamin or extra vitamin E experience a smaller decrease in important immune cells, a common side effect of chemotherapy, new research suggests.

Women who took a nutritional supplement, a multivitamin or extra vitamin E had a smaller drop in neutrophils（中性粒细胞）, white blood bold cells that help fight bacterial infections. However, women with relatively high levels of B-vitamin folate（叶酸）had a larger drop in neutrophils.

Study author Richard F. Branda cautioned that chemotherapy patients should first discuss taking supplements with their doctors, because some supplements may interfere with treatment. For instance, cod liver oil and St. John's Wort may interfere with blood thinning drugs, hormone treatment or chemotherapy.

Previous research has also shown that an herbal dietary supplement that some men use to treat prostate cancer, called PC-SPES, may interfere with the anti-cancer activity of the chemotherapy drug paclitaxel, making it less effective. However, studies have also shown that vitamin E may enhance the benefits and reduce the side effects of chemotherapy, and many doctors now recommend vitamin therapy during treatment.

To investigate whether supplements help reduce side effects from chemotherapy, Branda and his colleague asked 49 women with breast cancer to complete questionnaires detailing their use of supplements during chemotherapy. The authors found that more than 70 percent of women were taking at least one of 165 different types of supplements. On average, patients took three supplements. However, some women said they took up to 20 daily supplements during treatment. The most common supplements were multivitamins, vitamin E and calcium. Women who took multivitamins or vitamin E alone experienced a smaller decrease in their neutrophils during chemotherapy.

However, women with relatively high levels of the B-vitamin folate in their blood had a larger-than-average decrease in neutrophils, the authors report in the journal *Cancer*.

Branda, who is based at the University of Vermont in Burlington, explained that many cancer patients—and people without cancer—take supplements because they believe they are "natural", and could therefore only help them.

However, Branda noted that supplements typically consist of complex chemicals, which can have many possible effects on the metabolism of drugs and the functioning of cells.

"These effects may be beneficial or detrimental and need to be studied further," he said. For instance, based on the results with folate, Branda recommends that cancer patients avoid taking extra folate if they eat a balanced diet, because many foods are already fortified with folate, or folic acid.

1. Taking a multivitamin has been proven to be _____ for breast cancer patients.

   A. useless

   B. helpful

   C. detrimental

   D. effective

2. The study author suggested that chemotherapy patients _____.

   A. should take supplements every day

   B. should take multivitamins every two days

   C. should ask for their doctor's advice before taking supplements

   D. shouldn't discuss with their doctor

3. The most common supplements that breast cancer patients took during treatment were _____.

   A. multivitamins and vitamin B

   B. multivitamins, calcium and vitamin E

   C. vitamin B and calcium

   D. multivitamins, calcium and vitamin B

4. For breast cancer patients, taking multivitamins may lead to a _____ in neutrophils and white blood cells during chemotherapy.

   A. smaller decrease

   B. smaller increase

   C. larger decrease

   D. larger increase

5. Branda pointed out that _____.

   A. supplements have good effects on the functioning of cells

   B. supplements have negative effects on the functioning of cells

   C. supplements don't have any effect on the metabolism of drugs

   D. whether supplements have positive or negative effects on the metabolism of drugs needs to be confirmed

▶ Words & Expressions

supplement *n.*	补充物
chemotherapy *n.*	化学疗法
herbal *adj.*	草药的
on average	平均
metabolism *n.*	新陈代谢
detrimental *adj.*	有害的
fortify *v.*	加强，强化

▶ 文章大意

新研究显示，服用复合维生素或者补充维生素E的乳腺癌患者较不服用者重要免疫细胞减少的程度小。而重要免疫细胞的减少是化疗的一种常见副作用。

服用营养补充剂、复合维生素E或者额外的维生素E的女性，其机体用来抵御细菌感染的中性粒细胞和白细胞减少的程度较小，然而体内含有较高水平叶酸的女性则中性粒细胞减少的程度较大。

该研究报道的作者理查德•F. 布兰达博士告诫说，接受化疗的患者应该在与医生讨论后再服用补充剂，因为有些补充剂可能干扰治疗。例如，鲟鱼鱼肝油和金丝桃可能会干扰血液稀释药、激素治疗或化疗。

过去的研究也显示，一些人用来治疗前列腺癌的草药补充剂——PC-SPES——可能会干扰化疗药紫杉醇的抗癌作用，使其疗效降低。但是，一些研究也显示，维生素E能够增强化疗的疗效并降低副作用。现在很多医生推荐在化疗期间服用维生素。

为了研究补充剂是否有助于降低化疗的副作用，布兰达和他的同事以问卷的形式让49名乳腺癌患者详细列出了化疗期间服用过的补充剂。作者们发现，超过70%的女性至少服用165种不同补充剂中的1种，平均每人3种。一些女性说自己在治疗期间每天服用多达20种补充剂。最常服用的补充剂是复合维生素、维生素E和钙。服用复合维生素或者单独的维生素E的女性，化疗期间中性粒细胞减少的程度较小。

但是，血液中含有较高水平的B族维生素叶酸的女性，中性粒细胞减少的程度大于平均水平，作者们在《癌症》杂志中如此报道。

在柏林顿市佛蒙特大学工作的布兰达解释说，很多癌症患者（也有健康人），服用补充剂是由于他们相信这些补充剂是"天然的"，因此只会有好处。

但是，布兰达指出，补充剂通常含有复杂的化合物，这些化学物质可能会对药物代谢和细胞功能产生很多影响。"这些影响可能有益，也可能有害，需要进一步研究，"他说。例如，根据对叶酸的研究结果，布兰达建议那些膳食平衡的癌症患者不要再额外摄入叶酸，因为很多食物都已经富含叶酸。

答案、考点及解析

1. 【答案】B

   【考点】细节理解题

   【解析】根据taking multivitamin和breast cancer定位到第一段，可知服用复合维生素的乳腺癌患者较不服用者重要免疫细胞减少的程度小（smaller decrease in important immune cells），由此可知，这对乳腺癌患者来讲是有帮助的。effective是一个不太好区分的混淆项。服用复合维生素只能是减少化疗的side effect，并非对治疗癌症本身有效，所以helpful最合适。

2. 【答案】C

   【考点】细节定位题

   【解析】由study author回到原文定位到第三段第一句，作者认为化疗病人应该在服用复合维生素之前先与医生交流，C选项中ask for their doctor's advice 与discuss是同义改写。

3. 【答案】B

   【考点】细节定位题

   【解析】由most common回到原文定位到第五段倒数第二句话，可知本题正确答案为B。

4. 【答案】A

   【考点】细节定位题

   【解析】通过taking multivitamins和neutrophils定位到第五段最后一句：服用复合维生素或者单独的维生素E的女性，在化疗中中性粒细胞减少的程度较小。

5. 【答案】D

   【考点】细节定位题

   【解析】从选项得知，本题是在讨论补充剂的药效。通过命题顺序和题干关键词Branda回到原文定位到最后一段 "These effects may be beneficial or detrimental and need to be studied further"，可知D选项中分别用positive和negative对原文进行了改写，因此最佳答案为D。

Passage Two

Educators are seriously concerned about the high rate of dropouts among the doctor of philosophy candidates and the consequent loss of talent to a nation in need of Ph. D. s. Some have placed the dropouts' loss as high as 50 percent. The extent of the loss was, however, largely a matter of expert guessing. Last week a well-rounded study was published. It was based on 22,000 questionnaires sent to former graduate students who were enrolled in 24 universities and it seemed to show many past fears to be groundless.

The dropouts rate was found to be 31 percent, and in most cases the dropouts, while not completing the Ph. D. requirement, went on to productive work. They are not only doing well financially, but, according to the report, are not far below the income levels of those who went on to complete their doctorates.

Discussing the study last week, Dr. Tucker said the project was initiated because of the concern frequently expressed by graduate faculties and administrators that some of the individuals who dropped out of Ph. D. programs were capable of completing the requirement for the degree. Attrition at the Ph. D. level is also thought to be a waste of precious faculty time and a drain on university resources already being used to capacity. Some people expressed the opinion that the shortage of highly trained specialists and college teachers could be reduced by persuading the dropouts to return to graduate schools to complete the Ph. D.

"The results of our research," Dr. Tucker concluded, "did not support these opinions."

1. Lack of motivation was the principal reason for dropping out.

2. Most dropouts went as far in their doctoral program as was consistent with their levels of ability or their specialities.

3. Most dropouts are now engaged in work consistent with their education and motivation.

Nearly 75 per cent of the dropouts said there was no academic reason for their decision, but those who mentioned academic reason cited failure to pass the qualifying examination, uncompleted research and failure to pass language exams. Among the single most important personal reasons identified by dropouts for non-completion of their Ph. D. program, lack of finances was marked by 19 per cent.

As an indication of how well the dropouts were doing, a chart showed 2% in humanities were receiving $ 20,000 and more annually while none of the Ph. D.'s with that background reached this figure. The Ph. D.'s income in the $ 7,500 to $ 15,000 bracket with 78% at that level against 50% for the dropouts. This may also be an indication of the fact that top salaries in the academic fields, where Ph. D. s tend to rise to the highest salaries, are still lagging behind other fields.

As to the possibility of getting dropouts back on campus, the outlook was glum. The main condition which would have to prevail for at least 25 % of the dropouts who might consider returning to graduate school would be to guarantee that they would retain their present level of income and in some cases their present job.

1. The author states that many educators feel that _____.

    A. steps should be taken to get the dropouts back to campus

    B. the dropouts should return to a lower quality school to continue their study

    C. the Ph. D. holder is generally a better adjusted person than the dropout

    D. the high dropouts' rate is largely attributable to the lack of stimulation on the part of faculty members

2. Research has shown that _____.

    A. dropouts are substantially below Ph. D. s in financial attainment

    B. the incentive factor is a minor one in regard to pursuing Ph. D. studies

    C. the Ph. D. candidate is likely to change his field of specialization if he drops out

    D. about one-third of those who start Ph. D. work do not complete the work to earn the degree

3. Meeting foreign language requirements for the Ph. D. _____.

    A. is the most frequent reason for dropping out

    B. is more difficult for the science candidate than for the humanities candidate

    C. is an essential part of many Ph. D. programs

    D. does not vary in difficulty among universities

4. After reading the article, one would refrain from concluding that _____.

    A. optimism reigns in regard to getting Ph. D. dropouts to return to their pursuit of the degree

    B. a Ph. D. dropout, by and large, does not have what it takes to learn the degree

    C. colleges and universities employ a substantial number of Ph. D. dropouts

    D. Ph. D. s are not earning what they deserve in nonacademic positions

5. It can be inferred that the high rate of dropouts lies in _____.

   A. salary for Ph. D. too low

   B. academic requirement too high

   C. salary for dropouts too high

   D. 1,000 positions

▶ Words & Expressions

dropout *n.*	辍学者，中途退学者
well-rounded *adj.*	全面的
attrition *n.*	缩/减员；磨损
drain *n.*	枯竭
bracket *v.*	把……视为同类
lag behind other fields	落后于其他领域
glum *adj.*	阴郁的

▶ 文章大意

教育工作者非常关注博士生辍学的高比率；这对需要博士生的国家是一个人才方面的严重损失。一些国家的博士辍学率高达50%。然而，如此高的辍学率很大程度上只是专家的推测。上周发布了一项全面的调查报告，该调查报告是以22 000份调查问卷分送给以前在24所大学就读的博士生为基础的，似乎表明过去的许多担心害怕是没有根据的。

研究发现辍学率为31%，大多数情况下，辍学者尚未完成博士学位学业，就去从事生产性工作。根据一项报告，他们不仅赚到了钱，而且收入水平并不比那些完成博士学位的人低多少。

经过对上周这次调查研究讨论之后，图赫尔博士说道，发起这项调查是因为高校的教师和管理者经常关注的一个问题是有些未完成博士课程的辍学者有能力完成博士学位。博士水平人员的缩减被认为是宝贵的教授时间的浪费和已经被使用到极限的大学资源的枯竭。有些人建议高级专家和大学教师短缺现象可以通过劝说辍学者返回校园完成博士学位来减少。

图赫尔博士得出结论，此项研究结果并不支持以上观点：

1. 缺乏动力是辍学的主要原因。

2. 大多数辍学者在博士课程上已经达到和他们的能力水平和专业水平相一致的水平。

3. 大多数辍学者现在从事的工作和他们所受的教育和动机相一致。

约75%的辍学者说，他们决定辍学并不是出于学术原因，而出于学术原因的辍学者提出：难以通过资格考试，难以完成研究，未能通过语言考试。19%的辍学者一致认为不能完成博士生课程的最主要的个人原因是缺乏经济来源。

作为辍学者干得不错的证明，统计图表说明2%的人文学科辍学者年收入为20 000多美元，没有一个有同样背景的博士生达到这个数目。在7 000至15 000美元年收入者中，博士生为78%，辍学者仅为50%。这也可能表明这样一个事实：在博士能挣到最高工资的学术领域中，高工资仍然落后于其他领域的工资。

至于让辍学者返回校园的可能性，前景不乐观。至少有25%的辍学者可能考虑返回研究生院就读，条件是保证他们保持现有的收入水平，有些还要求保留他们目前的工作。

答案、考点及解析

1. 【答案】A

   【考点】细节理解题

   【解析】A项"许多教育工作者感到应采取步骤让辍学者回校学习。"与第三段最后一句话内容相符："Some people expressed the opinion that the shortage of highly trained specialists and college teachers could be reduced by persuading the dropouts to return to graduate schools to complete the Ph. D." B项"辍学者应回到稍低级的学校去完成学业。" C项"有博士学位的人一般比辍学者具有较好的适应性。" D项"高辍学率的主要原因在于教师方面缺乏刺激鼓励。"这三项在文章中均没有提到。

2. 【答案】D

   【考点】细节理解题

   【解析】选项D"约三分之一开始就读博士学位的人没有完成学业取得学位。"与第二段第一句内容相符："The dropouts rate was found to be 31 percent, and in most cases the dropouts, while not completing the Ph. D. requirement, went on to productive work." A项"辍学者的经济收入比博士生低许多。"是错误的说法，这可以从倒数第二段得知："作为辍学者干得真不错的证明，统计图表说明2%人文学科的辍学者年收入为20 000多美元，没有一个同样背景的博士生达到这个数目。" B项"在博士学习中刺激因素较小。" C项"博士在读生如果中途退学很可能改变其专业领域。"这两项在文中均没有提到。

3. 【答案】C

   【考点】细节理解题

   【解析】选项C"博士生应达到外语要求的水平是许多博士生课程的一个基本组成部分。"在第五段中有所体现："约75%的辍学者说，他们决定辍学并不是出于学术的原因，而出于学术原因的辍学者提出：难以通过资格考试，难以完成研究，未能通过语言考试。"由此看出外语是博士生课程的基本组成部分。其他选项均不符合原文意思。A项"它是辍学最频繁的原因。"B项"它对理科博士生比文科博士应考生更难。"D项"它在大学中的难度并没有不同。"

4. 【答案】A

【考点】推理题

【解析】题干问的是：读完这篇文章，人们不会有哪种结论。可在第五段和最后一段找到答案。第五段提到：（1）缺乏动力是辍学的主要原因。（2）大多数辍学者在博士生课程上已经达到和他们的能力水平和专业水平相一致的水平。（3）大多数辍学者现在从事的工作和他们所受的教育和动机相一致。最后一段提到："The main condition which would have to prevail for at least 25 % of the dropouts who might consider returning to graduate school would be to guarantee that they would retain their present level of income and in some cases their present job." B项"博士生辍学者，大体而论，并不具备得到学位所需要的一切。"C项"学院和大学雇用了许多辍学者。"D项"博士生在非学术岗位上没有挣到他们应得的钱。"B、C两项在文章中没有提到；根据第六段最后一句可知：博士生在学术领域中没有挣到足够的钱，故D项说法错误。

5. 【答案】A

【考点】推理题

【解析】由倒数第二段"This may also be an indication of the fact that top salaries in the academic fields, where Ph. D. s tend to rise to the highest salaries, are still lagging behind other fields." 可知A项"博士生的工资太低"是对的。B项"学术要求太高"只是某些因学术原因辍学者的强调点。C项"辍学者工资太高"说法错误，文中表达"辍学者工资比博士生高"，而并非绝对值高。D项"1 000个职位"在文内没有提到。

Passage Three

Obesity is a complex disease for which no single cause of cure exists. You gain weight when you take in more calories than you burn off. But obesity is influenced by many other factors as well: family history, the type of work you do, race, and environment.

Overeating is easy in our culture today. Portions at fast-food and other restaurants are "supersized" to the point that one meal can provide an entire day's worth of calories. Food is also a focal point of social activity. Gathering of family and friends, work events, and holidays are usually centered around food. And eating can be a comfort when you are depressed or stressed.

Next, people are less active than ever. Some people hate to exercise and others may not have the time. Also, many of the conveniences we use, such as the remote control for the television, elevators, and cars, cut activity out of our lives.

Even making small changes like walking your dog makes a difference. Letting the dog out the door burns 2 calories. Walking the dog for 30 minutes burns 123 calories. Taking the car to a car wash uses 18 calories. Washing and waxing it yourself burn 300.

Other things can affect our weight, such as family history or genetics. If one of your parents is obese, you are 3 times as likely to be obese as someone with parents of healthy weight.

Your family's and friends' lifestyles can also affect your weight. If your family or friends eat a lot of high-fat or snack foods, eat at irregular times, and skip meals, you probably will too. And if they are not physically active, you may not be either.

Other things influence your weight and whether you are physically active, including:

Low self-esteem. Being overweight or obese may lower your self-esteem and lead to eating as a way to comfort yourself. Repeated failure at dieting also can affect your self-esteem and make it even more difficult to lose weight.

Emotional concerns. Emotional stress, anxiety, or illnesses such as depression or chronic pain can lead to overeating. Some people eat to calm themselves, to avoid dealing with unpleasant tasks or situations, or to dampen negative emotions.

Trauma. Distressing events, such as childhood sexual, physical, or emotional abuse; loss of a parent during childhood; or marital of family problems, can contribute to overeating.

Alcohol. Alcohol (beer and mixed drinks) is very high in calories. Drinking alcohol may cause you to gain more weight around your stomach.

Medicines or medical conditions. Some medical conditions and medicines may also cause weight gain. Examples include having Cushing's syndrome or hypothyroidism or taking antidepressants or corticosteroids.

How obesity affects your health depends on many things, including your age, gender, where you carry your body fat, and how physically active you are. For example, if you are an older woman who is physically active and you will be less likely to have the problems related to obesity than a younger man who is not physically active.

Risk for disease. If you are obese, you are more likely to develop type 2 diabetes, high blood pressure, coronary artery disease, stroke, and sleep apnea, among other conditions. If you lose weight, your risk for these conditions is reduced.

Where you carry body fat is important. If fat accumulates mostly around your stomach (sometimes called apple-shaped), you are at greater risk for type 2 diabetes, high blood pressure, high cholesterol, and coronary artery disease than people who are lean or people with fat around the hips (sometimes called pear-shaped).

▶ Words & Expressions

focal point	焦点
convenience n.	便利
remote control	遥控器
wax v.	（给车）打蜡
self-esteem n.	自尊
dampen v.	减压，缓冲
hypothyroidism n.	甲状腺功能减退
antidepressant n.	抗抑郁病药

1. _____ is not an affecting factor of obesity.

 A. Family history and the race you belong to

 B. Environment and your job

 C. Reading habit

 D. Your lifestyle

2. According to the author, why modern men are less active?

 A. Some people hate to exercise.

 B. Some may not have the time.

 C. The extensive use of some conveniences such as remote controls.

 D. All of the above.

3. Which of the following statements is not true?

 A. Weight loss can decrease the risk of many diseases.

 B. Beer as well as some medications can cause weight gain.

 C. The fat which accumulated around your hip is not so harmful.

 D. Snack food is not a healthy food in general.

4. According to the text, _____ doesn't belong to trauma contributing to overeating.

    A. traffic accident injury

    B. the death of a parent during childhood

    C. awful spouse relationship

    D. sexual abuse when young

5. What can be inferred from the text?

    A. A weight-loss plan should combine different measures altogether.

    B. Obesity is a complex disease which is curable.

    C. Only the fat put around your stomach is harmful.

    D. A physically inactive young man may be at greater risks for obesity problems than an active over-weighted older woman.

▶ 文章大意

肥胖症是一种复杂的疾病，没有单一的病因或疗法。当你摄入的热量超过你所消耗的热量，你的体重就会增加。但是肥胖症也受其他很多因素的影响：家族史、工作类型、种族和环境。

吃得过饱在我们当今的文化中很普遍。快餐店和其他餐馆提供的饮食分量均为"特大号"，以至于一顿就提供了一整天所需要的热量。食物也是社会活动的一个重点。家人和朋友的聚会、工作场合和假日往往以食物为中心。而且当你感到沮丧或是处于重压之下时，吃东西可能是一种安慰。

其次，人们的活动比以前减少了。一些人讨厌锻炼，而其他人可能没有时间。而且，我们使用的一些便利设备，如电视遥控器、电梯和轿车，把体力活动从我们的生活里删减了。

即使做一些小的改变（像遛遛你的狗）都能起些作用。例如，把狗带出门消耗2卡路里，遛狗30分钟消耗123卡路里，把车送去洗消耗18卡路里，自己洗车并上蜡消耗300卡路里。

其他的东西也能影响我们的体重，比如家族史或遗传因素。如果你的父母中有一人肥胖，那么与那些父母都是正常体重的人相比你发胖的概率几乎是他们的三倍。

你的家人和朋友的生活方式也能影响你的体重。如果你的家人或朋友吃高脂肪或快餐，进食不规律，并误餐，你就有可能也这样。而且如果他们不爱体力劳动，你可能也一样。

其他一些影响你体重以及你是否精力旺盛的因素包括：

缺乏自尊。由于超重或肥胖会降低你的自尊并导致你把进食当作安慰自己的一种手段。反复的节食失败也会影响你的自尊并让减肥变得更加困难。

情绪问题。情绪上的压力、焦虑，或是疾病（如抑郁症或慢性疼痛）能导致过度饮食。

一些人通过进食来使自己平静下来，避免处理不愉快的工作或处境，或缓解消极情绪。

创伤。令人痛苦的事件，如儿童时期受到性的、身体的或情绪上的虐待，童年时失去父亲或母亲，或是婚姻、家庭问题，会导致过度饮食。

酒类。酒类（啤酒或混合饮料）的热量很高。饮酒会使你的胃部周围重量增加。

药物或疾病状态。一些疾病状态和药物也可能引起体重增加。例子包括库欣综合征或甲状腺功能减退，或者是服用抗抑郁药或皮质激素。

肥胖症如何影响你的健康取决于很多因素，包括你的年龄、性别、体内脂肪储存的部位，以及你爱不爱活动。比方说，如果你是一位经常进行体力活动的年长女性，你患有与体重相关的健康问题的风险就比一个年轻而不爱活动的男性要低。

疾病的风险。如果你身体肥胖，在某些条件下，你就有较大可能患2型糖尿病、高血压、冠心病、中风及睡眠呼吸暂停症。如果你减肥，你陷于这些状况的风险就会降低。

你的脂肪储存在哪里很重要。如果你的脂肪主要堆积在你的腹部（有时被称为苹果形），你得2型糖尿病、高血压、高胆固醇、冠心病的风险就要比那些瘦子或脂肪在臀部（有时被称为梨形）的人大得多。

答案、考点及解析

1. 【答案】C

   【考点】细节定位题（排除题）

   【解析】根据affecting factors回到原文定位到第一段，可知"family history, the type of work you do, race, and environment"都是影响因素，而reading habit没有提及。

2. 【答案】D

   【考点】细节定位题

   【解析】根据less active定位到文章第三段，可知"有些人讨厌锻炼""有些人没有时间"和"广泛使用便利装置"都是人们变得不太爱动的原因。

3. 【答案】C

   【考点】细节理解题（排除题）

   【解析】该题只能通过选项定位后再一一进行对比排除。从倒数第二段可知，减轻体重可以减少患病风险，A选项是正确的；从倒数第四和第五段可知，饮酒和药物都有可能导致体重增加，B选项是正确的。从文中最后一句可知，苹果形身材比起脂肪聚集在臀部周围的人患2型糖尿病、高血压、高胆固醇、冠心病的风险大，但并未说后者就无害，因此C选项属于过度推理；从第六段中可知，如果你的家人和朋友爱吃高脂肪含量的食物或者小吃，你变胖的概率就很高，可知通常来讲

snack是不健康的食物。

4. 【答案】A

　　【考点】细节定位题

　　【解析】通过trauma定位到第十段，导致overeating的创伤包括"令人痛苦的事件，比如童年受到性的、身体的及情绪上的虐待""童年时失去父母或者其他婚姻家庭问题"等，不包含A选项（交通事故带来的伤害）。

5. 【答案】A

　　【考点】细节理解题

　　【解析】A选项（减肥计划应该结合不同的方法）与文章首句"肥胖是一种复杂的疾病，没有单一的病因或疗法"是一致的。B选项（肥胖是一种能够治疗的疾病）仍可对应该句，但文中并未提及是否可治愈。C选项（只有在腹部累积的脂肪才是有害的）对应文章最后一句，脂肪在哪儿只会影响罹患某些疾病的概率，并非只有在腹部才有害。D选项（不运动的年轻人比爱运动的超重老龄女性有更大的肥胖问题）对应第13段中的"一个保持规律运动的年长女性比不太运动的年轻人罹患肥胖相关疾病的概率小"，该选项错误。

Passage Four

If you smoke and you still don't believe that there's a definite link between smoking and bronchial troubles, heart disease and lung cancer, then you are certainly deceiving yourself. No one will accuse you of hypocrisy. Let us just say that you are suffering from a bad case of wishful thinking. This needn't make you too uncomfortable because you are in good company. Whenever the subject of smoking and health is raised, the governments of most countries hear no evil, see no evil and smell no evil. Admittedly, a few governments have taken timid measures. In Britain for instance, cigarette advertising has been banned on television. The conscience of the nation is appeased, while the population continues to puff its way to smoky, cancerous death.

You don't have to look very far to find out why the official reactions to medical findings have been so lukewarm. The answer is simply money. Tobacco is a wonderful commodity to tax. It's almost like a tax on our daily bread. In tax revenue alone, the government of Britain collects enough from smokers to pay for its entire educational facilities. So while the authorities point out ever so discreetly that smoking may, conceivable, be harmful, it doesn't do to shout too loudly about it.

This is surely the most short-sighted policy you could imagine. While money is eagerly collected in vast sums with one hand, it is paid out in increasingly vaster sums with the other. Enormous amounts are spent on cancer research and on efforts to cure people suffering from the disease. Countless valuable lives are lost. In the long run, there is no doubt that everybody would be much better-off if smoking were banned altogether.

Of course, we are not ready for such a drastic action. But if the governments of the world were honestly concerned about the welfare of their peoples, you'd think they'd conduct aggressive anti-smoking campaigns. Far from it! The tobacco industry is allowed to spend staggering sums on advertising. Its advertising is as insidious as it is dishonest. We are never shown pictures of real smokers coughing up their lungs early in the morning. That would never do. The advertisement always depicts virile, clean-shaven young men. They suggest it is manly to smoke, even positively healthy! Smoking is associated with the great open-air life, with beautiful girls, true love and togetherness. What utter nonsense!

For a start, governments could begin by banning all cigarette and tobacco advertising and should then conduct anti-smoking advertising campaigns of their own. Smoking should be banned in all public places like theatres, cinemas and restaurants. Great efforts should be made to inform young people especially of the dire consequences of taking up the habit. A horrific warning — say, a picture of a death's head — should be included in every packet of cigarettes that is sold. As individuals, we are certainly weak, but if governments acted honestly and courageously, they could protect us from ourselves.

1. Why do a few governments take timid measures toward smoking?

    A. Because they are afraid of people.

    B. Because diseases cost a lot.

    C. Because they are afraid of the cutting down of their revenue.

    D. Because they are afraid of manufacturers.

2. The tone of this passage is _____.

    A. critical   B. ironical

    C. distaste   D. amusing

3. What does the sentence "because you are in good company" mean?

    A. You are backed by the government.

    B. You are not alone.

    C. You have good colleagues.

D. Governments are blind to evils of smoking too.

4. What is the main idea of this passage?

   A. World governments should conduct serious campaigns against smoking.

   B. World governments take timid measures against smoking.

   C. Smoking is the most important source of income to many countries.

   D. Tobacco industry spends a large sum of money on medical research.

5. All of the following statements are correct EXCEPT _____.

   A. governments collect a great amount of money from the tobacco industry

   B. most governments hold ambiguous attitudes toward new findings about the harm of smoking

   C. some governments have taken radical measures against smoking

   D. advertisements by tobacco industry are quite dishonest

▶ Words & Expressions

bronchial *adj.*	支气管的
hypocrisy *n.*	虚伪
lukewarm *adj.*	冷淡的，漠然的
conceivable *adj.*	可以想象的
a wishful thinking	根据愿望的想法，不顾事实的想法
puff *v.*	喷
puff its way to	一路吞云吐雾地走向（指抽烟抽到死）
insidious *adj.*	阴险的，狡猾的
virile *adj.*	年富力强的
dire *adj.*	可怕的，悲惨的

▶ 文章大意

假如你吸烟，依然认为吸烟和支气管炎、心脏病、肺癌等毫无关系，那你是自欺欺人。可没有人会说你虚伪。我们可以说你是患上了一厢情愿病。你无须太难受，因为你有好伙伴。每当提出吸烟和健康相关的问题时，大多数国家的政府对其恶果听而不闻、视而不见、嗅而不觉。不得不承认，一些政府采取了软弱无力的政策。比如，在英国，香烟广告只是禁止在电视上播放。政府的良心得到了告慰，然而，人们还是一路吞云吐雾直到患癌死亡。

你不用看得很远就能发现为什么官方对医学成果的反应如此冷淡，答案就是钱。烟草是征税的最奇妙的商品，几乎就像日用面包的税收。光烟草税收一项，英国政府就从抽烟者身上征收到足以支付所有教育设施的费用。所以在当局那么谨慎地指出吸烟有害时，可以想象，喊叫得太响是不行的。

这无疑是你能想象到的最缺乏远见的政策。一方面急切地收敛大笔金钱，另一方面还要不断地花费更大一笔钱。很大一笔钱花在了癌症研究和治愈癌症患者身上。不计其数的宝贵生命终止了。从长远来看，毫无疑问，如果抽烟能够完全禁止的话，每个人的生活都将会过得更好。

当然，我们还没做好准备迎接如此巨大的行动，但是，如果世界各国政府都能够诚心诚意地关心其国民福利的话，你能想到各国政府会发起有力的禁烟运动。事实并非如此！烟草工业是允许在广告上花费惊人巨款的。其广告的阴险正如其欺骗性一样。我们从来都不会在广告上看到抽烟者在清晨咳肺的真实画面，从来都不会。广告上描绘的从来都是胡子刮得干干净净的年轻男子。这些广告暗示吸烟展现了男子气概，甚至是有益健康的，吸烟是和美好的户外生活、美女、真爱及聚会联系在一起的。纯属一派胡言！

作为起步，政府可以从禁止烟草广告开始，然后开展抵制吸烟的广告运动。一切公共场合，如戏院、电影院、餐馆等应禁止吸烟。应竭尽全力告诫青年，尤其是告诫他们染上恶习的严重后果。在零售的每包烟盒上应有令人胆战心惊的警告：例如，一幅骷髅头画像。作为个人，我们力量薄弱，可是如果政府真诚地鼓舞人心去行动起来，他们可以保护我们。

答案、考点及解析

1. 【答案】C

   【考点】细节理解题

   【解析】通过why和government定位到第二段中 "You don't have to look very far to find out why the official reactions to medical findings have been so lukewarm. The answer is simply money." A项 "他们害怕人民。" 和D项 "他们害怕厂商。" 在文中没有提到。B项错在说因为疾病花费很大，所以一些政府采取软弱无力的禁烟措施，而是因为采取了软弱政策，所以疾病花费很大。本题题干和原文有同义替换：government和official，timid和lukewarm。

2. 【答案】A

   【考点】态度题

   【解析】从文章第一段中的 "you are deceiving yourself" "the governments of most countries hear no evil, see no evil and smell no evil"，第二段中的 "official reactions… lukewarm"，第三段中的 "the most short-sighted policy" 和第四段的 "what utter nonsense"，都不难看出作者对于政府的烟草政策是批判的、不满意的。而讽

刺、厌恶和有趣都不符合文章的态度。

3. 【答案】D

【考点】细节理解题

【解析】答案可以通过上下文理解得出来，第一段提到 "This needn't make you too uncomfortable because you are in good company."；下文进行解释，"每当提出吸烟和健康有关的问题时，大多数国家的政府对其恶果听而不闻、视而不见、嗅而不觉。" 由此可见，A，B，C三项不正确。

4. 【答案】A

【考点】主旨大意题

【解析】前面四段讲的都是现象：（1）政策软弱；（2）烟草的税收高，所以未被禁止；（3）这项政策的后果是疾病花费大于烟草税收；（4）烟草广告泛滥毒害人，唯一的解救办法就是禁烟。最后一段是结论，也是画龙点睛的主题和标题。B项 "世界各国政府采取的禁烟政策软弱无力。" C项 "吸烟是许多国家的重要收入。" D项 "烟草工厂在医疗研究上花了大笔费用。" 这三项都不是本文的主题。

5. 【答案】C

【考点】多项细节排除题

【解析】A选项在第二段中的the government of Britain collects enough from smokers to pay for its entire educational facilities及第四段都有体现。B选项见第二段：You don't have to look very far to find out why the official reactions to medical findings have been so lukewarm. D选项从第四段中的 "Its advertising is as insidious as it is dishonest." 可以推断出。只有C选项在文中没有正确的呼应，第二段虽然提及烟草行业税收对政府的重要性，但并未表明政府已采取有效措施宣传烟草危害及推动禁烟。

Passage Five

Until about five years ago, the very idea that peptide hormones might be made anywhere in the brain besides the hypothalamus was astounding. Peptide hormones, scientists thought, were made by endocrine glands and the hypothalamus was thought to be the brains' only endocrine gland. What is more, because peptide hormones cannot cross the blood-brain barrier, researchers believed that they never got to any part of the brain other than the hypothalamus, where they were simply produced and then released into the bloodstream.

But these beliefs about peptide hormones were questioned as laboratory after laboratory found that antiserums to peptide hormones, when injected into the brain, bind in places other than the hypothalamus, indicating that either the hormones or substances that cross-react with the antiserums are present. The immunological method of detecting peptide hormones by means of antiserums, however, is imprecise. Cross-reactions are possible and this method cannot determine whether the substances detected by the antiserums really are the hormones, or merely close relatives. Furthermore, this method cannot be used to determine the location in the body where the detected substances are actually produced.

New techniques of molecular biology, however, provide a way to answer these questions. It is possible to make specific complementary DNAs (cDNAs) that can serve as molecular probes seek out the messenger RNAs (mRNAs) of the peptide hormones. If brain cells are making the hormones, the cells will contain these mRNAs. If the products the brain cells make resemble the hormones but are not identical to them, then the cDNAs should still bind to these mRNAs, but should not bind as tightly as they would to mRNAs for the true hormones. The cells containing these mRNAs can then be isolated and their mRNAs decoded to determine just what their protein products are and how closely the products resemble the true peptide hormones.

The molecular approach to detecting peptide hormones using cDNA probes should also be much faster than the immunological method because it can take years of tedious purifications to isolate peptide hormones and then develop antiserums to them. Roberts, expressing the sentiment of many researchers, states: "I was trained as an endocrinologist. But it became clear to me that the field of endocrinology needed molecular biology input. The process of grinding out protein purifications is just too slow."

If, as the initial tests with cDNA probes suggest, peptide hormones really are made in brain in areas other than the hypothalamus, a theory must be developed that explains their function in the brain. Some have suggested that the hormones are all growth regulators, but Rosen's work on rat brains indicates that this cannot be true. A number of other researchers propose that they might be used for intercellular communication in the brain.

1. Which of the following titles best summarizes the text?

   A. Is Molecular Biology the Key to Understanding Intercellular Communication in the Brain?

   B. Molecular Biology: Can Researchers Exploit Its Techniques to Synthesize Peptide Hormones?

C. The Advantages and Disadvantages of the Immunological Approach to Detecting Peptide Hormones

D. Peptide Hormones: How Scientists Are Attempting to Solve Problems of Their Detection and to Understand Their Function?

2. The text suggests that a substance detected in the brain by use of antiserums to peptide hormones may _____.

A. have been stored in the brain for a long period of time

B. play no role in the functioning of the brain

C. have been produced in some part of the body other than the brain

D. have escaped detection by molecular methods

3. According to the text, confirmation of the belief that peptide hormones are created in the brain in areas other than the hypothalamus would force scientists to _____.

A. reject the theory that peptide hormones are made by endocrine glands

B. revise their beliefs about the ability of antiserums to detect peptide hormones

C. invent techniques that would allow them to locate accurately brain cells that produce peptide hormones

D. develop a theory that accounts for the role played by peptide hormones in the brain

4. Which of the following is mentioned in the text as a drawback of the immunological method of detecting peptide hormones?

A. It cannot be used to detect the presence of growth regulators in the brain.

B. It cannot distinguish between the peptide hormones and substances that are very similar to them.

C. It uses antiserums that are unable to cross the blood-brain barrier.

D. It involves a purification process that requires extensive training in endocrinology.

5. The idea that the field of endocrinology can gain from developments in molecular biology is regarded by Roberts with _____.

A. incredulity

B. derision

C. indifference

D. enthusiasm

◉ Words & Expressions

peptide hormones	肽激素
hypothalamus *n.*	下丘脑
astounding *adj.*	令人惊讶的
endocrine gland	内分泌腺
antiserums *n.*	抗血清
specific *adj.*	特定的，特别的
complementary *adj.*	互补的
resemble *v.*	看起来像
identical *adj.*	相同的
tedious *adj.*	冗长的
endocrinologist *n.*	内分泌学家

◉ 文章大意

肽激素除了下丘脑能制造，在大脑中任何其他的地方都能够制造。大约五年前仅这一想法本身就是令人惊诧的。科学家认为，肽激素是由内分泌腺制造的，而下丘脑被认为是大脑中唯一的内分泌腺。而且，由于肽激素无法穿过血脑障碍，研究人员认为它们从不曾到过除下丘脑以外的大脑任何其他部位，肽激素仅在下丘脑制造出来，然后被释放到血管中。

但是关于肽激素的这种观点已经遭到质疑。一次又一次的实验发现，肽激素的抗血清一旦被注射到大脑中，它就会在下丘脑以外的地方凝结起来。这就说明这些地方或是有肽激素存在，或是有与抗血清发生交叉反应的其他物质存在。但是，通过抗血清来检验肽激素的免疫学方法是不精确的。交叉反应可能会发生，而且以这种手段无法确认用抗血清检测的特质确实是肽激素还是仅是与其近似的亲缘物质。另外，这种方法不能用来确定被测物质在人体内产生的部位。

然而，分子生物学的新技术为解决这些问题提供了一个新途径。科学家可以制造出一种特别的互补DNA (cDNA)，作为分子探子查找出肽激素的信使RNA (mRNA)。如果脑细胞正在制造肽激素，那么它应该包含这些信使RNA。如果脑细胞制造的产物与肽激素相似但并不完全相同，那么这些互补DAN仍然会和这些信使RNA黏结，但不会像和真正肽激素的信使RNA结合得那么紧密，这些包含信使RNA's的细胞能被分开。研究者可以将信使RNA解码，以确定其蛋白质产物究竟是什么及这些产物在多大程度上类似于真正的肽激素。

采用cDNA探子这一分子生物学方法检测肽激素同时也比免疫学方法快得多，因为如果用免疫学方法，分离肽激素需要几年枯燥乏味的提纯过程，然后还需培养出它们的抗血清。罗伯茨的一番话表达了许多研究人员的心声，他说："我是作为一名内分泌学家接受训练的，但情况对我来说很清楚，内分泌学领域需要分子生物学的输入，靠碾磨来制造蛋白质纯化物的过程实在是太慢了。"

如果正如用cDNA探子所做的最初测试表明的那样，肽激素确实是由大脑中下丘脑以外的部位制造出来的，则有必要建立一套理论来解释它们在大脑中的作用。某些学者指出肽激素是生长调节剂，但罗森对老鼠大脑所做的实验表明事实并非如此。很多其他的研究人员指出肽激素或许被用于大脑内细胞与细胞间的信息传输。

答案、考点及解析

1. 【答案】D

   【考点】中心主旨题

   【解析】全文从头至尾讨论的是peptide hormones在人体内产生的部位，所以有关全文中心主旨内容的答案应该包含peptide hormones。从各段的主题句进行分析，第一至四段主要讲如何detect（探测）肽激素（peptide hormones）所产生的位置，第五段主要讲有关肽激素的function。可见本题的正确选项应该是D。在解题时一定要搞清楚原文所涉及的对象并且抓住每段的主题句以及它们之间的相互关系。

2. 【答案】C

   【考点】细节理解题

   【解析】通过substance detected in the brain by use of antiserums可定位到第二段中的"...the immunological method of detecting peptide hormones by means of antiserums, however, is imprecise."由此可知，以前测试的方法是不精确的。该段接着解释了不精确的原因：可能发生交叉反应、该方法无法确定被测物质在人体内产生的部位。因此C选项"该物质在身体其他部位产生而不是脑部"是正确答案。

3. 【答案】D

   【考点】细节推导题

   【解析】通过本题题干中的peptide hormones are created in the brain in areas other than the hypothalamus可确定在尾段的第一句。尾段第一句主要就肽激素的function进行论述，可见本题的正确选项应该是D，选项D中的role就等于原文中的function。考生在解题时一定要善于抓住主句中的重要信息。

4. 【答案】B

   【考点】细节理解题

   【解析】根据本题题干中的the immunological method可确定在第二段的第二句，而本题

的确切答题点在第二段的第三句的后半部分。从第二段第三句的后半部分可以推
导出本题的正确答案是B。在解题时一定要注意一般概括句和具体陈述句之间的
相互关系。

5. 【答案】D

【考点】细节推导题

【解析】根据本题题干中的人名Roberts可将本题的答案迅速确定在倒数第二段引号部分
的第二句话，即But一词引导的句子。从该句中的needed一词可以看出本题的正
确选项应该是D。考生在解题时一定要学会深入理解原文的字面含义。

Passage Six

A study published in the *New England Journal of Medicine* estimated that there are an average of 30 in-flight medical emergencies on U.S. flights every day. Most of them are not grave; fainting, dizziness and hyper ventilation are the most frequent complaints. But 13% of them — roughly four a day — are serious enough to require a pilot to change course. The most common of the serious emergencies include heart trouble (46%), strokes and other neurological problems (18%), and difficult breathing (6%).

Let's face it: plane riders are stressful. For starters, cabin pressures at high altitudes are set at roughly what they would be if you lived at 5,000 to 8,000 feet above sea level. Most people can tolerate these pressures pretty easily, but passengers with heart disease may experience chest pains as a result of the reduced amount of oxygen flowing through their blood. Low pressure can also cause the air in body cavities to expand — as much as 30%. Again, most people won't notice anything beyond mild stomach cramping. But if you've recently had an operation, your wound could open. And if a medical device has been implanted in your body — a splint, a tracheotomy tube or a catheter — it could expand and cause injury.

Another common in-flight problem is venous thrombosis — the so-called economy-class syndrome. When you sit too long in a cramped position, the blood in our legs tends to clot. Most people just get sore calves. But blood clots, left untreated, could travel to the lungs, causing breathing difficulties and even death. Such clots are readily prevented by keeping blood flowing; walk and stretch your legs when possible.

Whatever you do, don't panic. Things are looking up on the in-flight-emergency front. Doctors who come to passengers' aid used to worry about getting sued; their fears have lifted somewhat since the 1998 *Aviation Medical Assistance Act* gave them "good Samaritan" protection. And thanks to more recent legislation, flights with at least one attendant are starting to install emergency medical kits with automated defibrillator to treat heart attacks.

Are you still wondering if you are healthy enough to fly? If you can walk 150 ft. or climb a flight of stairs without getting winded, you'll probably do just fine. Having a doctor close by doesn't hurt, either.

1. Heart disease takes up about _____ of the in-flight medical emergencies on US flights.

    A. 13%   B. 46%   C. 18%   D. 6%

2. According to Paragraph 2, the expansion of air in body cavities can result in _____.

    A. heart attack   B. chest pain

    C. stomach cramping   D. difficult breathing

3. We can learn from Paragraph 3 that deep venous thrombosis usually happens because _____.

    A. the economy class is not spacious enough

    B. there are too many economy-class passengers

    C. passengers are not allowed to walk during the flight

    D. the low pressure in the cabin prevents blood flowing smoothly

4. According to 1998 *Aviation Medical Assistance Act*, doctors who came to passengers' aid _____.

    A. do not have to be worried even if they give the patients improper treatment

    B. will not be submitted to legal responsibility even if the patients didn't recover

    C. are assisted by advanced emergency medical kits

    D. will be greatly respected by the patient and the crew

5. The phrase "getting winded" (Para. 5) is closest in meaning to _____.

    A. falling over   B. being out of breath

    C. spraining the ankle   D. moving in a curving line

Words & Expressions

estimate v.	估计
emergency n.	紧急情况
grave adj.	严重的

hyperventilation *n.*	过度换气
neurological *adj.*	神经的
altitude *n.*	高度
cramp *n.*	痉挛
splint *n.*	夹板
tracheotomy *n.*	气管切开术
catheter *n.*	导管
venous *adj.*	静脉的
thrombosis *n.*	血栓形成
syndrome *n.*	综合征
clot *v./n.*	（形成）血栓
sore *adj.*	酸疼的
aviation *n.*	航空
good Samaritan	乐善好施者
legislation *n.*	立法
defibrillator *n.*	除颤器

▶ 文章大意

　　一项刊登在《新英格兰医学杂志》上的研究估计，美国的航班平均每天发生30起飞行中的医疗急症。大多数情况并不严重，最常见的症状包括晕厥、头晕目眩及过度换气。但是其中13%——每天约4起——症状非常严重，因而迫使飞行员改变航向。最常见的严重突发状况包括心脏病（46%）、中风和其他神经系统疾病（18%）以及呼吸困难（6%）。

　　让我们面对现实吧：飞机乘客很紧张。对初次乘坐飞机的人而言，高空机舱内设置的压力大约相当于海拔5 000～8 000英尺的气压水平。大多数人能轻松地承受这样的压力，但是有心脏病的乘客可能会因为流经血液的氧气减少而感觉胸痛。低气压也可能导致体腔内的空气膨胀——最大时可膨胀30%。此外，大多数人除了轻微的胃部痉挛外不会有其他感觉。但如果你刚动过手术，伤口可能会裂开。如果你体内植入了医疗器材——如夹板、气管切开套管或导管——这些东西可能会膨胀，并导致受伤。

　　飞行中常见的另一种毛病是深静脉血栓的形成——即所谓的经济舱综合征。长时间坐在狭窄的位置上，腿部的血液容易结块。大部分人只会感觉小腿酸痛。但血栓不经治疗，可能转移至肺部，引起呼吸困难，甚至死亡。保持血液通畅，尽可能多走动并伸展腿部，就可以轻松预防血栓。

　　无论做什么都不要惊慌。飞行中急症的状况正在好转。过去抢救乘客的医生曾担心会被起诉，自从1998年颁布的《航空医疗救助法案》为医生们提供了"乐善好施"称号的保护，大致消除了医生们的担心。最近的立法规定，至少有一名护理人员的航班开始配备急救医疗包，内有治疗心脏病突发的自动电击除颤器。

你还在怀疑自己身体是否足够健康去乘坐飞机吗？如果你走150英尺的路，或爬上一段楼梯而不气喘吁吁，那你可能没问题。当然，身边有个医生也不是什么坏事。

答案、考点及解析

1. 【答案】D

   【考点】计算题

   【解析】根据各选项中的百分比数值，可以定位到文章第一段，根据第一段最后一句，心脏病占飞行中医疗重症的46%；而根据倒数第二句，重症在美国所有飞行中的医疗急症中占13%。结合这两句可知，13%×46%，即心脏病在所有急症中应占约6%，因此D项为本题答案。

2. 【答案】C

   【考点】细节因果题

   【解析】第二段第四句提到"体腔内空气膨胀"，对应题干，可知答案在此。接下来的三句分别列出了这种现象可能导致的三种病症，其中C项（stomach cramping）在第五句中提到，为本题答案。A项引起的原因没有提到；根据第二段第三句，B项是由血液中含氧量低导致的；D项在第三段提及，由血栓引起。

3. 【答案】A

   【考点】细节题

   【解析】第三段最后一句建议乘客有机会就多运动或伸展腿部，由此可以推断该段第二句中的cramped表明经济舱空间狭窄，因此A项为本题答案。B项虽然为客观情况，但无法从原文推断得出，故可排除；第三段最后一句表明乘客可以离开座位走动，C项与此矛盾；D项与题干提到的病症没有直接联系。

4. 【答案】B

   【考点】细节推理题

   【解析】根据专有名词定位到第四段。该段第三句提到，医生担心他们给予病人的医疗援助一旦出现意外就会遭到起诉，而这种害怕从1998年法案颁布后，在某种程度度上就消失了。由此可推断，在出现意外时，该法案让医生避免承担法律责任，B项为正确答案。

5. 【答案】B

　　【考点】语义理解题

　　【解析】最后一段第二句指出了测试身体是否足够健康去乘坐飞机的方法，结合全文中提到的飞机中气压低、含氧量低的特点，可以推断getting winded应指"气喘吁吁"。正确答案为B。

Passage Seven

That experiences influence subsequent behavior is evidence of an obvious but nevertheless remarkable activity called remembering. Learning could not occur without the function popularly named memory. Constant practice has such an effect on memory as to lead to skillful performance on the piano, to recitation of a poem, and even to reading and understanding these words. So-called intelligent behavior demands memory, remembering being a primary requirement for reasoning. The ability to solve any problem or even to recognize that a problem exists depends on memory. Typically, the decision to cross a street is based on remembering many earlier experiences.

Practice (or review) tends to build and maintain memory for a task or for any learned material. Over a period of no practice, what has been learned tends to be forgotten; and the adaptive consequences may not seem obvious. Yet, dramatic instances of sudden forgetting can seem to be adaptive. In this sense, the ability to forget can be interpreted to have survived through a process of natural selection in animals. Indeed, when one's memory of an emotionally painful experience leads to serious anxiety, forgetting may produce relief. Nevertheless, an evolutionary interpretation might make it difficult to understand how the commonly gradual process of forgetting survived natural selection.

In thinking about the evolution of memory together with all its possible aspects, it is helpful to consider what would happen if memories failed to fade. Forgetting clearly aids orientation in time, since old memories weaken and the new tend to stand out, providing clues for inferring duration. Without forgetting, adaptive ability would suffer, for example, learned behavior that might have been correct a decade ago may no longer be. Cases are recorded of people who (by ordinary standards) forgot so little that their everyday activities were full of confusion. This forgetting seems to serve the survival of the individual and the species.

Another line of thought assumes a memory storage system of limited capacity that provides adaptive flexibility specifically through forgetting. In this view, continual adjustments are made between learning or memory storage (input) and forgetting (output). Indeed, there is evidence that the rate at which individuals forget is directly related to how much they have learned. Such data offers gross support of contemporary models of memory that assume an input-output balance.

1. From the evolutionary point of view, _____.

   A. forgetting for lack of practice tends to be obviously maladaptive

   B. if a person gets very forgetful all of a sudden he must be very adaptive

   C. the gradual process of forgetting is an indication of an individual's adaptability

   D. sudden forgetting may bring about adaptive consequences

2. According to the passage, if a person never forgot _____.

   A. he would survive best

   B. he would have a lot of trouble

   C. his ability to learn would be enhanced

   D. the evolution of memory would stop

3. From the last paragraph we know that _____.

   A. forgetfulness is a response to learning

   B. the memory storage system is an exactly balanced input-output system

   C. memory is a compensation for forgetting

   D. the capacity of a memory storage system is limited because forgetting occurs

4. In this passage, the author tries to interpret the function of _____.

   A. remembering　　B. forgetting　C. adapting　D. experiencing

5. What will the passage talk about next?

   A. The importance of learning.

   B. How forgetfulness functions.

   C. How adaptive ability develops.

   D. Other schools about thinking.

▶ 文章大意

　　过去的经历会影响日后的行为，这就表明存在着一种明显然而却非凡的脑力活动——记忆。若没有这种被广泛称之为"记忆"的作用，学习就不可能发生。不断的练习实践对记忆产生了影响，从而成就了钢琴上的熟练弹奏、背诵诗歌，甚至阅读和理解这些文字。所谓的智力行为需要记忆能力，因为它是推理的基本要求。用于解决问题或者甚至是辨别出有问题存在的能力有赖于记忆。举例来说，一个穿过街道的决定是根据对许多以往经历的回忆而做出的。

练习（或者复习）有助于建立和保持对一项任务或任何学习过的材料的记忆。如果我们不及时复习或练习已学过的东西的话，过一段时间，我们可能会忘记它，这种情况所造成的适应性（adaptive）后果也许不太明显。然而，突然失去记忆力却会对适应带来明显后果。从这点看，遗忘可以被看作是动物在自然选择过程中遗留给人的一种能力。的确，当一个人对一件情感上很痛苦的经历的记忆导致严重的焦虑时，遗忘可以带来解脱。然而，进化论的解释可能会使人很难理解通常逐渐的遗忘过程是如何经自然选择生存下来的。

在思考记忆的进化过程及其他相关方面时，考虑下面这个问题是很有益处的，即，如果记忆不能渐渐消失将会出现什么情形。遗忘明显有助于时间的定位，因为旧的记忆淡化了，使新的记忆清晰醒目，为推断某事的持续时间提供了线索。没有遗忘，适应性能力就会受损；例如，十年前所学的正确行为现在也许不再被认为正确。案例记载了这样一些人，他们（按一般人的标准）忘记的事情太少以至于日常生活充满了困惑。因此，遗忘似乎有助于个人以及人类的生存。

另一条思路是，假设人的记忆存储系统储量是有限的，它专门通过遗忘来提供适应之灵活性。依此观点，学习或记忆储存（输入）与遗忘（输出）之间始终在不断地调节。的确，有证据显示个人遗忘的比率与他们学得的知识量的多少直接相关。这样的数据为认为输入—输出平衡的现代记忆模式提供了总体上的支持。

答案、考点及解析

1. 【答案】D

【考点】细节推理题

【解析】通过evolutionary point of view可定位到第二段。该段第二、三句指出，如果我们不及时复习或练习已学过的东西的话，过一段时间，我们可能会忘记，这种情况所造成的适应性（adaptive）后果也许不太明显。然而，突然失去记忆力却会对适应带来明显后果。A项意为：由于缺乏练习所造成的遗忘明显不利于生存适应。这与第二段第二句的意思相反。B项意为：如果一个人突然（all of a sudden）变得健忘，他肯定是非常适应生活的。这与第二段第三句表达的内容相反。C项意为：逐渐的遗忘过程证明了人的（较强的）适应能力。第二段第四句指出，遗忘可以被看作动物在自然选择（natural selection）过程中遗留给人的一种能力。第三段最后一句指出，遗忘（指逐渐的遗忘）似乎对每个个体或整个物种来说有其生存价值。由此可见，逐渐的遗忘过程是人在物种间的生存竞争过程中形成的，它是人适应外部世界的结果。C项则将人的适应能力看作逐渐遗忘过程的结果，这显然颠倒了逻辑关系。

2. 【答案】B

【考点】细节推理题

【解析】用never forget定位到第三段（if memory failed to fade），第三段第三、四句指出，没有遗忘过程，人就无法适应。例如，十年前正确的做法现在未必合适，所以应该忘记它。对遗忘很少的人的调查也表明：他们的日常活动缺乏头绪。A项意为：他适于生存。这与事实相反。C项意为：他的学习能力会得到加强。这也与事实相反，事实是：所学的东西在大脑中会无头绪可寻。D项意为：记忆力的进化就会停止，文中并未讲记忆力的进化，而是在讨论记忆与遗忘的平衡关系。

3. 【答案】A

【考点】段落大意题

【解析】文章最后一段指出，对记忆力也可以做另一种解释：记忆存储系统的总量是有限的，遗忘使该系统具有了灵活性。这种看法认为：在学习或存储（输入）与遗忘（输出）之间有一个不断调整的过程。事实上，有证据表明：遗忘率与学习的东西的量直接相关，这对现代记忆模式—— 输入—输出平衡—— 提供了证据。B项意为：记忆存储系统是一个输入—输出完全平衡的系统。根据原文，有一种理论认为或推测（assume）记忆存储系统是一个输入—输出平衡的系统，但也仅是假设而已，另外，exactly太绝对。C项意为：记忆力是对遗忘的补偿。严格地讲，forgetting与remembering都是memory的组成部分，是部分与整体之间的关系。D项意为：记忆的存储系统总量有限，这是由遗忘造成的。原文只是说遗忘使记忆存储系统更具适应性，没有说它造成了记忆存储系统的有限性。

4. 【答案】B

【考点】主旨题

【解析】本题答案容易在remembering和forgetting之间迷失。文章第一段讲到记忆对学习的重要性，第二段前几句承接第一段，到了yet之后话锋一转，开始谈forgetting对人类适应性的重要意义，最后得出遗忘是人类生存的重要现象。综合起来看，remembering为导入，文章重点实则为forgetting，故正确答案为B。

5. 【答案】D

【考点】语篇关系题

【解析】根据最后一段的逻辑标志词Another line of thought assumes...可知，该段在讨论另一个关于思维流派的观点，因此接下来文章极有可能阐述其他不同的观点。故D为最佳答案。

Passage Eight

Valeta Young, 81, a retiree from Lodi, Calif., suffers from congestive heart failure and requires almost constant monitoring. But she doesn't have to drive anywhere to get it. Twice a day she steps onto a special electronic scale, answers a few yes or no questions via push buttons on a small attached monitor and presses a button that sends the information to a nurse's station in San Antonio, Texas. "It's almost a direct link to my doctor," says Young, who describes herself as computer illiterate but says she has no problems using the equipment.

Young is not the only patient who is dealing with her doctor from a distance. Remote monitoring is a rapidly growing field in medical technology, with more than 25 firms competing to measure remotely — and transmit by phone, Internet or through the airwaves — everything from patients' heart rates to how often they cough.

Prompted both by the rise in health-care costs and the increasing computerization of health-care equipment, doctors are using remote monitoring to track a widening variety of chronic diseases. In March, St. Francis University in Pittsburgh, Pa., partnered with a company called BodyMedia on a study in which rural diabetes patients use wireless glucose meters and armband sensors to monitor their disease. And last fall, Yahoo began offering subscribers the ability to chart their asthma conditions online, using a PDA-size respiratory monitor that measures lung functions in real time and e-mails the data directly to doctors.

Such home monitoring, says Dr. George Dailey, a physician at the Scripps Clinic in San Diego, "could someday replace less productive ways that patients track changes in their heart rate, blood sugar, lipid levels, kidney functions and even vision."

Dr. Timothy Moore, executive vice president of Alere Medical, which produces the smart scales that Young and more than 10,000 other patients are using, says that almost any vital sign could, in theory, be monitored from home. But, he warns, that might not always make good medical sense. He advises against performing electrocardiograms remotely, for example, and although he acknowledges that remote monitoring of blood-sugar levels and diabetic ulcers on the skin may have real value, he points out that there are no truly independent studies that establish the value of home testing for diabetes or asthma.

Such studies are needed because the technology is still in its infancy and medical experts are divided about its value. But on one thing they all agree: you should never rely on any remote testing system without clearing it with your doctor.

1. How does Young monitor her health conditions?

    A. By stepping on an electronic scale.

    B. By answering a few yes or no questions.

    C. By using remote monitoring service.

    D. By establishing a direct link to her doctor.

2. Which of the following is not used in remote monitoring?

    A. The car.   B. The telephone.

    C. The Internet.   D. The airwaves.

3. The word "prompted" (Line 1, Paragraph 3) most probably means _____.

    A. made   B. reminded   C. aroused   D. driven

4. Why is Dr. Timothy Moore against performing electrocardiograms remotely?

    A. Because it is a less productive way of monitoring.

    B. Because it doesn't make good medical sense.

    C. Because its value has not been proved by scientific study.

    D. Because it is not allowed by doctors.

5. Which of the following is true according to the text?

    A. Computer illiterate is advised not to use remote monitoring.

    B. The development of remote monitoring market is rather sluggish.

    C. Remote monitoring is mainly used to track chronic diseases.

    D. Medical experts agree on the value of remote monitoring.

▶ Words & Expressions

retiree *n.*	退休者
congestive *adj.*	拥挤的，充满的
illiterate *n./adj.*	文盲；不识字的
prompt *v./adj.*	促使；迅速的

▶ 文章大意

　　81岁高龄的瓦勒塔·扬是来自加利福尼亚劳地的退休老人，她身患充血性心力衰竭，需要长时间的监测。但她不必外出求医。每天她到一台电子秤上称两回，通过电子秤上的一台小型监视器上的按钮回答一些答案为"是"或"否"的问题，然后再按一个按钮把信息送到得克萨斯州圣安东尼奥的一个护士台。"这跟直接同我的医生联系差不多，"扬说道。她说自己是个电脑盲，但使用这台设备并没有问题。

扬并不是远程就医的唯一病人。远程监测是目前医学技术快速发展的一个领域，有超过25家公司正在竞争远程监测业务——并且通过电话、互联网或者电视广播来发送——包括病人的心律、咳嗽频率在内的各种测量信息。

由于医疗保健成本的增加和医疗保健设备的不断计算机化，医生们目前正在运用远程监测来跟踪各种慢性疾病，而且监测范围也在不断扩大。三月，宾夕法尼亚州匹兹堡的圣弗朗西斯大学和一家名为BodyMedia的公司联合进行了一项研究，让居住在农村的糖尿病患者使用无线血糖仪和绑在胳膊上的传感器来监测他们的病情。此外，雅虎在去年秋季也开始为用户提供了解他们哮喘情况的在线绘图服务，用户使用的是一个和掌上电脑差不多大小的呼吸监视器，它可以实时测量他们的肺部功能并且直接将数据通过电子邮件发送给医生。

圣迭戈斯克里普斯诊所的医生乔治·戴利说，这种家庭监测"将会取代那些效果略差的方法，让病人记录自己的心律、血糖、血脂水平、肾功能，甚至视力方面的变化"。

阿勒尔医疗公司是生产扬和其他一万多位病人所使用的那种小型秤的企业。该公司的执行副总裁蒂莫西·莫尔医生认为，从理论上讲，任何重大病兆都可以在家里监测到。但是，他警告说，那种做法并不总是可行的。比如，他反对做远程心电图，虽然他承认远程监控血糖水平和糖尿病性皮肤溃疡也许会有实际价值，但他指出并没有真正独立的研究证实家庭测试糖尿病或者哮喘的价值。

由于该技术尚处于初期，医学专家对其价值存在分歧，因而有必要进行这类研究。但医学专家都一致同意：在没有得到医生的许可时，决不能依赖任何远程测试系统。

🔍 答案、考点及解析

1. **【答案】** C

   【考点】 细节定位题

   【解析】 文中第一段讲Young在家中每天上两回电子秤，通过电子秤上的一台小型监视器上的按钮回答一些答案为"是"或"否"的问题，然后再按一个按钮把信息送到得克萨斯州圣安东尼奥的一个护士台。第二段开头说，Young并不是远程就医的唯一病人，可见她是通过远程监护服务来监测自己的健康情况的。

2. **【答案】** A

   【考点】 细节排除题

   【解析】 通过命题顺序和选项可定位到第二段最后一句。第一段提到Young的身体监护时说"she doesn't have to drive anywhere to get it"。第二段提到各种测量数据是通过"phone, Internet or through the airwaves"传送的，可见汽车是不用于远程监护的。

3. 【答案】D

   【考点】猜词题

   【解析】根据上下文，"医疗保健成本的增加和医疗保健设备的不断计算机化"显然和医生们开始利用远程监测有着因果联系，成本的增加和设备信息化是原因，主句中的"利用远程监测"是结果。所以prompted表示"促使"，D项意义最为接近。arouse通常都表示"引起或者唤起某种情感"。

4. 【答案】B

   【考点】细节因果题

   【解析】用人名定位到第五段。文中第五段提到Dr. Timothy Moore时说，"他警告说，那种做法并不总是make good medical sense。"接下来就以他反对performing electrocardiograms remotely为例，说没有truly independent studies证明其价值。故答案为B。

5. 【答案】C

   【考点】细节判断题

   【解析】文章第二段第二行提到医生们正在利用远程监测跟踪a widening variety of chronic diseases。可见远程监测主要用于跟踪慢性疾病。这个答案也可以从文中提到的应用远程监测的充血性心力衰竭、糖尿病、哮喘等疾病推断出来。A项"电脑不能使用远程监测"，文中未提及；B项"远程监测市场发展非常缓慢"，这与原文正好相反；D项"医学专家在远程监测价值上达到一致"，这与第五段相悖。

Passage Nine

One of the many theories about alcoholism is the learning and reinforcement theory, which explains alcoholism by considering alcohol ingestion as reflex response to some stimulus and as a way to reduce an inner-drive state such as fear or anxiety. Characterizing life situations in terms of approach and avoidance, this theory holds that persons tend to be drawn to pleasant situations or repelled by unpleasant ones. In the latter case, alcohol ingestion is said to reduce the tension or feelings of unpleasantness and to replace them with the feeling of euphoria generally observed in most persons after they have consumed one or more drinks.

Some experimental evidence tends to show that alcohol reduces fear in an "approach-avoidance" situation. Conger trained one group rats to approach a food goal and, using aversive conditioning, trained another group to avoid electric shock. After an injection of alcohol the pull away from the shock was measurably weaker, while the pull toward food was unchanged.

The obvious troubles experienced by alcoholic persons appear to contradict the learning theory in the explanation of alcoholism. The discomfort, pain, and punishment they experience should presumably serve as a deterrent to drinking. The fact that alcoholic persons continue to drink in the face of family discord, loss of employment, illness, and other sequels of repeated bouts is explained by the proximity of the drive reduction to the consumption of alcohol; that is, alcohol has the immediate effect of reducing tension while the unpleasant consequences of drunken behavior come only later. The learning paradigm, therefore, favors the establishment and repetition of the resort to alcohol.

In fact, the anxieties and feelings of guilt induced by the consequences of excessive alcohol ingestion may themselves become the signal for another bout of alcohol abuse. The way in which the cue for another bout could be the anxiety itself is explained by the process of stimulus generalization: Conditions or events occurring at the time of reinforcement tend to acquire the characteristics of stimuli. When alcohol is consumed in association with a state of anxiety or fear, the emotional state itself takes on the properties of a stimulus, thus triggering another drinking bout.

The role of punishment is becoming increasingly important in formulating a cause of alcoholism based on the principles of learning theory. While punishment may serve to suppress a response, experiments have shown that in some cases it can serve as a reward and reinforce the behavior. Thus if the alcoholic person has learned to drink under conditions of both reward and punishment, either type of condition may precipitate renewed drinking.

Ample experimental evidence supports the hypothesis that excessive alcohol consumption can be learned. By gradually increasing the concentration of alcohol in drinking water, psychologists have been able to induce the ingestion of larger amounts of alcohol by an animal than would be normally consumed. Other researchers have been able to achieve similar results by varying the schedule of reinforcement; that is, by requiring the animal to consume larger and larger amounts of the alcohol solutions before rewarding it. In this manner, animals learn to drink enough to become dependent on alcohol in terms of demonstrating withdrawal symptoms.

1. The main purpose of the text is to _____.

    A. introduce some existing theories about alcoholism

    B. show the most effective new treatment of alcoholism

C. explain the application of an approach to alcoholism

D. help alcoholics and others know the cause of alcoholism

2. The description of Conger's experiment with two groups of rats was intended to _____.

A. show that alcohol drinking does not affect appetite

B. confirm the findings of other academic researchers

C. show people that alcohol can minimize fear

D. disprove the learning and reinforcement theory

3. We can learn from Paragraph 3 that _____.

A. the learning theory sometimes contradicts itself in some fields

B. drinking alcohol can solve the problem of family discord

C. tension reduction usually appears first after drinking alcohol

D. alcoholics can't recall the unhappy consequence of alcoholism

4. The author provides enough information to answer the question of _____.

A. why alcoholics continue to drink despite the unhappy consequences

B. how Conger explained the behavior of alcoholics by shock therapy

C. under what circumstances an alcoholic benefits from anxiety attacks

D. which treatment is the best one of alcoholism in the world now

5. It can be inferred from the text that _____.

A. the behavior of alcoholics contradicts the approach-avoidance theory

B. the behavior of most alcoholics often proves the learning theory

C. punishment may become the stimulus for another time of drinking

D. frequent excessive drinking makes alcoholics indifferent to punishment

▶ Words & Expressions

alcoholism n.	酗酒
reinforcement n.	加强，增援
discord n./v.	分歧，纠纷
abuse n./v.	滥用，虐待

▶ 文章大意

关于酗酒的众多理论中，有一个是学习和强化理论，它认为饮酒是对某些刺激的反射反应，以此作为减少如恐惧或焦虑之类的内部驱动状态的方法。这个理论基于趋近与回避的策略来定义生活环境，它认为，人们倾向于被吸引到愉快的状况，或远离令人不快的状况。在后一种情况中，酒精摄入据说可以减轻不适感和紧张感，取而代之的是兴奋感，这种现象在大多数饮酒后的人身上都有所体现。

一些实验证据表明，酒精可以在"趋近—回避"情境中减少恐惧。康格训练了一组老鼠接近食物目标，用条件反射原理来训练另一组老鼠，使之对电击产生厌恶，从而远离之。注射酒精后，老鼠躲避电击的动力有了很大的减弱，但趋近食物的动力没有改变。

酗酒者经历的显而易见的麻烦，似乎与学习理论对酗酒的解释相矛盾。他们所经历的不适、痛苦和惩罚，想必对饮酒应该有威慑作用。事实上，面对家庭不和谐、失业、生病以及其他一连串容易复发的后果，饮酒者仍然继续酗酒，是因为他们想用酒精来一醉解千愁。也就是说，酒精具有减轻紧张感的直接效果，而醉酒行为的不愉快后果仅在后来才出现。因此，根据学习和强化理论，借酒浇愁与酗酒的习惯便很容易养成。

事实上，过量酒精摄入的后果所带来的焦虑和内疚感本身就可能成为下次酗酒的动因。焦虑本身居然都可以成为下次酗酒的导火索，可以用刺激泛化的过程来解释：发生在强化时的条件和事件会获得这种刺激的特征。当饮酒同时伴随着焦虑或恐惧时，情绪状态本身就具备刺激的性质，从而引发再次饮酒。

根据学习理论阐述的原则，惩罚在酗酒成因中的作用越来越重要。虽然惩罚可能有助于抑制一种反应，但实验表明，在某些情况下，它也可以作为一种奖励来强化一种行为。因此，要是人学会了在奖励和惩罚两种情况下喝酒，那么不管哪种情况都会引发他们再次喝酒。

充足的实验证据支持了过量饮酒可以被习得的假设。通过逐步增加饮用水的酒精浓度，心理学家能够诱导动物摄取比正常需要的更多的酒精。其他研究人员也可以通过改变强化方案来获得类似的结果；也就是说，让动物消耗越来越多的酒精溶液，然后对其给予奖励。以这种方式，动物习得了大量饮酒，从而形成对酒精的依赖（即表现出了断瘾症状）。

🔍 答案、考点及解析

1. 【答案】D

   【考点】主旨题

   【解析】文章首先提到了有关酗酒的诸多理论，随后具体介绍了学习和强化理论对酗酒的解释，指出，该理论认为，人们往往被吸引到令人愉快的情境，或者厌恶不愉快的情境；事实上，过度饮酒所导致的忧虑与负疚感可能本身就成为另一次酗酒的导火索。这说明，本文主要是在解释酗酒的原因。D项"帮助酗酒者和其他人了解酗酒的原因"是对本文的概括，为正确答案。

2. 【答案】C

【考点】细节理解题

【解析】题干中的Conger出自文章第二段第二句话中，表明本题与第二段有关。第二段首先提到，一些实验证据表明，酒精减轻了恐惧，接着列举了康格所做的实验，指出，给老鼠注射酒精后，它们远离电击的动力明显减弱，而接近食物的动力却保持不变。这说明，描述康格用老鼠所做的实验是想表明，酒精可以降低恐惧。C项"证实酒精将恐惧降到最低点"是对该段中alcohol reduces fear in an "approach-avoidance" situation这句话的改写，为正确答案。

3. 【答案】C

【考点】归纳题

【解析】第三段分号后的句子提到，酒精对减缓压力有立竿见影的效果，而酗酒行为导致的不愉快后果只是随后才发生。C项"压力减缓在饮酒后首先出现"是对文中这句话的改写，为正确答案。

4. 【答案】A

【考点】细节理解题

【解析】文章前两段介绍了有关酗酒的学习理论，随后的段落解释了酗酒者继续饮酒的原因，指出饮酒者在面临家庭不和谐、失业以及疾病时继续饮酒，过度饮酒所导致的忧虑与负罪感可能本身就成为另一次酗酒的导火索，如果饮酒者学会了在奖赏和惩罚这两种情况下饮酒，那么任何一种情况都可能引发反复饮酒。这说明，作者在本文回答了"酗酒者为什么继续饮酒"这个问题。A项"虽然有令人不愉快的后果，但酗酒者为什么继续饮酒"是对作者观点的概括，为正确答案。

5. 【答案】C

【考点】推理题

【解析】文章前面的段落解释了酗酒者继续饮酒的原因，最后一段提到，虽然惩罚可以用来抑制反应，但是，惩罚可以当作一种奖赏，并且强化饮酒这种行为。由此可知，奖赏和惩罚都可能引发反复饮酒。C项"惩罚可能成为另一次饮酒的刺激因素"是对文中either type of condition may trigger renewed drinking这句话的改写，为正确答案。

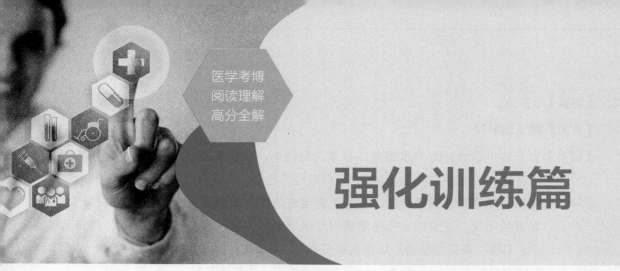

医学考博
阅读理解
高分全解

强化训练篇

第一节　医学类文章20篇精练全解

Passage One

People who sleep fewer than six hours a night are more likely to die early, researchers have found in a study they claim provides "unequivocal（毫无疑问的，确实的）evidence" of a link between sleep deprivation and premature death. They discovered that people who slept for less than six hours each night were 12 per cent more likely to die prematurely — before the age of 65 — than those who slept the recommended six to eight hours a night.

The team from the University of Warwick and Federico II University Medical School in Naples analyzed 16 studies involving a total of 1.3 million people before reaching their conclusions. They pointed out that previous studies had shown that sleep deprivation was associated with heart disease, high blood pressure, obesity, Type 2 diabetes, and high cholesterol.

However, the researchers also found that sleeping too much was linked to an early death. Those who slept for more than nine hours a night were 30 per cent more likely to die early, the research published in the journal *Sleep* found. That directly contradicts research published in the same journal last week which suggested that people who slept for ten hours or longer a night were more likely to live to 100. This was thought to be because people who lived into extreme old age were healthier and therefore slept better.

However, the authors of the latest research contradicted this and suggested that long sleep was a sign of underlying illnesses such as depression and low levels of physical activity. Some cancer is also associated with sleeping for longer. Professor Francesco

Cappuccio, leader of the Sleep, Health and Society Programme at the University of Warwick and Consultant Physician at the University Hospitals Coventry and Warwickshire NHS Trust, said: "*Whilst* short sleep may represent a cause of ill-health, long sleep is believed to represent more an indicator of ill-health."

"Consistently sleeping six to eight hours per night may be optimal for health. The duration of sleep should be regarded as an additional behavioral risk factor, or risk marker, influenced by the environment and possibly amenable to change through both education and counseling as well as through measures of public health aimed at favorable modifications of the physical and working environments."

1. According to the passage, which one has the least possibility to die early?

    A. Sleep less than six hours per night.

    B. Sleep more than six hours per night.

    C. Sleep between six to eight hours per night.

    D. Sleep more than nine hours per night.

2. When someone is lack of sleep for a long time, he is apt to have some kinds of diseases EXCEPT _____.

    A. heart disease
    B. high blood pressure
    C. fatness
    D. tuberculosis

3. What can we infer from the passage?

    A. The longer hours we sleep, the healthier we would be.

    B. The shorter hours we sleep, the healthier we would be.

    C. People who sleep between six to eight hours wouldn't die early.

    D. If someone tends to sleep long hours, then it indicates that there is something wrong with his body.

4. What does "whilst" (Line 6, Para.4) probably mean?

    A. Although.
    B. Furthermore.
    C. Because.
    D. Since.

5. Which is the best title of the passage?

    A. Sleep and Health
    B. Long Hours' Sleep Leads to Early Death
    C. Don't Sleep Too Long
    D. The Deterioration of Our Health Status

Passage Two

Imagine eating everything delicious you want — with none of the fat. That would be great, wouldn't it?

New "fake fat" products appeared on store shelves in the United States recently, but not everyone is happy about it. Makers of the products, which contain a compound called olestra, say food manufacturers can now eliminate fat from certain foods. Critics, however, say the new compound can rob the body of essential vitamins and nutrients（营养物）and can also cause unpleasant side effects in some people. So it's up to consumers to decide whether the new fat-free products taste good enough to keep eating.

Chemists discovered olestra in the late 1960s, when they were searching for a fat that could be digested by infants more easily. Instead of finding the desired fat, the researchers created a fat that can't be digested at all.

Normally, special chemicals in the intestines（肠）"grab" molecules of regular fat and break them down so they can be used by the body. A molecule of regular fat is made up of three molecules of substances called fatty acids.

The fatty acids are absorbed by the intestines and bring with them the essential vitamins A, D, E, and K. When fat molecules are present in the intestines with any of those vitamins, the vitamins attach to the molecules and are carried into the bloodstream.

Olestra, which is made from six to eight molecules of fatty acids, is too large for the intestines to absorb. It just slides through the intestines without being broken down. Manufacturers say it's that ability to slide unchanged through the intestines that make olestra as valuable as a fat substitute. It provides consumers with the taste of regular fat without any bad effects on the body. But critics say olestra can prevent vitamins A, D, E, and K from being absorbed. It can also prevent the absorption of carotenoids（类胡萝卜素）, compounds that may reduce the risk of cancer, heart disease, etc.

Manufacturers are adding vitamins A, D, E, and K as well as carotenoids to their products now. Even so, some nutritionists are still concerned that people might eat unlimited amounts of food made with the fat substitute without worrying about how many calories they are consuming.

1. We learn from the passage that olestra is a substance that _____.

    A. contains plenty of nutrients

    B. renders foods calorie-free while retaining their vitamins

C. makes foods easily digestible

D. makes foods fat-free while keeping them delicious

2. The result of the search for an easily digestible fat turned out to be _____.

    A. commercially useless

    B. just as anticipated

    C. somewhat controversial

    D. quite unexpected

3. Which of the following is NOT true about the fatty acid?

    A. The fatty acid is made up of three molecules of substances.

    B. The fatty acid can be absorbed by the intestines.

    C. The fatty acid brings the essential vitamins A, D, E and K to the intestines.

    D. Olestra is made from six to eight molecules of fatty acids.

4. Olestra is different from ordinary fats in that _____.

    A. it passes through the intestines without being absorbed

    B. it facilitates the absorption of vitamins by the body

    C. it helps reduce the incidence of heart disease

    D. it prevents excessive intake of vitamins

5. Why are nutritionists concerned about adding vitamins to olestra?

    A. It may lead to the over-consumption of vitamins.

    B. People may be induced to eat more than is necessary.

    C. The function of the intestines may be weakened.

    D. It may trigger a new wave of fake food production.

Passage Three

On the face of things, a fall in the number of people infected with HIV (the virus that causes AIDS) from 39.5m to 33.2m over the course of a single year, as reported in this year's AIDS epidemic update from the World Health Organisation (WHO) and UNAIDS, should be cause for rejoicing. Indeed, it is, for it means there are fewer people to treat, and fewer to pass the infection on, than was previously thought. But the fall is not a real fall. Rather, it is due to a change in the way the size of the epidemic is estimated.

If you factor in that change, the number of infected individuals has actually risen since last year, by 500,000. Yet even that is not necessarily bad news in the paradoxical world of AIDS. As treatment programmes are rolled out around the world, death rates are falling.

According to the revised figures, the lethal peak, of 2.2m a year, was in 2005. Now the figure is 2.1m. Since the only way for an infected person to drop out of the statistics in reality (as opposed to by sleight of statistical hand) is for him to die, such increased survivorship inevitably pushes up the total size of the epidemic.

The best news of all, however, is that the new figures confirm what had previously been suspected — that the epidemic has peaked. The highest annual number of new infections around the world was 3.4m in 1998. That figure has now fallen to 2.5m.

Both the change in the death rate and the change in the infection rate are partly a consequence of the natural flow and ebb of any epidemic infection. But they are also a reflection of the hard graft of public-health workers in many countries, who have persuaded millions of people to modify or abandon risky behaviour, such as having unprotected sex, as they have also created the medical infrastructure needed to distribute anti-retroviral drugs that can keep symptoms at bay in those who do become infected.

The revision of the figures is mainly a result of better data-collection methods, particularly in India (which accounts for half the downward revision) and five African countries (which account for another fifth). In India many more sampling points have been established, and in all countries better survey methods, relying on surveyors knocking on doors rather than asking questions at clinics, have gathered data from more representative samples.

Skeptics will feel vindicated by the revision. They have suspected for a while that the older survey methods were biased, and that the inflation thus produced was tolerated because it helped twang the heart-strings of potential donors. However, the structures for collecting and distributing money to combat AIDS are now well established, and accurate data are crucial if that money is not to be misdirected. The new information also means that the goal of treatment for all who need it will be easier and cheaper to achieve. The WHO and UNAIDS are planning to publish a report on the matter early next year, but Paul De Lay, UNAIDS's director of evidence, monitoring and policy, says that the financial requirements for 2010 will probably be about 5% less than previously estimated, and that by 2015 that figure will have risen to 10%. Good news for everyone, then, donors and sufferers alike.

1. Though the number of infected individuals has risen, it is still worth rejoicing because _____.

    A. the number of people who are dying from AIDS has decreased

    B. the total size of the epidemic is shrinking to a significant extent

C. it is only a rise in the sense of statistics, instead of a real number

D. in the paradoxical world of AIDS bad news can turn out to be good news

2. About the changes in the death rate and the infection rate of HIV, which of the following statements is NOT true?

A. Any epidemic will naturally have such changes.

B. They are mainly caused by the new statistic methods.

C. They clearly mirror the essential achievements of public-health workers.

D. The death rate has been greatly suppressed due to massive implementation of treatment programmes.

3. The word "vindicated" (Line 1, Paragraph 6) most probably means _____.

A. confused   B. clarified

C. doubting   D. annoyed

4. By 2015, the financial requirements will _____.

A. have risen by 10% more than what was previously estimated

B. be 10% of what was previously estimated

C. be 10% less than previously estimated

D. be 15% less than previously estimated

5. Towards the revision, the author's attitude can be said to be _____.

A. negative   B. positive

C. indifferent   D. neutral

Passage Four

Infertility is normally seen as a private matter. If a couple are infertile and wish they were not, that is sad. But there is understandable resistance in many countries to the idea that treatments intended to deal with this sadness — known collectively as assisted reproductive technologies, or ARTs — should be paid for out of public funds. Such funds are scarce, and infertility is not a life-threatening condition.

However, two papers presented to the "State of the ARTs" conference held earlier this month in Lyon argue that in Europe, at least, there may be a public interest in promoting ARTs after all. The low fertility rate in many of that continent's more developed countries means their populations are ageing and shrinking. If governments want to change this, ARTs — most significantly in-vitro fertilisation (IVF) — could offer at least part of a way to do so.

As the conference heard, IVF does seem to be keeping up the numbers in at least one country. Tina Jensen of the University of Southern Denmark has just finished a study of more than 700,000 Danish women. She found that young women in Denmark have a significantly lower natural conception rate than in past decades. That is partly, but not entirely, because they are having their children later in life. The rest of the cause is unknown, though reduced sperm quality in men may be a factor. Whatever the cause, she also found that the effect has been almost completely compensated for by an increasing use of ARTs. Denmark's native population is more or less stable, but some 3.9% of babies born there in 2003 were the result of IVF. The comparable figure for another northern European country, Britain, was 1.5%.

Without IVF, then, the number of Danes would be shrinking fast. That may not have something to do with the fact that in Denmark the taxpayer will cover up to six cycles of IVF treatment. In Britain, by contrast, couples are supposed to be entitled to three cycles. In practice, many of the local trusts that dish the money out do not pay for any cycles at all. Jonathan Grant, the head of the Cambridge branch of the Rand Corporation (an American think-tank), believes this is shortsighted. His paper showed that if Britain supported IVF at the Danish level then its birth rate would probably increase by about 10,000 a year.

The cost of offering six cycles to couples (and doing so in practice, rather than just in theory) would be an extra £250m-430m a year. That is not trivial, but Dr. Grant reckons it is cheaper than other ways of boosting the birth rate. Some countries, for example, have tried to bribe women into having more children by increasing child benefits. According to his calculations, raising such benefits costs between £50,000 and £100,000 a year for each additional birth procured. Ten thousand extra births each year would thus cost between £500m and £1 billion.

There are, of course, some disadvantages to promoting IVF. In particular, women who use it tend to be older than those who conceive naturally, and that can lead to congenital problems in their children. But if the countries of Europe do wish to keep their populations up, making IVF more widely available might be a good way of doing so.

1. According to the text, the public's opinion on the infertility treatments is that_____.

   A. the treatments should be paid for out of public funds

   B. the treatments are not so compulsory as they consume the limited public funds

C. the treatments are not necessarily only paid for out of public funds

D. the public is not obliged to pay for such treatments of no urgent nature

2. According to the study conducted by Tina Jensen, which of the following statements is TRUE?

A. ARTs have reversed the tendency of the decreasing population in Denmark.

B. Danes' problem of low natural conception has been completely counterbalanced by the widely use of ARTs.

C. The population of Denmark is not decreasing after the adoption of ARTs.

D. IVF has played an essential role in Denmark in terms of keeping up the number of its population.

3. From the paper of Dr. Grant, it can be inferred that _____ .

A. the cost of offering six cycles of IVF to couples is not high at all

B. IVF treatment is an economical way of solving population shrinking

C. Britain does not promote adopting IVF to boost the birth rate

D. encouraging women to bear more babies by bonus is not so efficient to solve the problem of population shrinking

4. The word "congenital" (Line 2, Paragraph 6) most probably means _____ .

A. innate   B. instinctive

C. cerebral   D. acquired

5. According to the text, the author's attitude towards promoting in-vitro fertilization can be said to be _____ .

A. supportive   B. opposing

C. ambiguous   D. objective

Passage Five

Back in 2000, Steve Ballmer, Microsoft's chief executive, described a grand vision for the future of health care. One day, he said, everyone would have a secure and private website on the Internet on which their doctors could post their "scans, lab results, test results, visit minutes", and to which the owner could grant certain people access, to view some or all of that information. His ideas met with guffaws from the old lags of the industry, who have seen many fancy schemes for electronic medical records fall flat. America's health sector is simply too balkanised and too paper-based to stitch together easily in digital form. Even Mr. Ballmer conceded back then that he was searching for the "holy grail" of healthcare.

And yet, after years of frustration and furious development work, Microsoft now believes it has realised Mr. Ballmer's dream. On October 4th, the software giant was poised to unveil its new health-information product at a big event in Washington, DC. It is called the Health Vault, in keeping with Microsoft's promise to make storing data on the Internet just as secure as keeping it in a bank. Health Vault will store all its customers' health data, ranging from test results to doctors' reports to daily measurements of weight or blood pressure, online. Individuals then have access to those records anytime, anywhere, via the Internet — a great boon for those who travel a lot. Medical offices and hospitals who sign up for the service could easily send test results in digital form to the vault, and patients could authorise them in turn to have access to various, carefully circumscribed bits of their personal data.

Microsoft was also set to announce this week that several dozen manufacturers, hospitals and charities have signed up for Health Vault. Big names including the American heart, diabetes and lung associations, the New York-Presbyterian Hospital, and Omron and Texas Instruments, in addition to various firms devoted to the craze for "wellness", are all now on board, and are expected to announce products and services shortly. If the software giant has really found a hacker-proof way of storing records online, then the benefits of Health Vault are clear. But use of the vaults will be free both for the individuals that sign up for them and for the vendors and doctors that provide services based on the information they contain. So how will Microsoft make any money?

Sean Nolan of Microsoft explains that the business model depends on one thing: targeted search. Microsoft is betting that people will use its Health Vault Search to find out about their ailments. This service relies on an approach known as "vertical search" which attempts to provide more relevant results than generalist search engines like "Google" and "Yahoo!" by specialising in a particular field. The firm's recent acquisition of Medstory, a vertical-search engine focusing on health care, has given it a boost in this area.

Health Vault's search engine would definitely work better than those of rival sites if it could examine users' health records and past queries, and thus provide the responses that are most relevant to each individual's situation. But in order to attract any users in the first place, Microsoft has promised to enforce strict privacy rules. These would preclude such data-mining.

1. The old lags of the industry did not think highly of Ballmer's scheme because _____.

    A. Ballmer's scheme sounded too fantastic and far-fetched to be true

    B. Ballmer lacked technology proof to back up his ideas

    C. they had witnessed too many failures of attempts to realize such schemes

    D. America's health sector is too stubborn and is reluctant to change for the digital

2. Which of the following statements is NOT true of Health Vault?

    A. Individuals can have access to the medical records of anybody anytime via the Internet.

    B. Those who travel a lot will greatly benefit from services of Health Vault.

    C. Hospitals who sign up for the service could improve their efficiency by Health Vault.

    D. Health Vault is software invented by Microsoft.

3. The main problem of Health Vault is _____.

    A. that it will be difficult for Vault to make profit during the beginning phase

    B. that the software may be trapped in the dilemma of customer privacy and convenient data search

    C. that it has to adopt the "vertical search" which is not the company's strength

    D. that Microsoft does not have powerful search engines as Google and Yahoo! do

4. Microsoft will make money in Health Vault by _____.

    A. attracting customers with the enforcement of strict privacy rules

    B. providing a charging platform for the communication of patients and hospitals

    C. cooperating with big hospitals and charities by providing useful customer information

    D. providing highly specialized service with high efficiency

5. Compared with Google and Yahoo!, the advantage of Health Vault Search is _____.

    A. that its technology far more advanced than that of the other two

    B. that it is more effective for those who need special information

    C. that it specializes on the information of ailment diagnosis

    D. that its business model is more promising and profitable

Passage Six

Vegetarians would prefer not to be compelled to eat meat. Yet the reverse compulsion (强迫) is hidden in the proposals for a new plant-based "planetary diet". Nowhere is this more visible than in India.

Earlier this year, the EAT-Lancet Commission released its global report on nutrition and called for a global shift to a more plant-based diet and for "substantially reducing consumption of animal source foods". In countries like India, that call could become a tool to aggravate an already tense political situation and stress already undernourished populations.

The EAT report presumes that "traditional diets" in countries like India include little red meat, which might be consumed only on special occasions or as minor ingredients in mixed dishes. In India, however, there is a vast difference between what people would wish to consume and what they have to consume because of innumerable barriers around class, religion, culture, cost, geography, etc. Policymakers in India have traditionally pushed for a cereal-heavy "vegetarian diet" on a meat-eating population as a way of providing the cheapest sources of food.

Currently, under an aggressive Hindu nationalist government, Muslims, Christians, disadvantaged classes and indigenous communities are being compelled to give up their traditional foods. None of these concerns seem to have been appreciated by the EAT-Lancet Commission's representative, Brent Loken, who said "India has got such a great example" in sourcing protein from plants.

But how much of a model for the world is India's vegetarianism? In the *Global Hunger Index 2019*, the country ranks 102nd out of 117. Data from the *National Family Health Survey* indicate that only 10 percent of infants of 6 to 23 months are adequately fed.

That is why calls for a plant-based diet modeled on India risk offering another whip with which to beat already vulnerable communities in developing countries. A diet directed at the affluent West fails to recognize that in low-income countries undernourished children are known to benefit from the consumption of milk and other animal source foods, improving cognitive functions, while reducing the prevalence of nutritional deficiencies as well as mortality.

EAT-Lancet claimed its intention was to "spark conversations" among all Indian stakeholders. Yet vocal critics of the food processing industry and food fortification strategies have been left out of the debate. But the most conspicuous omission may well be the absence of India's farmers.

The government, however, seems to have given the report a thumbs-up. Rather than addressing chronic hunger and malnutrition through an improved access to wholesome and nutrient-dense foods, the government is opening the door for company-dependent solutions, ignoring the environmental and economic cost, which will destroy local food systems. It's a model full of danger for future generations.

1. What is more visible in India than anywhere else according to the passage?

   A. People's positive views on the proposals for a "planetary diet".

   B. People's reluctance to be compelled to eat plant-based food.

   C. People's preferences for the kind of food they consume.

   D. People's unwillingness to give up their eating habits.

2. What would the EAT-Lancet Commission's report do to many people in countries like India?

   A. Radically change their dietary habits.

   B. Keep them further away from politics.

   C. Make them even more undernourished.

   D. Substantially reduce their food choices.

3. What do we learn from the passage about food consumption in India?

   A. People's diet will not change due to the EAT-Lancet report.

   B. Many people simply do not have access to food they prefer.

   C. There is a growing popularity of a cereal-heavy vegetarian diet.

   D. Policymakers help remove the barriers to people's choice of food.

4. What does the passage say about a plant-based diet modeled on India?

   A. It may benefit populations whose traditional diet is meat-based.

   B. It may be another blow to the economy in developing countries.

   C. It may help narrow the gap between rich and poor countries.

   D. It may worsen the nourishment problem in low-income countries.

5. How does the Indian government respond to the EAT-Lancet Commission's proposals?

   A. It accepts them at the expense of the long-term interests of its people.

B. It intends them to spark conversations among all Indian stakeholders.

C. It gives them approval regardless of opposition from nutrition experts.

D. It welcomes them as a tool to address chronic hunger and malnutrition.

Passage Seven

For a Nobel laureate, the molecular biologist Max Perutz made a lot of mistakes. His science was strewn with assertions that were not supported by the sparse evidence he had gathered. No matter. He was eventually right about the important things — and gentleman enough to concede his errors.

With bloody-minded persistence, Perutz mastered the painstaking task of analysing images of haemoglobin, the component of blood that carries oxygen. This was by no means feat: a molecule of haemoglobin consists of thousands of atoms and, at the time, only simple structures of tens of atoms had been mapped. It was for this work that Perutz was awarded the Nobel prize in chemistry in 1962. But his triumphal announcement of the correct structure of haemoglobin was by no means his first solution to the problem: he had previously claimed all sorts of unlikely arrangements, backing down each time a colleague spotted a fatal flaw.

Even when he did finally hold the secret to why blood supports life, he did not piece together the evidence to produce the ultimate result. Indeed, Perutz was furious when a junior researcher saw how the final piece fitted and could not resist popping it into its slot, completing what Perutz viewed as his jigsaw puzzle. Nevertheless, it was Perutz who had gathered all the pieces and who ensured, in the end, that they were correctly assembled.

Perutz was long the outsider. Of Jewish descent, he was a lapsed Catholic by religion. He left his native Austria in 1936, two years before Hitler annexed it. The outbreak of war saw him expelled to Canada as an enemy alien. On returning to Cambridge, he was not welcomed by his college. It was only after he won the Nobel Prize that he felt accepted as an Englishman, despite having been naturalised as a British subject 20 years earlier.

As a scientist, too, Perutz was always on the fringe. His field of endeavour, X-ray crystallography, was neither physics nor maths nor chemistry nor biology but a combination of these. As often happens to researchers working in interdisciplinary areas of science, his progress was impeded by an establishment that sought to promote existing subjects. He lived from grant to grant, each lasting a matter of months. Nevertheless, he managed to establish the unit in which James Watson and Francis Crick elucidated the double helix structure of DNA. A decade later, a whole institute was established under him.

Georgina Ferry's biography captures not only the scientific advances made by Perutz but also his curious personal qualities. A skinny, sickly and, for much of his life, skint individual, Perutz is an unlikely hero. He was demanding — his diet required him to eat black bananas, even in February — and he was unselfconscious in ensuring that his elaborate needs were met. He was also naive in insisting that scientific reasoning would trump political thought and religious teaching.

Ms Ferry portrays his foibles sympathetically. Perutz used to complain that, although he was famous, few people knew what it was he had achieved. By combining scientific with personal anecdotes, her book goes a good way towards redressing that balance.

1. Max Perutz won the Nobel prize though he made a lot of mistakes because _____.

   A. his important contribution outweighed those marginal mistakes

   B. he made assertions not based on the sparse evidence he had gathered

   C. he could always reach the correct conclusion in the end

   D. he was brave enough to admit his mistakes and strived for improvement

2. Which of the following statements is TRUE of Perutz's task of analyzing the structure of hemoglobin?

   A. Perutz successfully worked out the structures of all the different arrangements of atoms of hemoglobin.

   B. It is not Perutz who had first provided an answer to the correct structure of hemoglobin.

   C. It is in fact Perutz's colleague who had sorted out the solution to the problem of hemoglobin's structure.

   D. Perutz had worked diligently on the divergences between himself and his colleague in analyzing the structure of hemoglobin.

3. Perutz was very angry with the junior researcher who popped the final piece into its slot because _____.

   A. the researcher asserted that what Perutz viewed was only jigsaw puzzle

   B. the researcher pointed out that Perutz did not piece together the evidence to prove the final result

   C. the researcher passed off the secret to why blood supports life as his own idea

   D. the researcher pieced together the evidence to work out the final result

4. Perutz's progress was interrupted by an establishment because _____.

   A. the subject he studied did not belong to any of the conventional disciplines

   B. his study threatened existing subjects by promoting interdisciplinary areas of science

   C. that establishment prevented him from receiving adequate and long-term funds

   D. he was diverted to the cause of setting up a brand new institute

5. The word "redressing" (Paragraph 7) most probably means _____.

   A. remedying   B. rectifying

   C. re-adjusting   D. reversing

Passage Eight

A boy or a girl? That is usually the first question asked when a woman gives birth. Remarkably, the answer varies with where the mother lives. In rich countries the chances of being a boy are about 5% higher than in poor ones. Equally remarkably, that figure has been falling recently. Several theories have been put forward to explain these observations. Some argue that smoking plays a role, others that diet may be important. Neither of these ideas has been supported by evidence from large studies. But new research points to a different factor: stress.

Strange as it might seem, the terrorist attacks of September 11th 2001 shed light on the enigma. Studies noting the sex of babies conceived in New York during the week of the attacks found a drop in the ratio of males to females. That is consistent with earlier studies, which revealed a similar shift in women who became pregnant during floods and earthquakes and in time of war. Moreover, a study carried out eight years ago by researchers at the University of Aarhus, in Denmark, revealed that women who suffered the death of a child or spouse from some catastrophic illness around the time they conceived were much more likely to give birth to girls than to boys.

Taken together, these results suggest that acute stress to a woman at the time of conception shifts the sex ratio towards girls. However, Carsten Obel, a researcher at Aarhus who was not involved in the earlier study, wondered if the same might be true of chronic stress too. In a paper just published in Human Development, he shows that it is.

Dr. Obel used a set of data collected between 1989 and 1992. During that period 8,719 expectant mothers were asked to fill in questionnaires that inquired, among other things, about their level of stress. Dr. Obel found that the more stressed a mother had been, the less chance she had of having given birth to a boy. Only 47% of children born to women in the top quartile of stress were males. That compared with 52% for women in the bottom quartile. Dr. Obel suspects the immediate cause is that male pregnancies are more likely to miscarry in response to stress than female pregnancies are, especially during the first three months. However, that is difficult to prove. More intriguing, though, is the ultimate cause, for he thinks it might be adaptive, rather than pathological.

That is because the chances are that a daughter who reaches adulthood will find a mate and thus produce grandchildren. A son is a different matter. Healthy, strapping sons are likely to produce lots of grandchildren, by several women — or would have done in the hunter-gatherer societies in which most human evolution took place. Weak ones would be marginalised and maybe even killed in the cut and thrust of male competition. If a mother's stress adversely affects the development of her fetus then selectively aborting boys, rather than wasting time and resources on bringing them to term, would make evolutionary sense.

That, in turn, would explain why women in rich countries, who are less likely to suffer from hunger and disease, are more likely to give birth to sons. That this likelihood is, nevertheless, falling suggests that rich women's lives may be more stressful than they used to be.

1. The author begins the passage by _____.
   A. presenting an argumentation
   B. explaining a phenomenon
   C. raising a question
   D. making a comparison

2. The ratio of giving birth to a boy is falling in rich countries because _____.
   A. the terrorist attacks of September 11th 2001 exerted huge negative impact
   B. women are facing greater pressure now than in the past
   C. women are under new pressure now which they seldom faced in the past
   D. male pregnancies are more easily to miscarry

3. Which of the following can explain Dr. Obel's opinion that the ultimate cause is adaptive rather than pathological?
   A. 47% of children born to women in the top quartile of stress were males while 52% in the bottom quartile.
   B. Women in rich countries are more likely to give birth to boys.
   C. Women selectively abort boys rather than waste time and resources on bringing

them to term for fear of male competition.

    D. Women who suffer from calamity in conception are more likely to give birth to girls.

4. Women in the hunter-gatherer societies are more likely to give birth to daughters because _____.

    A. they agree that giving birth to daughters is beneficial in the evolutionary sense

    B. sons are likely to produce lots of grandchildren with several women

    C. they think it is a better practice for a daughter to produce grandchildren with only one mate

    D. they think bringing sons to term is wasting time and resources

5. From this passage, we may draw a conclusion that _____.

    A. acute stress is more likely to cause women to choose aborting boys than chronic stress

    B. stress to a woman at the time of conception, whether acute or chronic, will shift the sex ratio towards girls

    C. more girls will be born in the future because today's women, in both rich and poor countries, suffer from increasing pressure

    D. chronic stress is more decisive in influencing the women's pregnancies

Passage Nine

Everyone is interested in whether different foods or nutrients affect our odds of getting diseases like cancer or of developing risk factors for those diseases, such as too much weight or high blood pressure. But there are many barriers to studying dietary change, which is why we still have no easy answers to the question of what, exactly, we should eat to be at our healthiest. It's also why you can be forgiven for often feeling whipsawed by headlines: Is coffee good or bad? What about alcohol, garlic, or chocolate?

This week researchers reported in the Journal of the American Medical Association that breast cancer survivors who cram their diets with fruits and vegetables are no more likely to escape a recurrence than women who stick to the usual five-a-day recommendation. Does that mean fruits and vegetables don't protect against cancer? No—just that in this specific group of women with breast cancer, the extra greens and additional apples didn't seem to help.

We asked researchers to explain why studies involving dietary changes are so hard to do—and what consumers should keep in mind when they read about them. Here's what the experts said:

Most diet studies take place in the real world. That means study subjects are keeping diaries of what they eat as they go rather than having their intake strictly controlled by someone else. You can give them meal advice, counseling, and how-to books up to their ears, but at the end of the day, they are on their own when it comes to what they put in their mouths. It's easier to get people to add something — like garlic, in the form of tasty sandwich spreads, or dark chocolate — than to take something away; no wonder a recent study comparing low-fat and low-carb diet plans found that almost no one was sticking to them by the end.

In studies focusing on diet, including the recent study on breast cancer recurrence, the amount of calories subjects reported eating would have caused them to lose far more weight than they actually did lose. The misreporting isn't necessarily vicious, but the inaccuracies add up. Say you're phoned about your daily intake on a day when it was someone's birthday at work and you had a slice of cake. You may not report it, thinking that a typical day wouldn't include the cake ... forgetting yesterday's "special occasion" piece of pizza, and the Big Gulp of the day before. Or, despite the portion size guides you get, you characterize your bagel from the deli as a 4-ounce standard serving when a 4-ounce bagel hasn't been sighted in any major city for a decade.

"You can't put a camera in everyone's belly and see exactly what they ate," says Christopher Gardner, a nutrition scientist at the Stanford Prevention Research Center who has recently published research on garlic and diet plans. You can get around this in some studies by taking objective measurements. Weight, for example, or if you're assessing intake of fruits and veggies, you can measure the level of pigments called carotenoids in the blood. In the breast cancer study, blood tests showed that the study subjects actually did eat more fruits and veggies (carotenoid concentration was 73 percent higher in those women after one year and 43 percent higher after four years). But objective measures can't definitively nail down whether someone is eating nutrients in certain proportions.

1. One can be forgiven for feeling whipsawed by those headlines because _____.

    A. there is no solid and convincing scientific hypothesis on these subjects

    B. the question about what the healthiest food is has no answers

    C. opinions on these subjects are quite contradictory

D. there is no authoritative answer to these questions

2. Which of the following statements is TRUE of the conclusion of the study on breast cancer recurrence?

A. Women who stick to the five-a-day recommendation are less likely to have a recurrence.

B. Women who eat extra greens and vegetables are less likely to escape a recurrence.

C. Women could not depend on fruit diet to avoid the breast cancer recurrence.

D. Fruits and vegetables are no good to women with breast cancer.

3. From the results of the studies focusing on diet, it can be inferred that _____.

A. the amount of calories set in diet could not help people to lose weight

B. people are reluctant to take part in such studies

C. it is difficult to get valuable conclusion from these studies

D. this kind of studies is not objective enough

4. The fact that a 4-ounce bagel hasn't been sighted in any major city for a decade implies that _____.

A. you should re-examine the standard size of the food you intake

B. you tend to give an inaccurate report of your actual diet

C. you fail to cooperate with the doctor by false record of your daily food

D. you make a mistake in noting down the size of standard serving

5. The limitation of the objective measurements mentioned in the last paragraph is that _____.

A. they could only assess the proportion of fruits and veggies study subjects have taken

B. they could not have the subjects follow exactly the food proportion of their diet

C. they could not identify the levels of all the nutrients in patients' blood

D. they could not tell the exact proportions of nutrients study subjects have eaten

Passage Ten

Cancer has always been with us, but not always in the same way. Its care and management have differed over time, of course, but so, too, have its identity, visibility, and meanings. Pick up the thread of history at its most distant end and you have cancer the crab—

so named either because of the spreading out from a tumor or because its pain is like the pinch of a crab's claw. Premodern cancer is a lump, a swelling that sometimes breaks through the skin in ulcerations producing foul-smelling discharges. The ancient Egyptians knew about many tumors that had a bad outcome, and the Greeks made a distinction between benign tumors (oncos) and malignant ones (carcinos). In the second century A.D., Galen reckoned that the cause was systemic, an excess of melancholy or black bile, one of the body's four "humors", brought on by bad diet and environmental circumstances. Ancient medical practitioners sometimes cut tumors out, but the prognosis was known to be grim. Describing tumors of the breast, an Egyptian papyrus from about 1600 B.C. concluded: "There is no treatment."

The experience of cancer has always been terrible, but, until modern times, its mark on the culture has been light. In the past, fear coagulated around other ways of dying: infectious and epidemic diseases (plague, smallpox, cholera, typhus, typhoid fever); "apoplexies" (what we now call strokes and heart attacks); and, most notably in the nineteenth century, "consumption" (tuberculosis). The agonizing manner of cancer death was dreaded, but that fear was not centrally situated in the public mind—as it now is. This is one reason that the medical historian Roy Porter wrote that cancer is "the modern disease par excellence", and that Mukherjee calls it "the quintessential product of modernity".

At one time, it was thought that cancer was a "disease of civilization", belonging to much the same causal domain as "neurasthenia" and diabetes, the former a nervous weakness believed to be brought about by the stress of modern life and the latter a condition produced by bad diet and indolence. In the eighteenth and nineteenth centuries, some physicians attributed cancer—notably of the breast and the ovaries—to psychological and behavioral causes. William Buchan's wildly popular eighteenth-century text *Domestic Medicine* judged that cancers might be caused by "excessive fear, grief, religious melancholy". In the nineteenth century, reference was repeatedly made to a "cancer personality", and, in some versions, specifically to sexual repression. As Susan Sontag observed, cancer was considered shameful, not to be mentioned, even obscene. Among the Romantics and the Victorians, suffering and dying from tuberculosis might be considered a badge of refinement; cancer death was nothing of the sort. "It seems unimaginable," Sontag wrote, "to aestheticize" cancer.

1. According to the passage, the ancient Egyptians _____.

    A. called cancer the crab

    B. were able to distinguish benign tumors and malignant ones

C. found out the cause of cancer

    D. knew about a lot of malignant tumors

2. Which of the following statements about the cancers of the past is best supported by the passage?

    A. Ancient people did not live long enough to become prone to cancer.

    B. In the past, people did not fear cancer.

    C. Cancer death might be considered a badge of refinement.

    D. Some physicians believed that one's own behavioral mode could lead to cancer.

3. Which of the following is the reason for cancer to be called "the modern disease"?

    A. Modern cancer care is very effective.

    B. There is a lot more cancer now.

    C. People understand cancer in radically new ways now.

    D. There is a sharp increase in mortality in modern cancer world.

4. "Neurasthenia" and diabetes are mentioned because _____.

    A. they are as fatal as cancer

    B. they were considered to be "disease of civilization"

    C. people dread them very much

    D. they are brought by the high pressure of modern life

5. As suggested by the passage, with which of the following statements would the author most likely agree?

    A. The care and management of cancer have development over time.

    B. The cultural significance of cancer shifts in different times.

    C. Cancer's identity has never changed.

    D. Cancer is the price paid for modern life.

Passage Eleven

In patients with Huntington's disease, it's the part of the brain called the basal ganglia that's destroyed. While these victims have perfectly intact explicit memory systems, they can't learn new motor skills. An Alzheimer's patient can learn to draw in a mirror but can't remember doing it: a Huntington's patient can't do it but can remember trying to learn. Yet another region of the brain, an almond-size knot of neural tissue seems to be crucial in forming and triggering the recall of a special subclass of memories that is tied to strong emotion, especially fear. These are just some of the major divisions. Within the category implicit memory, for example, lie the subcategories of associative memory—the phenomenon that famously led Parlov's dogs to salivate at the sound of a bell which they had learned to associate with food and of habituation, in which we unconsciously file away unchanging features of the environment so we can pay closer attention to what's new and different upon encountering a new experience.

Within explicit, or declarative memory, on the other hand, there are specific subsystems that handle shapes, textures such as faces, names—even distinct systems to remember nouns vs. verbs. All of these different types of memory are ultimately stored in the brain's cortex, within its deeply furrowed outer layer—a component of the brain dauntingly more complex than comparable parts in other species. Experts in brain imaging are only beginning to understand what goes where, and how the parts are reassembled into a coherent whole that seems to be a single memory is actually a complex construction. Think of a hammer, and your brain hurriedly retrieves the tool's name, its appearance, its function, its heft and the sound of its clang, each **extracted** from a different region of the brain. Fail to connect person's name with his or her face, and you experience the breakdown of that assembly process that many of us begin to experience in our 20s and that becomes downright worrisome when we reach our 50s. It was this weakening of memory and the parallel loss of ability to learn new things easily that led biologist Joe Tsien to the experiments reported last week. "This age-dependent loss of function," he says, "appears in many animals, and it begins with the onset of sexual maturity".

What's happening when the brain forms memories—and what fails with aging, injury and disease—involves a phenomenon known as "plasticity". It's obvious that something in the brain changes as we learn and remember new things, but it's equally obvious that the organ doesn't change its overall structure or grow new nerve cells wholesale. Instead, it's the connections between new cells—and particularly the strength of these connections that are altered by experience. Hear a word over and over, and the repeated firing of certain cells in a certain order makes it easier to repeat the firing pattern later on. It is the pattern that represents each specific memory.

1. Which of the following symptoms can be observed in a person who suffers from the Huntington's disease?

   A. He cannot remember what he has done but can remember trying to learn.

   B. He cannot do something new but he can remember doing it.

   C. He suffers from a bad memory and lack of motor skills.

   D. He suffers from a poor basal ganglia and has intact explicit memory.

2. According to the passage, which of the following memories has nothing to do with implicit memory?

   A. Associating a signal with an action.

   B. Recognizing of new features.

   C. Focusing on new environment.

   D. Remembering a familiar face of a friend.

3. Which of the following may happen to a patient who suffered from damages to his explicit memory?

   A. When he is in a new environment, he is always frightened.

   B. When he plays football, he cannot learn new tricks.

   C. When he sees a friend, it's hard for him to remember his name.

   D. When he finds a hammer, he cannot tell anything about it.

4. The word "extract" in the second paragraph means _____.

   A. obtain   B. remove   C. pull   D. derive

5. We can draw a conclusion from the passage that _____.

   A. scientists have found the mechanism underlying the memorizing activities

   B. more research must be done to determine the brain structure

   C. some researchers are not content with the findings

   D. it is obvious that something in the brain changes as we learn and remember

Passage Twelve

The animal dissection requirement of biology classes has been getting under the skin of students for generations, and there have always been some who asked to be excused from the requirement. Now, a growing number of technological alternatives are making it possible for students to swap that scalpel for a computer mouse. There are laws in nearly a dozen states — including California, Florida, New Jersey, and New York — protecting a student's choice to learn about animal anatomy sans scalpel. Some students choosing to opt out feel we should be kinder to our web-footed friends. Others are just queasy at the thought of rubbery frog bodies and the smell of formaldehyde.

"Dissection is icky. There's a yuck factor," admits Brian Shmaefsky, a board member with the National Association of Biology Teachers. "And a teacher has to weigh the benefits with the cost of students being offended to the point that it interferes with learning."

Virtual blades. So for cases in which a real dissection would be too slimy, it's time to try some toad tech. While the first computer-based alternatives to dissection emerged in the 1980s, modern frog dissection software can be found at different websites. These software programs use creative clicking, high-powered zoom functions, and video clips to teach anatomy. Froguts software, for example, lets students trace incision lines with a computer mouse and snip through skin with a virtual blade. There are even sound effects like a "slish" for slicing frog flesh, or a "shwoosh" for pinning down skin flaps. (Schools currently pay about $300 for a one-year software license, though some organizations will lend programs out free of charge.)

Earlier this year, a graduate student from Simon Fraser University in Vancouver designed the first-ever haptic (the Greek word for "touch") frog dissection program, which uses a penlike tool to create a sensation similar to cutting into real flesh. The hand-held device connects to a computer, and students move the device through the air while watching the results of their actions on a computer screen.

With Digital Frog — a popular program that's had approximately 1,500 frog demo downloads since January and is currently in use in 2,000 schools — students can add or subtract those amphibious organs with a mere mouse click. They can then assess their learning with sporadic frog anatomy quizzes.

"Repetition is helpful. The fact that a student can review sections of a program over and over again is important," says Martin Stephens, vice president for animal research issues at the Humane Society of the United States. "In dissections, the animal's organs are all shriveled and discolored. You look for things and can't find them because body parts have changed drastically since the animal was killed. But on a computer screen, layers can be digitally peeled away." Other experts think the dissection technology has its limits. Gerry Wheeler, executive director of the National Science Teachers Association, says that artificial simulations don't give as enriching an experience as the real thing. Still others worry the programs are depriving kids of experiential learning.

1. The word "swap" (Paragraph 1) most probably means _____.

   A. exchange   B. throw away

   C. reject   D. refuse

2. Some students ask to be excused from the requirement of biology classes because of the following reasons EXCEPT that _____.

   A. dissection consists of disgusting procedures and unpleasant smells

   B. they are entitled to reject dissection requirement given the legal regulation

   C. they are offended when fulfilling the requirements of animal dissection

   D. they insist that people should treat animals more as friends instead of simply objects

3. Brian Shmaefsky's statement implies that _____.

   A. he indeed supports the students' animal protection movement

   B. he thinks the animal dissection should be banned

   C. he thinks the animal dissection may not be good for students to learn biology effectively

   D. he always evaluate the teaching effect by weighing reluctant factors of cost and effect

4. Compared with the real dissection, the dissection on computer has the following advantages EXCEPT _____.

   A. it has authentic sound effect like a "slish" or "shwoosh"

   B. there is a sensation of always dealing with fresh and recognizable organs

   C. the process can be repeated so that students can gather better insight of the animal structure

   D. students can take quizzes with the software to evaluate the learning effect

5. The author's attitude towards the toad tech can be said to be _____.

   A. supportive   B. doubtful

   C. objective   D. biased

Passage Thirteen

We sometimes think humans are uniquely vulnerable to anxiety, but stress seems to affect the immune defenses of lower animals too. In one experiment, for example, behavioral immunologist（免疫学家）Mark Laudenslager, at the University of Denver, gave mild electric shocks to 24 rats. Half the animals could switch off the current by turning a wheel in their enclosure, while the other half could not. The rats in the two groups were paired so that each time one rat turned the wheel it protected both itself and its helpless partner from the shock. Laudenslager found that the immune response was depressed below normal in the helpless rats but not in those that could turn off the electricity. What he has demonstrated, he believes, is that lack of control over an event, not the experience itself, is what weakens the immune system.

Other researchers agree. Jay Weiss, a psychologist at Duke University School of Medicine, has shown that animals who are allowed to control unpleasant stimuli don't develop sleep disturbances or changes in brain chemistry typical of stressed rats. But if the animals are confronted with situations they have no control over, they later behave passively when faced with experiences they can control. Such findings reinforce psychologists' suspicions that the experience or perception of helplessness is one of the most harmful factors in depression.

One of the most startling examples of how the mind can alter the immune response was discovered by chance. In 1975 psychologist Robert Ader at the University of Rochester School of Medicine conditioned（使形成条件反射）mice to avoid saccharin（糖精）by simultaneously feeding them the sweetener and injecting them with a drug that while suppressing their immune systems caused stomach upsets. Associating the saccharin with the stomach pains, the mice quickly learned to avoid the sweetener. In order to extinguish this dislike for the sweetener, Ader re-exposed the animals to saccharin, this time without the drug, and was astonished to find that those mice that had received the highest amounts of sweetener during their earlier conditioning died. He could only speculate that he had so successfully conditioned the rats that saccharin alone now served to weaken their immune systems enough to kill them.

1. Laudenslager's experiment showed that the immune system of those rats who could turn off the electricity _____.
   A. was strengthened
   B. was not affected
   C. was altered
   D. was weakened

2. Laudenslager has demonstrated that it is the _____ that weakens the immune system.
   A. mild electric shocks
   B. saccharin

C. depressed mind   D. lack of control over an event

3. According to the passage, the experience of helplessness causes rats to _____.

    A. try to control unpleasant stimuli

    B. turn off the electricity

    C. behave passively in controllable situations

    D. become abnormally suspicious

4. The reason why the mice in Ader's experiment avoided saccharin was that _____.

    A. they disliked its taste   B. it affected their immune systems

    C. it led to stomach pains   D. they associated it with stomachaches

5. The passage tells us that the most probable reason for the death of the mice in Ader's experiment was that _____.

    A. they had been weakened psychologically by the saccharin

    B. the sweetener was poisonous to them

    C. their immune systems had been altered by the mind

    D. they had taken too much sweetener during earlier conditioning

Passage Fourteen

Humans are fascinated by the source of their failings and virtues. This preoccupation inevitably leads to an old debate: whether nature or nurture moulds us more. A revolution in genetics has poised this as a modern political question about the character of our society: if personalities are hard-wired into our genes, what can governments do to help us? It feels morally questionable, yet claims of genetic selection by intelligence are making headlines.

This is down to "hereditarian (遗传论的)" science and a recent paper claimed "differences in exam performance between pupils attending selective and non-selective schools mirror the genetic differences between them". With such an assertion, the work was predictably greeted by a lot of absurd claims about "genetics determining academic success". What the research revealed was the rather less surprising result: the educational benefits of selective schools largely disappear once pupils' inborn ability and socio-economic background were taken into account. It is a glimpse of the blindingly obvious— and there's nothing to back strongly either a hereditary or environmental argument.

Yet the paper does say children are "unintentionally genetically selected" by the school system. Central to hereditarian science is a tall claim: that identifiable variations in genetic sequences can predict an individual's aptness to learn, reason and solve problems. This is problematic on many levels. A teacher could not seriously tell a parent their child has a low genetic tendency to study when external factors clearly exist. Unlike-minded academics say the inheritability of human traits is scientifically unsound. At best there is a weak statistical association and not a causal link between DNA and intelligence. Yet sophisticated statistics are used to create an intimidatory atmosphere of scientific certainty.

While there's an undoubted genetic basis to individual difference, it is wrong to think that socially defined groups can be genetically accounted for. The fixation on genes as destiny is surely false too. Medical predictability can rarely be based on DNA alone; the environment matters too. Something as complex as intellect is likely to be affected by many factors beyond genes. If hereditarians want to advance their cause it will require more balanced interpretations and not just acts of advocacy.

Genetic selection is a way of exerting influence over others, "the ultimate collective control of human destinies", as writer H. G. Wells put it. Knowledge becomes power and power requires a sense of responsibility. In understanding cognitive ability, we must not elevate discrimination to a science: allowing people to climb the ladder of life only as far as their cells might suggest. This will need a more sceptical eye on the science. As technology progresses, we all have a duty to make sure that we shape a future that we would want to find ourselves in.

1. What did a recent research paper claim?

   A. The type of school students attend makes a difference to their future.

   B. Genetic differences between students are far greater than supposed.

   C. The advantages of selective schools are too obvious to ignore.

   D. Students' academic performance is determined by their genes.

2. What does the author think of the recent research?

   A. Its result was questionable.

   B. Its implication was positive.

   C. Its influence was rather negligible.

   D. Its conclusions were enlightening.

3. What does the author say about the relationship between DNA and intelligence?

    A. It is one of scientific certainty.

    B. It is not one of cause and effect.

    C. It is subject to interpretation of statistics.

    D. It is not fully examined by gene scientists.

4. What do hereditarians need to do to make their claims convincing?

    A. Take all relevant factors into account in interpreting their data.

    B. Conduct their research using more sophisticated technology.

    C. Gather gene data from people of all social classes.

    D. Cooperate with social scientists in their research.

5. What does the author warn against in the passage?

    A. Exaggerating the power of technology in shaping the world.

    B. Losing sight of professional ethics in conducting research.

    C. Misunderstanding the findings of human cognition research.

    D. Promoting discrimination in the name of science.

Passage Fifteen

Often people with deep vein thrombosis do not have any symptoms. In these people, this condition is usually suspected only after a blood clot is discovered in the lung. Once diagnosed with deep vein thrombosis, treatment begins if it is likely that the blood clot will grow or that a piece of the clot might break loose and flow to the lungs.

If you have a blood clot in your upper leg vein, you will usually need to take anticoagulant medication for 3 to 6 months, and possibly longer. After 3 to 6 months, your doctor may recommend that you continue Warfarin on an ongoing basis to prevent deep vein clots from recurring. Typically, if you have a blood clot in the lower deep leg veins, you will need to take anticoagulant medication for 6 to 12 weeks fan monitor the blood clot with ultrasound.

The main goal of treatment is to prevent the blood clot from growing or moving to the lungs. If a blood clot in the deep veins of the leg breaks loose and travels to the lungs, it can cause pulmonary embolism. Pulmonary embolism occurs in 25% of cases of untreated, diagnosed deep leg vein thrombosis. In people who receive treatment for deep vein thrombosis, the rate of pulmonary embolism falls drastically. Blood clots in the lung occur more often in people with deep vein blood clots in the upper rather than the lower leg veins. Only about 20% of blood clots in the veins of the calf will become larger and extend into the upper leg or groin veins. Blood clots that extend into the upper leg veins usually require with anticoagulant medication to prevent pulmonary embolism.

The recurrence rate for deep vein thrombosis varies depending on what caused the blood clot and how it was treated. Recurrence is most common in people who have continuing risk factors such as cancer or inherited blood-clotting problems and in people who have more than one blood clot in the leg. Recurrence is lowest in people who have a short-term risk factor, such as surgery or temporary inactivity. In 30% to 50% of people who have had deep vein thrombosis with symptoms, a condition called post thrombotic syndrome may develop within 8 years. This condition can cause pain, swelling, discoloration, and sores on the leg.

1. Once diagnosed with deep vein thrombosis, the patient will be given the treatment to

    _____.

    A. dissolve the existing blood clots

    B. break loose the existing blood clots

    C. prevent the new clots from forming

    D. prevent the existing blood clots from growing and moving to the lungs

2. If a patient is found a clot in his lower deep leg vein, he will have to _____.

    A. take anticoagulant medication for 3 to 6 months

    B. monitor his blood clot with ultrasound with no need for medication

    C. take anticoagulant medication for 6 to 12 weeks

    D. need continuous use of Warfarin

3. According to Paragraph 3, Pulmonary embolism is most likely to occur when _____.

    A. blood clots are found in the upper leg veins

    B. more than one blood clot is found in the leg

    C. blood clots appear in the lower leg veins

    D. proper treatment was given to patients with deep vein thrombosis

4. The recurrence rate for deep vein thrombosis may be the lowest among people

    _____.

    A. who have had a family history of blood-clotting problems

B. who have been diagnosed with deep vein thrombosis after undergoing the mastectomy due to breast cancers

C. whose deep vein thrombosis are caused by temporary sedentary work

D. who have more than one clot in the leg

5. The author of this passage focuses on the _____ of deep vein thrombosis.

A. treatment   B. early diagnosis

C. treatment and prevention   D. treatment and prognosis

Passage Sixteen

After 25 years battling the mother of all viruses, have we finally got the measure of HIV? Three developments featured in this issue collectively give grounds for optimism that would have been scarcely believable a year ago in the wake of another failed vaccine and continuing problems supplying drugs to all who need them.

Perhaps the most compelling hope lies in the apparent "cure" of a man with HIV who had also developed leukemia. Doctors treated his leukemia with a bone marrow transplant that also vanquished the virus. Now US Company Sangamo Biosciences is hoping to emulate the effect patients being cured with a single shot of gene therapy, instead of taking antiretroviral drugs for life.

Antiretroviral therapy (ART) is itself another reason for optimism. Researchers at the World Health Organization have calculated that HIV could be effectively eradicated in Africa and other hard-hit places using existing drugs. The trick is to test everyone often, and give those who test positive ART as soon as possible. Because the drugs rapidly reduce circulating levels of the virus to almost zero, it would stop people passing it on through sex. By blocking the cycle of infection in this way, the virus could be virtually eradicated by 2050.

Bankrolling such a long-term program would cost serious money — initially around $3.5 billion a year in South Africa alone, ring to $85 billion in total. Huge as it sounds, however, it is peanuts compared with the estimated $1.9 trillion cost of the Iraq war, or the $700 billion spent in one go propping up the US banking sector. It also looks small beer compared with the costs of carrying on as usual, which the WHO says can only lead to spiraling cases and costs.

The final bit of good news is that the cost of ART could keep on falling. Last Friday, GlaxoSmithKline chairman Andrew Witty said that his company would offer all its medicines to the poorest countries for at least 25 per cent less than the typical price in rich countries. GSK has already been doing this for ART, but the hope is that the company may now offer it cheaper still and that other firms will follow their lead.

No one doubts the devastation caused by AIDS. In 2007, 2 million people died and 2.7 million more contracted the virus. Those dismal numbers are not going to turn around soon — and they won't turn around at all without huge effort and investment. But at least there is renewed belief that, given the time and money, we can finally start riddling the world of this most fearsome of viruses.

1. Which of the following can be most probably perceived beyond the first paragraph?

   A. The end of the world.   B. A candle of hope.

   C. A Nobel Prize.   D. A quick fix.

2. According to the passage, the apparent "cure" of the HIV patient who had also developed leukemia would _____.

   A. make a promising transition from antiretroviral medication to gene therapy

   B. facilitate the development of effective vaccines for the infection

   C. compel people to draw an analogy between AIDS and leukemia

   D. would change the way we look at those with AIDS

3. As another bit of good news, _____.

   A. HIV will be virtually wiped out first in Africa

   B. the cycle of HIV infection can be broken with ART

   C. the circulating levels of HIV have been limited to almost zero

   D. the existing HIV drugs will be enhanced to be more effective in 25 years

4. The last reason for optimism is that _____.

   A. governments will invest more in improving ART

   B. the cost of antiretroviral therapy is on the decline

   C. everybody can afford antiretroviral therapy in the world

   D. the financial support of ART is coming to be no problem

5. The whole passage carries a tone of _____.

   A. idealism   B. activism

   C. criticism   D. optimism

Passage Seventeen

European Union environmental officials have determined that two kinds of genetically modified corn could harm butterflies, affect food chains and disturb life in rivers and streams, and they have proposed a ban on the sale of the seeds, which are made by DuPont Pioneer, Dow Agrosciences and Syngenta. The preliminary decisions are circulating within the European Commission, which has the final say. Some officials there are skeptical of a ban that would upset the powerful biotechnology industry and could exacerbate tensions with important trading partners like the United States. The seeds are not available on the European market for cultivation.

In the decisions, the environment commissioner, Stavros Dimas, contends that the genetically modified corn, or maize could affect certain butterfly species, specifically the monarch, and other beneficial insects. For instance, research this year indicates that larvae of the monarch butterfly exposed to the genetically modified corn "behave differently than other larvae". In the decision concerning the corn seeds produced by Dow and Pioneer, Mr. Dimas calls "potential damage on the environment irreversible". In the decision on Syngenta's corn, he says that "the level of risk generated by the cultivation of this product for the environment is unacceptable".

A decision by the European Union to bar cultivation of the genetically modified crops would be the first of its kind in the trade bloc, and would intensify the continuing battle over genetically modified corn. Banning the applications for corn crops also would mark a bold new step for European environmental authorities, who are already aggressively pursuing regulations on emissions from cars and aircraft, setting it at odds with the United States and angering industries.

"These products have been grown in the U.S. and other countries for years," said Stephen Norton, a spokesman for the United States trade representative. "We are not aware of any other case when a product has been rejected after having been reviewed and determined safe by European food safety authorities," he said.

Barbara Helfferich, a spokeswoman for Mr. Dimas, declined to comment on the specifics of the procedure because commissioners had not yet made a final decision. But she said that the European Union was within its rights to make decisions based on the "precautionary principle" even when scientists had found no definitive evidence proving products can cause harm. She said that the decisions by Mr. Dimas could go before the commission within a few weeks, but she said that no date had been set. In the decisions, Mr. Dimas cited recent research showing that consumption of genetically modified "corn byproducts reduced growth and increased mortality of nontarget stream insects" and that these insects "are important prey for aquatic and riparian predators" and that this could have "unexpected ecosystem-scale consequences".

Although still preliminary, his decisions could drastically **tilt** the policy against future approvals of genetically modified crops, said Nathalie Moll, a spokeswoman for Europabio, an industry group with 80 members including Syngenta, Pioneer and Dow. Europabio says that the crops grown using the genetically modified corn are already imported into several European countries, including France and Germany, where they are used to feed animals like cows and chickens.

Rob Gianfranceschi, spokesman at the United States mission to the European Union in Brussels, said it was too early to comment on a decision that had not yet been formalized. But he made clear that the United States remained frustrated with European policies on genetically modified crops.

1. The preliminary decisions are made by _____.

    A. DuPont Pioneer, Dow Agrosciences and Syngenta

    B. European Union environmental officials

    C. European Commission

    D. Stavros Dimas

2. To the decisions, the European Commission officials' attitudes are _____.

    A. skeptical   B. controversial

    C. contradictory   D. divergent

3. About the decisions, which of the following statements is TRUE?

    A. The decisions aim to put a ban on the sale of the seeds of genetically modified corn due to political and biological concerns.

    B. The decisions are warmly embraced by all EU members but bitterly rejected by their trade partners.

    C. The decisions could probably be made even if no definitive evidence proving the products harmful is found.

    D. There is high possibility that the decisions would be approved by the European Commission.

4. Mr. Dimas cited many researches on the genetically modified corn in his decisions in order to _____.

    A. dispel some officials' doubt on his decisions

    B. enhance the strength of his decision-making

    C. demonstrate the latest achievement of his decisions

    D. assure that they can be presented before the commission with solid evidence

5. The word "tilt" (Line 1, Paragraph 6) most probably means _____.

    A. incline   B. affect

    C. include   D. evoke

Passage Eighteen

Once upon a time, the only ideologically acceptable explanations of mental differences between men and women were cultural. Any biologist who dared to suggest in public that perhaps evolution might work differently on the sexes, and that this might perhaps result in some underlying neurological inequalities, was likely to get tarred and feathered. Today, by contrast, biology tends to be an explanation of first resort in matters sexual. So it is salutary to come across an experiment which shows that a newly discovered difference which fits easily, at first sight, into the biological-determinism camp, actually does not belong there at all.

Writing in *Psychological Science*, a team led by Ian Spence of the University of Toronto describes a test performed on people's ability to spot unusual objects that appear in their field of vision. Success at spatial tasks like this often differs between the sexes (men are better at remembering and locating general landmarks; women are better at remembering and locating food), so the researchers were not surprised to discover a discrepancy between the two. The test asked people to identify an "odd man out" object in a briefly displayed field of two dozen otherwise identical objects. Men had a 68% success rate. Women had a 55% success rate.

Had they left it at that, Dr. Spence and his colleagues might have concluded that they had uncovered yet another evolved difference between the sexes, come up with a "Just So" story to explain it in terms of division of labour on the African Savannah, and moved on. However, they did not leave it at that. Instead, they asked some of their volunteers to spend ten hours playing an action-packed, shoot-'em-up video game, called "Medal of Honour: Pacific Assault". As a control, other volunteers were asked to play a decidedly non-action-packed puzzle game, called "Balance", for a similar time. Both sets were then asked to do the odd-man-out test again.

Among the Balancers, there was no change in the ability to pick out the unusual. Among those who had played "Medal of Honour", both sexes improved their performances. That is not surprising, given the different natures of the games. However, the improvement in the women was greater than the improvement in the men — so much so that there was no longer a significant difference between the two. Moreover, that absence of difference was long-lived. When the volunteers were tested again after five months, both the improvement and the lack of difference between the sexes remained. Though it is too early to be sure, it looks likely that the change in spatial acuity — and the abolition of any sex difference in that acuity — induced by playing "Medal of Honour" is permanent.

That has several implications. One is that playing violent computer games can have beneficial effects. Another is that the games might provide a way of rapidly improving spatial ability in people such as drivers and soldiers. And a third is that although genes are important, upbringing matters, too. In this instance, exactly which bit of upbringing remains unclear. Perhaps it has to do with the different games that boys and girls play. But without further research, that suggestion is as much of a "Just So" story as those tales from the savannah.

1. The "odd man out" object in the experiment of Ian Spence refers to _____.

   A. a weird man
   B. the different object
   C. an ugly guy
   D. something separated from others

2. In Ian Spence's experiment, the fact that men had higher success rate of identifying the "odd man out" object proves _____.

   A. that the biological-determinism is universal because men are better at remembering general landmarks than women
   B. the cultural conclusion that women are of no difference with men in terms of judging objects
   C. that it is an accepted conclusion that men have higher success rate at spatial tasks than women
   D. the biological discovery that men are genetically more intelligent than women

3. The word "control" (Paragraph 3) most probably means _____.

   A. contrast
   B. regulation
   C. monitor
   D. manipulation

4. Which of the following case is NOT true of game players' performances of identifying the "odd man out" object?

   A. There was no difference between men and women in identifying the "odd man out" object after playing the violent game.

   B. Women exceeds men at picking out the unusual object after playing the violent game.

   C. Men were the same as women at picking out the unusual object after playing "Balance".

   D. Women improved more greatly in identifying the "odd man out" object after playing "Medal of Honour".

5. From the game experiment by Ian Spence, the following conclusion can be drawn that _____.

   A. violent games should be widely promoted to improve people's ability of remembering and locating general landmarks

   B. the reason that boys have better spatial ability is mainly because they play much more violent games

   C. genes in determining the spatial ability can not be changed by acquired practice

   D. playing violent games could change people's congenital ability

Passage Nineteen

In recent years, the food industry has increased its use of labels. Whether the labels say "non-GMO（非转基因的）" or "no sugar", or "zero" carbohydrates, consumers are increasingly demanding more information about what's in their food. One report found that 39% of consumers would switch from the brands they currently buy to others that provide clearer, more accurate product information. Food manufacturers are responding to the report with new labels to meet that demand, and they're doing so with an eye towards giving their products an advantage over the competition, and bolstering profits.

This strategy makes intuitive sense. If consumers say they want transparency, tell them exactly what is in your product. That is simply supplying a certain demand. But the marketing strategy in response to this consumer demand has gone beyond articulating what is in a product, to labeling what is NOT in the food. These labels are known as "absence claims" labels, and they represent an emerging labeling trend that is detrimental both to the consumers who purchase the products and the industry that supplies them.

For example, Hunt's put a "non-GMO" label on its canned crushed tomatoes a few years ago — despite the fact that at the time there was no such thing as a GMO tomato on the market. Some diary companies are using the "non-GMO" label on their milk, despite the fact that all milk is naturally GMO-free, another label that creates unnecessary fear around food.

While creating labels that play on consumer fears and misconceptions about their food may give a company a temporary marketing advantage over competing products on the grocery aisle, in the long term this strategy will have just the opposite effect: by injecting fear into the discourse about our food, we run the risk of eroding consumer trust in not just a single product, but the entire food business.

Eventually, it becomes a question in consumers' minds: Were these foods ever safe? By purchasing and consuming these types of products, have I already done some kind of harm to my family or the planet? For food manufacturers, it will mean damaged consumer trust and lower sales for everyone. And this isn't just supposition. A recent study found that absence claims labels can create a stigma around foods even when there is no scientific evidence that they cause harm.

It's clear that food manufacturers must tread carefully when it comes to using absence claims. In addition to the likely negative long-term impact on sales, this verbal trick sends a message that innovations in farming and food processing are unwelcome, eventually leading to less efficiency, fewer choices for consumers, and ultimately, more costly food products. If we allow this kind of labeling to continue, we will all lose.

1. What trend has been observed in a report?

    A. Food manufacturers' rising awareness of product safety.

    B. Food manufacturers' changing strategies to bolster profits.

    C. Consumers' growing demand for eye-catching food labels.

    D. Consumers' increasing desire for clear product information.

2. What does the author say is manufacturers' new marketing strategy?

    A. Stressing the absence of certain elements in their products.

    B. Articulating the unique nutritional value of their products.

    C. Supplying detailed information of their products.

    D. Designing transparent labels for their products.

3. What point does the author make about non-GMO labels?

   A. They are increasingly attracting customers' attention.

   B. They create lots of trouble for GMO food producers.

   C. They should be used more for vegetables and milk.

   D. They cause anxiety about food among consumers.

4. What does the author say absence claims labels will do to food manufacturers?

   A. Cause changes in their marketing strategies.

   B. Help remove stigma around their products.

   C. Erode consumer trust and reduce sales.

   D. Decrease suport from food scientists.

5. What does the author suggest food manufacturers do?

   A. Take measures to lower the cost of food products.

   B. Exercise caution about the use of absence claims.

   C. Welcome new innovations in food processing.

   D. Promote efficiency and increase food variety.

Passage Twenty

There is nothing like the suggestion of a cancer risk to scare a parent, especially one of the over-educated, eco-conscious type. So you can imagine the reaction when a recent *USA Today* investigation of air quality around the nation's schools singled out those in the smugly （自鸣得意地）green village of Berkeley, Calif., as being among the worst in the country. The city's public high school, as well as a number of daycare centers, preschools, elementary and middle schools, fell in the lowest 10%. Industrial pollution in our town had supposedly turned students into living science experiments breathing in a laboratory's worth of heavy metals like manganese, chromium and nickel each day. This happens in a city that requires school cafeterias to serve organic meals. Great, I thought, organic lunch, toxic campus.

Since December, when the report came out, the mayor, neighborhood activists （活跃分子）and various parent-teacher associations have engaged in a fierce battle over its validity: over the guilt of the steel-casting factory on the western edge of town, over union jobs versus children's health and over what, if anything, ought to be done. With all sides presenting their own experts armed with conflicting scientific studies, whom should parents believe? Is there truly a threat here, we asked one another as we dropped off our kids, and if so, how great is it? And how does it compare with the other, seemingly perpetual health scares we confront, like panic over lead in synthetic athletic fields? Rather than just another weird episode in the town that brought you protesting environmentalists, this latest drama is a trial for how today's parents perceive risk, how we try to keep our kids safe — whether it's possible to keep them safe — in what feels like an increasingly threatening world. It raises the question of what, in our time, "safe" could even mean.

"There's no way around the uncertainty," says Kimberly Thompson, president of Kid Risk, a nonprofit group that studies children's health. "That means your choices can matter, but it also means you aren't going to know if they do." A 2004 report in the journal *Pediatrics* explained that nervous parents have more to fear from fire, car accidents and drowning than from toxic chemical exposure. To which I say: Well, obviously. But such concrete hazards are beside the point. It's the dangers parents can't — and may never— quantify that occur all of sudden. That's why I've rid my cupboard of microwave food packed in bags coated with a potential cancer-causing substance, but although I've lived blocks from a major fault line（地质断层）for more than 12 years, I still haven't bolted our bookcases to the living room wall.

1. What does a recent investigation by *USA Today* reveal?

   A. Heavy metals in lab tests threaten children's health in Berkeley.

   B. Berkeley residents are quite contented with their surroundings.

   C. The air quality around Berkeley's school campuses is poor.

   D. Parents in Berkeley are over-sensitive to cancer risks their kids face.

2. What response did *USA Today*'s report draw?

   A. A heated debate.　　　B. Popular support.

   C. Widespread panic.　　　D. Strong criticism.

3. How did parents feel in the face of the experts' studies?

   A. They felt very much relieved.

   B. They were frightened by the evidence.

   C. They didn't know who to believe.

   D. They weren't convinced of the results.

4. What is the view of the 2004 report in the journal *Pediatrics?*

   A. It is important to quantify various concrete hazards.

B. Daily accidents pose a more serious threat to children.

C. Parents should be aware of children's health hazards.

D. Attention should be paid to toxic chemical exposure.

5. Of the dangers in everyday life, the author thinks that people should have more to fear from _____.

    A. the uncertain   B. the quantifiable

    C. an earthquake   D. unhealthy food

第二节 答案与解析

Passage One

1. C。由 "Consistently sleeping six to eight hours per night may be optimal for health." 可知，睡眠时间在六到八小时之间对身体有好处，故答案为C。

2. D。由 "They pointed out that previous studies had shown that sleep deprivation was associated with heart disease, high blood pressure, obesity, type 2 diabetes, and high cholesterol." 可知，长期睡眠不足与心脏病、高血压、肥胖、Ⅱ型糖尿病和高胆固醇相关联。但是与肺结核无关，故答案为D。

3. D。由 "Whilst short sleep may represent a cause of ill-health, long sleep is believed to represent more an indicator of ill-health." 可知，睡眠过短可能是疾病产生的原因，但睡眠过长却更有可能是存在疾病的标志。故答案为D。

4. A。Whilst在文中是什么意思？A选项 "虽然，即使"；B选项 "而且，此外"；C选项 "因为"；D选项 "因为，既然"。根据语境可知whilst的意思应是 "虽然"，故答案为A。

5. A。全文都在探讨睡眠时间长短与健康的关系，故答案为A。最佳的标题是 "睡眠与健康"。

Passage Two

1. D。从第一、二段可知olestra是一种使食物既不含脂肪又保持其美味的物质。第二段中指出the new compound can rob the body of essential vitamins and nutrients（新的复合物能使体内的基本营养与维生素流失），所以A和B两项与原文不符，C项与第三段相悖。故答案为D。

2. D。根据第三段可知，研究人员本想寻找一种婴儿容易消化的脂肪，结果却发现了一种根本不能消化的脂肪，因此，结果是出人意料的。

3. A。根据题干中的fatty acid将本题定位到第四、五、六段。根据第四段末尾的"A molecule of regular fat is made up of three molecules of substances called fatty acids."可知a molecule of regular fat是由three molecules of substances组成的，而非fatty acids由three molecules of substances组成，所以A项错误。而B，C，D三项在接下来的第五段和第六段中均能找到相对应的句子。

4. A。根据第六段可知，olestra不同于一般的脂肪，它由六到八个脂肪酸分子组成，体积太大，肠胃无法吸收，与A项"它可以经过肠胃而不被分解"相符。

5. B。批评家担心olestra减少了人们对维生素的摄入，因此，食品制造商增加了维生素成分，这种做法又让营养学家担心会不会造成摄入量超出身体所需而造成不良后果。

Passage Three

1. A。本题针对的是文章的第一段和第二段。文章第二段提到，虽然感染的人数上升了，但并不是坏消息，因为随着全世界医疗水平的提高，艾滋病死亡率下降了。这个上升的数据对应的是死亡人数的减少，因此，选项中A符合题意。

2. B。选项A在第四段中提到，死亡率和感染率发生变化一部分原因是每种传染病都会有这样自然的起伏。第五段提到，数据的变化主要是由于采用了更好的数据收集方法，而不是统计方法。因此B是错误的，D是正确的。选项C在第四段中提到。那么，选项B是正确答案。

3. B。在第六段中，根据上下文可知，持怀疑态度者最开始怀疑旧的调查方法有偏颇，但是现在新的方法比较先进、科学，他们的疑虑应该打消了。因此，选项B最符合题意。

4. C。第六段中原文指出，到2010年财政需求可能要比先前估计的少5%，而到2015年这个数字将增加到10%。也就是说，到了2015年，财政需求要比先前估计的少10%。选项C为正确答案。

5. B。对于这次修订，作者在全文多次用了赞扬的语气，介绍了这样做的好处，因此，作者的态度是肯定的，正确答案为B选项。

Passage Four

1. B。题目问公众对不育症治疗的观点是什么。A选项的表述显然不符合题意。C选项的表述不如B选项确切。D选项的表述过于绝对，不能反映公众的意见。因此，选项中B最为符合。

2．D。根据第四段可知，没有体外受精，丹麦人口就会减少得更快，那么可以看出现在丹麦人口仍在减少，但是速度放缓了。因此，A，B，C选项是错误的。第四段提到了丹麦人口是稳定的。因此，答案为D选项。

3．A。根据第五段的金钱数据对比可以看出，体外受精比其他方法要经济，因此，选项中A符合题意。

4．A。根据上下文可知，这个方法可能会让女性衰老很快，也会让孩子出现一些先天性的问题。选项中A最为符合题意。

5．A。从文章中作者举的例子和分析可以看出，这个方法虽然有一定的缺点，但是对于解决目前欧洲人口减少的问题还是有积极作用的，因此是支持的态度，答案为A选项。

Passage Five

1．C。A选项是那些行业老古董们对这个方案的直接想法，而不是不看好的真正原因。B是错误的，因为在文章第一段Ballmer也谈到了一些技术上的实施。而D选项的相关内容文章中没有提及，属于干扰选项。因此，C选项是该题的正确答案。

2．A。第二段指出，个人可以随时随地在网上看到自己的记录，别人的记录是不能随便看的，这与A项的内容不相符；第二段指出，这对于经常旅行的人是个福音，他们会受益，与B项说法相符；第二段提到签约医院可以将化验结果以电子形式发到库中，病人也可以让医院查看自己的数据，这样效率肯定会大大增加，与C项内容一致；由第二段微软的宣告可以看出这是微软研发的软件，D项说法正确。因此，A是正确答案。

3．B。因为文章最后一段指出了"'健康库'搜索引擎如果可以查看用户的健康记录和历史询问的话，就一定会比其对手网站运行得更好，也可以根据各人的情况提供最接近的答复。但是为了吸引用户，微软承诺遵守严格的隐私规范"，因此这暗示了有这种两难境地的危险。故答案为B选项。

4．D。文章第三段末尾提到，健康库是让病人和医生免费查阅的，那么微软靠什么来赚钱呢？第四段就提出建立一个医学方面的专业引擎，通过该引擎来赚钱，而且该引擎只专注于一个方面，因此更加高效。由此可见，D选项为正确答案。

5．B。第四段提到，健康库可以提供比谷歌、雅虎等通用引擎更相关的结果，该引擎限定于某一专业领域。因此，该引擎的优势就在于更专业。由此可见，只有B选项更为符合题意。

Passage Six

1. B。根据题干中的visible和India定位到原文第一段。这个题看似简单，定位也不难，然而却不容易理清语义走向。该段第一句说素食主义者不想被强迫吃肉（即愿意吃素），yet将语义进行逆转：最近以植物为主的"行星饮食计划"暗含了反向（reverse）强迫，即强迫吃素（不愿意吃素）。Nowhere is this more visible than in India中用到了比较级的否定形式，相当于visible的最高级，也就是说，印度这种反向强迫是最明显的，即强迫吃素这种现象在印度是最明显的。其实本文主要讲的是尊重发展中国家的饮食习惯，无论吃素还是反向行之，都不要强迫他们改变。因此本题答案为B。

2. C。根据题干中的Lancet，India定位到第二段最后一句。EAT-Lancet呼吁全国践行以素食为基础的饮食，这不仅会恶化印度紧张的政治局势，还会给已经营养不良的人群带来压力，让情况变得更加糟糕。因此本题正确答案为C。

3. B。通过food consumption定位到第三段中含有consume的前两句。第二句指出，印度因为存在阶级、宗教、文化等很多障碍，人们想吃的食物和吃到的食物有很大差异。因此B选项是正确答案：很多印度人是没有机会接触自己想吃的食物的。

4. D。根据题干中的plant-based diet，modeled等定位到倒数第三、四段。以印度为模板推行以植物为主的饮食可能会给发展中国家的弱势群体带来再次伤害。众所周知，低收入国家营养不良的孩子是从牛奶和其他动物来源类饮食中获益的，因为这类饮食改善他们的认知功能，降低因营养不良导致的发病率和死亡率，所以可以推断素食饮食可能会令低收入国家的营养不良问题恶化。因此本题正确答案为D。

5. A。通过Indian government，respond to，proposals定位到原文最后一段。印度政府对这份report表示了赞赏（thumbs-up），但政府没有通过增加有益健康和营养丰富的食物来解决长期问题，而是依赖企业来解决问题，忽视了环境和经济成本，破坏了当地的食物体系，对后代来讲，这是一个非常危险的模式。因此，本题正确答案为A。

Passage Seven

1. C。根据第一段可知，尽管Perutz出了不少错，但都是小错，大事情上没有出错，最终才赢得了诺贝尔奖。因此，答案为C选项。A选项看似正确，但错在"marginal mistakes"这个提法，在文章中没有出现。小错可能也是一些关系核心的问题，而不是边缘性的。而B和D选项并不是他获得诺贝尔奖的根本原因。

2. A。第二段中提到了正是出于这个原因Perutz才获得了诺贝尔奖，A选项正确。第二段提到血红蛋白完整的结构是由他提供的，所以B项错误；第三段中提到是他的同事把一些材料总结起来得出了结论，但是之前Perutz已经得出了结论，所以C项错误；Perutz接受了同事的建议，并不是存在许多分歧，所以D项错误。因此A选项为正确答案。

3．D。根据第三段可知，这个同事发现最后的证据一致，忍不住将证据放在合适的地方，得出了最后的结论，其实Perutz早已得出了这个结论，因此，他非常生气。D选项符合这个意思。

4．A。根据第五段可知，Perutz研究的领域是边缘学科，是新的学科，所以提倡研究现有学科的机构阻挠了他的进展。因此，A选项最为符合题意。

5．C。根据上下文可知，Perutz过去抱怨说虽然自己名气很大，但是很少有人知道他所做出的成就是什么，所以现在这本书将科学和个人轶事结合在一起，就调整了这种平衡。因此，答案为C选项。

Passage Eight

1．A。作者在文章一开始就指出在富裕国家中妇女生男孩的比率比贫穷国家高出5%，但目前这个比率在下降，有许多人给出了自己的解释，但都未能被大型的研究所证明，而现在又有新的论点，就是压力的作用。接下来的几段就是对这个论点的证实。由此可见，作者是以提出一个论点的形式来开始这篇文章的。

2．B。题干要求找出富裕国家目前男孩出生率下降的原因，文章整篇都在讨论压力对于婴儿性别的作用，而且最后一段的最后一句话指出，目前这个比率下降可能是因为富裕国家妇女现在承受的压力要比以前多，但是没有说明有新的压力。因此，答案为B。

3．C。第四段中提到，Obel博士认为女性在面临压力时生女孩的概率更大，其根本原因应该是适应性的原因而不是生理性原因。而且Obel怀疑女性面临压力时如果怀孕的是男孩就更容易流产。因此，答案中C可以说明他的观点，A，B，D只是一些表象。

4．D。在原始狩猎社会中，女孩出生率较高的原因是因为妇女生育时面临的种种压力。四个选项中，D为正确答案；A选项显然是错误的，原始人不会以进化的观点去思考问题；B选项的说法只是一个现象，并不是题干的原因；C选项的说法与原文相反。

5．B。题干要求根据整篇文章推导出一个结论，本文主要讲述了压力对于婴儿出生性别的影响，分别用一些数据和事实证明突发压力和慢性压力都有一定的影响，从中可以得出结论，就是突发压力与急性压力都会使得女孩的出生率高一些。文中并没有进行比较，所以A，D两项错误；C的内容文中没有提到。因此，正确答案为B。

Passage Nine

1．D。根据第一段"But there are many barriers to studying dietary change, which is why we still have no easy answers to the question of what, exactly, we should eat to be at our healthiest" 可知，因为要进行摄入食物变化调查的障碍很多，因此在该问题上并没有一定的答案，选项中D最为符合题意。

2．A。根据第二段"breast cancer survivors who cram their diets with fruits and vegetables are no more likely to escape a recurrence than women who stick to the usual five-a-day recommendation"可知，该研究报道表明吃大量的蔬菜、水果并不能像医生推荐的每日主餐那样有效地让患有乳癌的妇女避免复发，那么A选项是正确的。虽然蔬菜、水果不能帮助妇女避免癌症复发，但还是对她们的身体有好处的，所以D选项说法错误。

3．D。根据第五段"the amount of calories subjects reported eating would have caused them to lose far more weight than they actually did lose"可知，这种研究的结果表明，受实验者报告自己摄入的卡路里数量本来可以让他们体重下降的幅度更大的，这和他们自己报告的情况不够真实有关。因此，这样的研究不够客观。故答案为D选项。

4．B。根据第五段可知，尽管吃了许多百吉饼，却报告说只吃了4盎司大的，那么可以看出报告有误。故答案为B选项。C选项错误的原因在于尽管报告有误，但是没有说明这就是不与医生合作。

5．D。根据最后一段可知，这种血液测量可以测出实验对象具体摄入的食物和蔬菜量，但是却不能确定人们是否摄入了一定量的营养物质。故答案为D选项。

Passage Ten

1．D。根据文章第一段中的"The ancient Egyptians knew about many tumors..., and the Greeks made a distinction...tumors (oncos) and malignant ones (carcinos)"可知，古埃及人知道许多有不良后果的肿瘤，而希腊人已经区分出良性肿瘤和恶性肿瘤了，所以答案为D。

2．D。文章中共有三处提及恐惧，但和癌症同时提到是在最后一段，威廉·巴契南认为过度恐惧会导致患癌症，但这并不等于说人们不惧怕癌症，故不选B。根据最后一段中的"Among the Romantics and the Victorians, suffering and dying from tuberculosis...cancer death was nothing of the sort"可知，在浪漫主义时期和维多利亚时期，受肺结核折磨甚至死于肺结核被认为是高雅的标志；患癌死亡就完全不同了，故排除C；通读全文，A项文中没有提到；根据最后一段中的"In the eighteenth and nineteenth centuries, some physicians attributed cancer—notably of the breast and the ovaries—to psychological and behavioral causes"可知，在十八、十九世纪，一些医生将癌症——尤其是乳腺癌和子宫内膜癌——的产生归咎到心理或行为方面，所以答案为D。

3．C。根据文章第二段最后两句话可知，癌症致死的极度痛苦的样子令人畏惧，但是恐惧并没有成为公众意识中的关注焦点，而现在不同了。医学史家罗伊·波特将其说成"现代疾病的典范"，慕克吉称其为"现代性最典型的产物"，这就是其中一方面的原因。所以C选项"现在，人们以全新的方式理解癌症"正确。

4. D。根据文章最后一段第一、二句话可知，人们曾经认为癌症是一种"文明病"，病因与神经衰弱症和糖尿病类似；前者是因现代生活的压力而产生的神经衰弱，后者是因饮食不良和懒惰而产生。在十八、十九世纪，一些医生将癌症——尤其是乳腺癌和子宫内膜癌——的产生归咎到心理或行为方面。这里提到神经衰弱症和糖尿病是为了说明癌症和它们类似，和心理和行为有关，故本题答案为D。

5. A。根据文章第一段第一、二句可知，癌症始终如影随形，但是方式却有变化。诊治处理方法当然也随着时代进步有变化，而其存在性质、表现和意义也发生了改变。作者在这两句话中隐藏了自己的观点。所以本题答案为A。

Passage Eleven

1. B。通过命题顺序定位到第一段，患者外显记忆系统毫发无伤，但无法学习新的技术，虽然能记住学习过程。因此本题正确答案为B，重点在new这个核心内容上。患者并非记不住所有做过的事。

2. D。根据第二段"Within explicit, or declarative memory, there are...shapes, textures such as faces, names..."可以判断remembering a familiar face of a friend属于explicit memory范畴。选项A，B，C均属于implicit memory的范畴，故本题答案为D。

3. C。从第三段首句对外显记忆的描述以及后面的"Fail to connect person's name with his or her face, ...becomes downright worrisome when we reach our 50s"可知，外显记忆系统受损会无法将人和名称对应起来。

4. A。hammer各个特征储存在大脑不同的位置，要想构成hammer的完整印象，我们需要从大脑不同部位中extract各自的名称，pull和remove都表示物理的拉动、拽动，而obtain则表示抽象的获得，故A是正确答案。

5. B。文中讲到关于人类记忆形成机制的研究并未结束，记忆衰退在很多动物身上也被发现，同时最后一段中讲到it's obvious...it's equally obvious...可知科学家们有了很大突破，但是具体的更深入的内容并未提及，这就暗示科学家们需要做更多的研究。故本题答案为B。

Passage Twelve

1. A。上文提到，有些学生要求不做这种解剖，那么现在有许多科技替代物使得这个成为现实，就是用计算机鼠标来替代解剖刀，下文也提到了用计算机程序来代替真正用解剖刀进行的实验。因此，正确答案为A选项。

2. B。文章第一段提到，一些学生选择不做是因为他们感到应该对这种动物友好些，另外是因为想到青蛙的身体、闻到甲醛的味道就感到恶心。因此，答案A，D是原因；答案B并不是他们不愿意做解剖的原因，而是因为他们不愿意做才有了相关法律保护他们的这种权利；选项C包含了A和D两个选项。因此，答案为B。

3. C。Brian Shmaefsky的话分为两部分：解剖黏糊糊的，比较讨厌；老师应该衡量一下，学生如果感觉受到了冒犯，甚至影响到了学习效果那就得不偿失了。前半句是为后半句做铺垫，又根据他是国家生物教师协会成员，那么他说的话应该是针对学生学习的，他觉得这种解剖有时会阻碍学生学习。选项C符合题意。选项D并不是他想要表达的意思；对于选项B他并没有表示出这一点来；而选项A在文章中则没有得到明确的体现。

4. A。题目要求找出计算机解剖相对于传统解剖的优点所在，选项A是计算机模仿实际解剖的声音效果，而这种声音本身在实际解剖中也存在，因此只是一种模仿，并不是计算机的高超之处。

5. A。在这篇文章中，作者介绍了生物课上解剖的替代物——计算机解剖程序，虽然在文章最后一段作者也提到了这种替代物的局限，但是从整篇文章来看作者都是一种赞赏的态度，列举了这种方法的优点。因此，其态度是支持的，选A。

Passage Thirteen

1. B。Laudenslager通过实验，发现半数的老鼠能切断电源，另外一半却不能。这说明不能切断电源的老鼠，其免疫力下降到了正常水平以下，而能切断电源的老鼠情况则不同，其免疫力不受影响。这与B意思相同。

2. D。答案在第一段的最后一句话"What he has demonstrated, he believes, is that lack of control over an event, not the experience itself, is what weakens the immune system"。可知，缺乏对事件的控制，削弱了免疫系统。故答案为D。

3. C。第二段中"But if the animals are confronted with situations they have no control over, they later behave passively when faced with experiences they can control."可知，无能为力的经验让老鼠在可控的环境下表现得十分被动。与C项内容相符。

4. D。Ader的实验是给老鼠喂糖精后立即注射一种可导致其肚子疼的药物，经过刺激，老鼠自然会把糖精与肚子疼联系起来而尽量避开。

5. C。之前吃过最多糖精的老鼠死亡说明老鼠受刺激后其免疫力大大下降，从而导致了死亡。A，B，D都不是老鼠死亡的原因。

Passage Fourteen

1. D。根据题干中的关键词recent，research paper定位到第二段第一句：近期一篇论文称，精英学校和普通学校的学生成绩差异反映了他们基因的不同。换言之，这项研究认为基因决定了学生的学习成绩。因此本题正确答案为D。

2. A。对于该论文研究结论的态度，作者毫不吝啬自己强烈的态度表达。第二段中的absurd claims，blindingly obvious等，作者认为这项研究成果是对显而易见的事实进行了简单总结，其结果是没有任何证据支持的。第三段中的tall claim（高谈阔论、夸大其词）同样在表达作者对研究结果的态度。因此本题答案为A，值得质疑的。

3. B。根据relationship，DNA and intelligence定位到第三段倒数第二句：DNA与智力最多只是在统计数据上有些关联，并不存在一种因果关系causal link。因此本题答案为B。

4. A。根据题干中的hereditarians，make their claims convincing定位到原文第四段最后一句。如果遗传论者想要继续推进自己的研究，必须提供更多公正客观的解释，而不仅仅是宣扬他们的论点。前一句中也提到智力很复杂，会受到除了基因之外的其他很多因素影响，需要考虑许多相关因素。因此本题正确答案为A。

5. D。最后一段中提到，在理解认知的过程中，我们不能elevate discrimination to a science,即不能将歧视上升到科学的层面，否则我们就只能在基因允许的范围内前进。我们需要用批判的目光看待科学。因此本题正确答案为D。

Passage Fifteen

1. D。答案在第三段第一句，大意是：给予病人治疗的主要目的是避免血栓形成并移动到肺部，故本题答案为D。

2. C。答案在第二段第三句，大意是：病人需要服用抗凝药6~12周，并且用超声检查来检测血栓，故正确答案为C。

3. A。答案在第三段第五句，大意是：肺血栓容易在大腿静脉血栓形成时发生，故正确答案为A。

4. C。答案在第四段第二、三句，大意是：静脉血栓复发率在有血栓遗传史的人群、患癌症人群以及多个血栓形成人群中较普遍，而在由短期危险因素造成血栓的人群中复发率是较低的，例如手术后和暂时性活动受限引起的血栓。因此可判断正确答案为C。

5. D。全文主要讲述对静脉血栓的治疗、发病概率和预后。不难判断正确答案为D。

Passage Sixteen

1. B。题干：下列哪一项是通过第一段可以得知的？根据第一段最后一句话可以得知针对HIV病毒，研究进展又带给我们希望，因而答案为B。

2. A。题干：根据文章可知，对已经患上白血病的HIV病毒病人表面上的治愈将_____。根据题干信息可定位到第二段最后一句，意思是希望仿效那些采用单一基因疗法治疗患者的疗效，而不是终身服用抗反转录病毒药物。因而答案为A。

3. B。题干：作为另一个好消息，_____。根据题干和第三段首句信息可以得知解题的有效信息就在第三段。首先，根据第三段第二句话可以排除选项A，因为原文信息中没有提到HIV病毒首先将在非洲被消灭；另外根据第四句话可排除选项C，因为原文信息是"因为药物能快速将病毒流行程度降到零，这就防止人们通过性传播病毒"；选项D在文章中没有相应的信息。

4. B。题干：乐观的最后一个原因是_____。根据题干信息，可定位至第五段首句，其含义与选项B吻合。

5. D。题干：通篇的语调是_____。根据每段的主题句内容以及上述细节题，可以得出全篇语气态度为乐观积极的，因而答案为D。

Passage Seventeen

1. D。本题具有一定的难度，文章一开头就提到欧盟环境官员确定了一些事实，并且建议要禁止销售转基因作物的种子。然后就提到决议在欧盟委员会中间流传。第六段也提到他的决议虽然是初步的但可能有很大影响。由此看来，该决议是Dimas先生提出的可能性大，答案为D。

2. D。这些决议仿佛在欧洲委员会中间得到了一些支持，那么可以推断这些官员所持的态度是有分歧的。选项D最为符合题意。

3. C。文章第五段Dimas先生的发言人谈到了选项C这一点，说即使没有确凿证据，欧洲委员会可以基于"预防原则"做出决定，所以这个选项是正确的；文章提到目前该决议还没有明确的说法，所以D选项错误。因此，答案为C。

4. D。Dimas先生在其拟定的决议中多次引用了关于转基因产品的研究，其目的是证实自己的决议是有根据的，这样就更有说服力。选项A错在他拟定决议在先，这些官员怀疑在后，拟订时不一定存在这种想法；B，C两项不是其主要的目的。因此，D最为恰当。

5. A。尽管他的决议还是初步的，但是却能够让政策倾向于反对未来批准转基因食品。答案中A最为符合。

Passage Eighteen

1. B。根据实验的内容 "The test asked people to identify an 'odd man out' object in a briefly displayed field of two dozen otherwise identical objects" 可知，是要求实验对象找出和其他物体不同的物体unusual object，因此，选项B为正确答案。

2. B。文章第三、四段在描述实验结果时，指出了 "Had they left it at that, Dr. Spence and his colleagues might have concluded that they had uncovered yet another evolved difference between the sexes" "Among the Balancers, there was no change in the ability to pick out the unusual. Among those who had played 'Medal of Honour', both sexes improved their performances" 由此可见在辨认异物时男女差别几乎不大，因此答案为B选项。

3. A。根据上下文 "As a control, other volunteers were asked to play a decidedly non-action-packed puzzle game, called 'Balance', for a similar time" 可知，这两个游戏是两种不同的游戏，作者这样做是为了有一个控制组与另一组进行参照和对比，因此选项A选项为正确答案。

4. B。根据第四段可知，玩暴力游戏后，女性与男性辨认异物的能力差不多，但是她们的提高程度大，因此，选项中B是错误的。

5. C。文章提到基因不能发生改变，而是能力发生了改变，因此C选项是正确的。A选项显然不正确，因为文章中没有提到violent games should be widely promoted。B选项在文章最后一段中有所暗示，Perhaps it has to do with the different games that boys and girls play，但这只是一个猜测，不是定论，所以B选项错误。D选项更是明显错误的结论。因此正确答案为C选项。

Passage Nineteen

1. D。用trend和report定位到第一段第三句。该句大意为：报告显示，39%的消费者会从他们目前购买的品牌转向提供更清晰、更精确产品信息的品牌。这表明消费者越来越追求清晰的产品信息。因此选项D为正确答案。

2. A。根据题干中的manufacturers' new marketing strategy定位到第二段倒数第二句，该句大意是：根据消费者的需求，生产厂商的营销策略不仅要清楚说明产品中含有什么，还要说明产品中不含有什么。选项A中的stressing对应定位句中的articulating和labeling，而absence of certain elements 对应原文中的what is NOT in the food，故本题正确答案为A。

3. D。用题干中的non-GMO labels定位到原文第三段最后一句：一些乳制品公司在他们的牛奶包装上贴上了"非转基因"的标签，但是实际上所有的牛奶都是非转基因食品，这类标签倒使得消费者产生了不必要的恐慌。选项D为原文的正确改写。

4. C。用absence claims labels定位到原文第五段第三、四句，第三句指出，对食品生产商来讲，使用"无添加"声明的标签会损害消费者的信任，导致产品销量下降。故选项C为正确答案。

5. B。按照命题顺序，同时根据题干中的author suggest等寻找答案，可以发现原文最后一段首句有答案：食品生产商应谨慎使用"无添加"标签。故选项B为正确答案。

Passage Twenty

1. C。由题干中的recent investigation by *USA Today*定位到原文第一段第二句。该句指出，最近，《今日美国》对全国学校周围的空气质量状况进行了调查，位于加利福尼亚州的伯克利绿色村庄被列入全国空气质量状况最差的地区之中。由此可见，伯克利校园周围的空气质量状况很差。

2. A。由题干中的response和*USA Today*定位到原文第二段第一句。该句提到报告公布之后引起的各方的反应，句中的a fierce battle over its validity实际上是指人们对报告结果的正确性展开了激烈的争论。答案A是对a fierce battle的同义转述。

3. C。由题干中的parents和the experts' studies定位到原文第二段第二句。该段开头指出，《今日美国》公布的调查报告引发了各方的激烈争论。第二句中接着指出："参与讨论的各方都介绍了一些支持各自观点的专家，但是这些专家的科学理论是相互矛盾的"，因此父母们感到非常困惑，不知道到底应该相信哪一方。

4. B。由题干中的the 2004 report in the journal *Pediatrics*定位到原文第三段第三句。由该句可知，2004年《儿科》杂志公布的一份报告曾解释说，与接触有毒化学物质相比，神经紧张的父母往往会更担心火灾、交通事故和溺水事件的发生。父母们担心的是孩子们容易遇到的日常事故，换言之，父母认为日常事故让孩子们面临严重的威胁。

5. A。由题干中的the author think和people have more to fear from定位到原文最后两句。文章第三段前面部分提到，父母往往会担心日常事故的发生，随后指出这些突发的危险都是父母无法估量的。随后又列举了自己的两个例子：清理包装袋上覆盖着的一种可能致癌的物质的微波食品和不固定书橱。这都是在防备一些不确定的危险，可见作者认为人们更应该注意防备一些不确定的危险。

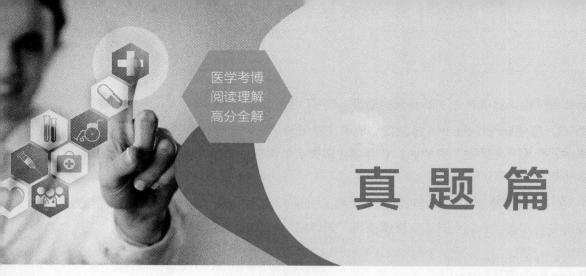

真 题 篇

2020年全国医学博士外语统一考试英语试题
（阅读部分）

Passage One

Gianluca Vialli, manager of Chelsea Football Club, expressed it explicitly enough: "The foot is the tool of the trade of the footballer." You might therefore expect footballers to take particularly good care of their feet. But results presented at a recent conference of dermatologists in Amsterdam suggest otherwise. Professional footballers seem as likely to suffer from fungal infections of the foot as other people.

One study, called Achilles Project, looked at 76, 475 pairs of feet belonging to people from 18 European countries. It found that 26% of the sample had Tinea pedis, better known as athlete's foot, while 30% had Onychomycosis, an infection that causes toenails to become thickened, discolored and distorted. The results showed that East European countries have consistently higher rates of infection. On average, 30% of Britons, Germans and Belgians had some form of fungal infection, compared with 85% of Russians, and less than 10% of Spaniards. Furthermore, adults under the age of 40 who took regular exercise had a 40% greater risk of fungal infection than those who did not.

Leisure centers and swimming pools were identified as potential health hazards to the very people who visit them to stay fit. Communal showers and changing rooms are perfect breeding-grounds for the highly infectious fungi that spread foot and nail infection: up to 1,500 fungally-infected skin fragments per square meter have been found in some leisure facilities. Sweaty socks and warm, damp sports shoes provide equally hospitable environments.

All of which goes some way to explaining the footballers. No doubt all that time spent in showers and changing-rooms is partly responsible. But Dr. Caputo, a dermatologist, also found another factor: footballers are often reluctant, for superstitious reasons, to discard their old boots. He found that players get attached to particular boots; if they score a goal with one, they will wear it again and again. The risk of athlete's foot may be a small price to pay for a goal.

61. What can we learn from the first paragraph?

    A. Footballers do not care for their feet as expected.

    B. Footballers' feet are more sensitive to fungal infections.

    C. Footballers usually care for their feet more than other people.

    D. Footballers' feet are more vulnerable than those of other people.

62. According to the passage, "Achilles Project" was designed to _____.

    A. serve as a global screening for foot infections

    B. collect a sample of infected athletes for research

    C. look into the conditions of feet in European countries

    D. find measures for reducing high rates of foot infections

63. From the description of Tinea pedis and Onychomycosis, we are sure that _____.

    A. Tinea pedis affects athletes more than Onychomycosis

    B. Tinea pedis and Onychomycosis are both fungal infections

    C. Tinea pedis is a more serious infection than Onychomycosis

    D. Tinea pedis is more sensitive to anti-fungal drugs than Onychomycosis

64. Which of the following can be safely inferred concerning the leisure centers and swimming pools?

    A. They could help people in one way and harm them in another.

    B. They do not spread infections as much as other public places.

    C. They do not perform adequate check-ups for their visitors.

    D. They are unlikely to spread fungal infection.

65. What did Dr. Caputo find about footballers?

    A. They play too much to keep their feet clean.

    B. They usually do not throw away comfortable boots.

C. They believe some shoes may bring them good luck.

D. They often stick to high-priced shoes for scoring goals.

Passage Two

A decade ago, most patients were informed over the phone or in person by the doctors. But in the past few years, hospitals and medical practices have urged patients to sign up for portals, which allow them rapid, round-the-clock access to their records. Lab tests are now released directly to patients.

The push for portals has been fueled by several factors: the widespread embrace of technology, incentive payments to medical practices and hospitals that were part of 2009 federal legislation to encourage "meaningful use" of electronic records, and a 2014 federal rule giving patients direct access to their results. Policymakers have long regarded electronic medical records as a way to foster patient engagement and improve patient safety.

Are portals delivering on their promise to engage patients? Or are these results too often a source of confusion and alarm for patients and the cause of more work for doctors because information is provided without adequate—or sometimes any—guidance?

Although what patients see online and how quickly they see it differs—sometimes even within the same hospital system—most portals contain lab tests, imaging studies, pathology reports and less frequently, doctors' notes. It is not uncommon for a test result to be posted before the doctor has seen it.

Katharine Treadway, an internist, knows what it's like to obtain shocking news from an electronic medical record. The experience, she said, has influenced the way she practices. More than a decade ago—long before most patients had portals—Treadway, with her husband's permission, pulled up the results of his MRI scan on a hospital computer while waiting to see the specialist treating his sudden, unbearable arm pain.

"It showed a massive tumor and widespread metastatic disease," Treadway recalled. She never suspected that her 59-year-old husband had cancer, let alone a highly aggressive and usually fatal form of advanced lymphoma.

Treadway, whose husband has been cancer-free for more than a decade, said she remembered intently checking the name and date of birth, certain she had the wrong patient, then rebooting the computer several times "like I was going to get a different answer".

66. What is the trend mentioned at the beginning of the passage?

    A. More lab tests are ordered through portals.

    B. More hospitals provide rapid, round-the-clock services.

    C. More medical consultations are conducted over the phone.

    D. More patients are encouraged to use portals for their medical information.

67. Which of the following is NOT mentioned as a contributing factor for the increasing use of portals?

    A. Popular acceptance of technology.

    B. Lower payments for the patients to obtain their results.

    C. Financial benefits for hospital use of electronic records.

    D. Legal requirement to provide patients with direct access to their results.

68. What concerns the author in respect to the increasing use of portals?

    A. Unsafe access to patients' personal information.

    B. Inadequate guidance for the patients to use portals.

    C. Improper delivery of the medical results to the patients.

    D. Different contents provided to the patients by different systems.

69. Which of the following statements is true about Dr. Treadway's husband?

    A. He was depressed by the diagnosis of his disease.

    B. He was screened for a highly aggressive and fatal cancer.

    C. He was mismatched with the electronic records of his MRI scan.

    D. He was informed of the results of his MRI scan via hospital portals.

70. The author cites Katharine Treadway's experience to _____.

    A. explain the hidden risk of portals being illegally accessed

    B. exemplify the potential risk of misinforming patients through portals

    C. illustrate the progress in the way information is delivered to the patients

    D. show the advantages of portals over phone in releasing patients' information

Passage Three

In planning for the health needs of these immigrant families, Francesca Weissman, a healthcare practitioner, asked two questions: (1) "What are the most urgent needs of this population?" and (2) "How can this population be induced to use the health services that are available?" In some respects, the second question is more important because persuading immigrant families to utilize services is a basic problem.

Building trust is a primary goal. Employing caregivers who can speak the clients' language will do much to lower ethnic barriers and reduce suspicion on the part of potential clients. Many traditional families are slow to develop personal relationships, and this holds true in the interactions with caregivers. Unless the families can communicate with caregivers, they cannot begin to trust them. Without trust, they are not likely to seek or even accept assistance.

Communication is a two-way channel. Caregivers, Francesca realized, have an obligation to become acquainted with the culture of the growing ethnic populations, and of their diverse subgroups. By becoming informed and by conveying respect, caregivers can make interactions with immigrant families less frightening and more productive. Awareness of the economic climate and other conditions in the place of origin helps caregivers recognize that the suspiciousness of immigrant families towards officials may not be wholly irrational.

A family approach to health care is recommended for immigrant groups. If the whole family can be involved in the healthcare program, the individual members are likely to be less fearful. Family-oriented programs may begin with practical advice about the neighborhood: locations of grocery stores, where to apply for food stamps, and how to look for work. Any programs developed for immigrant families must be offered at convenient times and places because they may not have the knowledge or resources to travel freely in their new community.

71. The passage begins by implying that immigrant families may not _____.

    A. be aware of their own health needs

    B. be willing to use the available services

    C. be entitled to the basic healthcare services

    D. be able to afford services other than the most basic

72. It is difficult to build trust between immigrant clients and caregivers because _____.

    A. caregivers have little overseas working experience

    B. caregivers may not speak the clients' native language

    C. caregivers have a strong sense of cultural superiority

    D. caregivers are averse to the clients' ethnic background

73. Which of the following can be inferred from Paragraph 3?

    A. Understanding different cultures is necessary in offering good services.

    B. Lack of information and respect is a common problem among caregivers.

    C. Ethnic populations are gaining significant influence in the healthcare system.

    D. It is unreasonable to emphasize specific conditions in immigrants' native homes.

74. Which of the following is important when the family approach is adopted?

    A. Sufficient resources should be guaranteed to ensure the success.

    B. The daily life of the family should be cared for first and foremost.

    C. Fear among family members should be relieved at the beginning stage.

    D. What is included in the programs should be both practical and practicable.

75. What does the passage mainly focus on in terms of services to immigrant families?

    A. How to establish an immigrant-friendly neighborhood.

    B. How to help immigrants enjoy available healthcare services.

    C. How to make an assessment of the existing healthcare services.

    D. How to assist caregivers in understanding immigrants' family influence.

Passage Four

This year marks the 100th anniversary of the deadliest event in U.S. history: the Spanish influenza epidemic of 1918. Although science and technology have advanced tremendously over the past century, the Pandemic peril remains; a recent exercise at the Johns Hopkins Center for Health Security showed that an epidemic of an influenza-like virus could kill 15 million Americans in a single year.

The medical community's response to this danger is, understandably, focused on research response — discovering new vaccines, therapeutics, and diagnostics and fighting ongoing epidemics, such as the current Ebola outbreak in Congo. But these urgent undertakings are not sufficient. If the world is to tackle many factors that raise our risk of a devastating pandemic, the medical community may have to enter theatres of operation beyond the laboratory bench and the treatment unit and publicly engage with controversial issues that some observers would consider nonmedical. Indeed, I believe that only such efforts can save us from the social trends, political movements, and policy failures that are elevating our risk of a pandemic. There are three aspects in particular where the medical community's intervention is urgently needed.

First is the rising tide of isolationism and xenophobia（排外）in many high-income nations, particularly the United States and European countries. The belief that isolating ourselves from the world can prevent the spread of diseases is irrational: we can build no wall high enough to keep out infectious diseases and disease-bearing vectors.

The second trend is the growing tide of antiscientific thinking and resistance to evidence-based medicine. In low-income countries, skepticism about vaccines is an everlasting challenge, but what we are seeing in the United States and Europe is something very different, and very dangerous. The growing refusal of parents in high-income countries to vaccinate their children is the tip of an iceberg that could sink us all in the event of an epidemic demanding rapid vaccine deployment and acceptance.

Finally, and perhaps most fundamentally, medical professionals can step into the public arena to take on unpleasant and contentious political issues such as climate change and isolationism. Many members of the medical community prefer to avoid becoming involved in controversial issues that seem to be outside the scope of medical concerns, but their voices are needed to confront such issues.

76. What does the author mainly do in the first paragraph?

    A. Warn the world against the upcoming influenza pandemic.

    B. Give credit to tremendous advances in science and technology.

    C. Remind the readers of the potential devastating pandemic perils.

    D. Reflect on the severity of the Spanish influenza epidemic of 1918.

77. To address the increasing risk of pandemics, the author suggests that the medical community _____.

    A. focus more on the urgent undertakings

    B. pay more attention to research and response

    C. make quicker response in fighting ongoing epidemics

    D. get more actively engaged with issues other than medical

78. According to Paragraph 3, what do the United States and European countries need to do to prevent infectious diseases and disease-bearing vectors?

    A. To build high walls.

    B. To maintain an open mentality.

C. To isolate themselves from each other.

D. To learn from other high-income nations.

79. What can be said of the second trend mentioned in Paragraph 4?

A. Skepticism about vaccines can be tackled easily.

B. Antiscientific thinking is not serious in low-income countries.

C. High-income countries should learn from low-income countries.

D. Parental resistance to vaccinating their children can be disastrous.

80. What can be inferred from the last paragraph?

A. Medical concerns are as controversial as nonmedical issues.

B. Medical professionals should be more concerned with medical issues.

C. More and more medical professionals are involved in controversial issues.

D. The medical community should play a more active role in controversial issues.

Passage Five

In medical terminology, the words history and physical almost always appear together in that order. As a physician, you do not engage a patient in the neurological examination until you've gathered the details of his or her debilitating headaches.

But at one time in our medical careers, we are instructed to perform the most thorough physical examination possible without learning so much as the patient's name. All we are given is an anatomy table number, an age, and a cause of death. We work our way through the anatomy lab — inspecting, searching, and feeling every muscle, bone, and organ — and we write our patients' histories ourselves.

To better understand the life of the woman who had donated her body for my education, I created the Obituary (讣告) Writing Program at Georgetown University during my first year of medical school. I worked with an obituary writer, Emily Langer, to develop a workshop to help interested medical students reflect on the lives that their corpses may have lived. She instructed us on the art of weaving disconnected memories into a single story. A series of creative writing prompts resulted in one student's story of a dramatic football injury occurring in the middle of a competitive match. This moment in his corpse's life was imagined from a pink prosthetic (假体的) hip beneath massive layers of muscle.

The first conversation with my donor's son lasted over an hour despite my initial fear that I would ask the wrong questions or offer the wrong words of sympathy. His mother was a small-town farm girl from Wisconsin. Dr. Carol Kennedy, Georgetown University School of Medicine, Class of 1972. She was a devout Catholic who considered being a physician a privilege and an opportunity to serve others. She wanted to continue to serve even after her death by donating her body to Georgetown University in order to educate future medical students like me.

We have finally put the history in its rightful place before the physical — students now interview the families of their donors before making the first cut in the anatomy lab. Our corpses are our first counterparts in the privileged patient-physician relationship, and now we are able to begin that partnership just as we hope to do throughout the rest of our medical careers.

81. The statement that "the words history and physical almost always appear together in that order" can be best interpreted as _____.

A. history taking is usually preceded by physical examination

B. history taking is usually taught before physical examination

C. history taking is usually overshadowed by physical examination

D. history taking is usually performed before physical examination

82. What is the teaching approach in the anatomy lab described in Paragraph 2?

A. Identifying the real cause of the patient's death.

B. Learning anatomy by taking patients' histories into account.

C. Training students how to do physical examination clinically.

D. Writing patients' histories based on the physical examination.

83. What can be said of the Obituary Writing Program created by the author at Georgetown University?

A. It helped students improve their writing skills.

B. It was aimed to arouse students' interest in anatomy.

C. It was a humane way of paying respect to body donors.

D. It was aimed to train the students' skills in physical examination.

84. What can be inferred from the information the author obtained about Dr. Carol Kennedy from his talk with her son?

A. She was born on a farm in the 1970s.

    B. She grew up in Georgetown as a devout Catholic.

    C. She was a graduate of the author's medical school.

    D. She donated her body as required by her religious belief.

85. Which of the following can be the best title of the passage?

    A. History Taking in the Anatomy Lab

    B. Writing Skills for Medical Students

    C. Dr. Carol Kennedy: a Devoted Georgetown Graduate

    D. Patient-physician Relationship: a Historical Review

Passage Six

There may be no better example of what is meant by preventive medicine than the strategy of Vaccination. A healthy person is given a tiny taste of a virus — flu or polio, say — that's too weak to cause illness but just enough to introduce the body to the pathogen. If the virus later shows up for real, the immune system is primed and waiting for it.

That's close to how a cancer vaccine works, but not precisely. Most experts see cancer vaccines as a hybrid of treatment and prevention. While it's true that the U. S. Food and Drug Administration has approved vaccines against cervical and liver cancer, both are designed to fight the viruses most responsible for causing the disease, as opposed to targeting cancer itself — human papilloma virus（HPV; 人乳头瘤病毒）in the case of cervical cancer and hepatitis B in the case of liver tumors.

Using vaccines to prevent nonviral cancers in someone who is disease-free is a whole different matter. For one thing, it's much more difficult to determine a person's chance of developing a particular type of cancer than it is to determine the likelihood of being exposed to, say, the influenza virus or chicken pox. What passes for "exposure" in the case of nonviral cancers is a combination of genes and environment and a range of other X factors that can vary from person to person. How do you vaccinate against your family legacy of breast cancer or your constant exposure to secondhand cigarette smoke?

But that doesn't mean the immune system can't be exploited in a different way. Cancer vaccines would ideally be used in patients whose disease has already been diagnosed and treated with surgery, chemotherapy or radiation. They would then be immunized as a way to prevent the cancer from coming back and spreading. Such metastases are actually the leading cause of death from cancer. "The charm of working with the immune system is that we can use the body's own defense mechanisms to possibly get to that last cancer cell or at least create a surveillance system that keeps that cancer under control," says an oncologist.

86. The first paragraph is meant to describe _____.

    A. the evolution of vaccination   B. the mechanism of vaccination

    C. the significance of vaccination   D. the popularization of vaccination

87. Which of the following is true of vaccines against cancer?

    A. They are both therapeutic and preventive.

    B. Vaccines against cervical cancer also work on liver cancer.

    C. Vaccines can replace other therapeutic modalities for cancer.

    D. They strictly follow the mechanism of traditional vaccination.

88. According to the passage, why is it difficult to use vaccines to prevent non-viral cancers?

    A. Because too many factors make it hard to determine the main causes.

    B. Because genetic makeup plays a dominant role in cancer development.

    C. Because the development of such vaccines requires enormous investment.

    D. Because literature is limited on the efficacy of vaccines for non-viral cancers.

89. From the context, what does the author suggest by saying "passes for 'exposure' "?

    A. The "exposure" in antiviral vaccination and anticancer vaccination is different.

    B. The "exposure" in cancer vaccination does not produce any long-term effect.

    C. "Exposure" is a useless concept when cancer is genetically-determined.

    D. Constant "exposure" to something may make the exposure ineffective.

90. We can conclude from the last paragraph that _____.

    A. vaccination is able to prevent the occurrence of cancer

    B. cancer vaccines may replace the conventional therapies

    C. cancer vaccines may control the cancer recurrences and metastases

    D. vaccination against cancer is possible in theory but almost impossible in reality

2020年全国医学博士外语统一考试英语试题（阅读部分）答案与解析

Passage One

61．D。主旨题。本文讲到脚部真菌感染的原因，除了种族、国籍、生活习惯等因素外，还有休闲场所里特殊的环境为真菌滋生提供了温床，足球运动员几乎全部中招。文末还提出，出于迷信原因，足球运动员会重复穿曾经进过球的鞋子，这加大了他们患病的概率。因此综合来看，D选项（足球运动员的脚部更容易感染真菌）是最佳选项。

62．C。排除题。Achilles Project出现在第二段首句，该项目调查了来自18个欧洲国家的76 475双脚，发现其中26%的样本有足部感染。文中并未提到这些脚均来自运动员，也没有提及如何避免真菌感染，而是在调查分析足部感染的各种因素。因此，排除A，B，D，正确答案为C。

63．B。细节题。文中讲到患Tinea pedis和 Onychomycosis的人数比例，以及不同国家患某些真菌感染的不同比例，可推断出的结论是Tinea pedis和 Onychomycosis是真菌感染的脚病，文中并未对二者的其他方面进行对比。

64．A。归纳题。从文中倒数第二段可知，休闲中心和游泳池是健身达人常去的地方，对这个人群的健康构成了潜在的威胁。从娱乐设施的检测可知，每平方米有1 500个被真菌感染的皮肤切片，这里是真菌的温床。因此A选项是正确答案：这些地方既给人们提供帮助（健身娱乐），也给人们带来危害（真菌感染相对严重）。其他三个选项明显与原文不符。

65．C。细节题。最后一段说："Dr. Caputo, a dermatologist, also found another factor: footballers are often reluctant, for superstitious reasons, to discard their old boots." 即运动员们出于迷信的原因，不愿意扔掉旧鞋。这里的迷信指：进过球的鞋子能带给他们好运。故本题正确答案为C。

Passage Two

66．D。细节题。第一段中是对照的行文结构：A decade ago…But in the past few years…，题干问的是trend（趋势），因此可判断But后为正确答案：患者被鼓励在门户网站上注册，以便随时获得records，故本题正确答案为D。

67. B。细节题。第二段讲到门户网站加速发展的原因：技术的广泛应用（embrace），医院因使用电子病历而获得奖励（incentive）、患者可直接获取检测结果的规定，只有B选项与原文背道而驰。

68. C。细节题。作者在第三段提出了疑问：门户网站是否兑现了让患者参与的承诺？或者这些结果是否过于频繁地使患者感到困惑和恐慌，并导致医生需要做更多工作，因为信息的提供没有足够的指导，有时甚至没有任何指导。C选项是最佳改写：医疗结果在传达给患者的时候没有得到正确充分的指导，即传达方式值得商榷。B选项是混淆项：作者质疑的是提供medical records的方式，而非使用portals的指导，不正确。

69. C。细节题。Dr. Treadway的丈夫因为胳膊疼痛在医院做MRI，她在丈夫的允许下，直接从医院电脑里获取了影像，结果显示她丈夫有巨大的肿瘤和转移性疾病，后来经过确认姓名和出生日期，发现该影像属于另一名患者（wrong patient）。在Treadway查看结果这个过程中，她的丈夫不知道自己的诊断结果，也并非是因为被确诊患癌后去做的扫描，而是医院搞错了患者和结果。故C选项是正确答案。

70. B。推理题。Dr. Treadway的经历正好印证了作者的担心：患者在没有得到正确指导的情况下直接获取医疗记录和检测结果所带来的潜在风险和令人不安的后果。A选项说违法使用门户网站的潜在风险，而文中作者并未谈及对门户网站使用的技术问题，该项是混淆项；C选项谈论信息传达方式的技术进步，与原文背道而驰；D选项说电话通知信息的优势，属于过度推理。B选项意为"举例说明通过门户网站向患者提供错误信息的潜在风险"，为正确答案。

Passage Three

71. B。细节题。第一段中讲到医疗保健从业者弗朗西斯卡·魏斯曼（Francesca Weissman）的两个担心，其中更重要的担心是：如何说服移民家庭去使用服务。由此可推理得知，移民家庭不愿意使用现成的医疗服务，而不是用不起或者无权使用。

72. B。细节题。第二段中提及："Unless the families can communicate with caregivers, they cannot begin to trust them. Without trust, they are not likely to seek or even accept assistance." 由此可推理得知，如果护理人员不能和移民家庭交流，无法建立相互之间的信任，移民家庭就不会接受帮助。而雇用会说客户本土语言的护理人员将大大降低种族障碍并减少潜在客户的怀疑，因此推理得知，语言是很大的障碍。

73. A。推理题。第三段讲到弗朗西斯卡意识到护理人员有义务熟悉移民的文化，了解他们原籍地的经济气候和其他条件，这些都有助于减少移民家庭的怀疑，提供更好的服务。A选项是最佳答案。B选项中的"缺乏信息和尊重"并不是存在于护理人员之间的一个普遍问题；C选项是个评价性和结论性的陈述，在该段没有提及；D选项说过分强调移民家庭的特殊情况是不合理的，与原文内容背道而驰，不正确。

74. D。细节题。文中最后一段讲到以家庭为导向的计划可以从关于社区的实用建议开始：杂货店的位置、在哪里申请食品券以及如何寻找工作，任何计划都必须在方便的时间和地点提供等，这些都可以推出正确答案为D"计划必须实际且实用"。

75. A。推理题。文中谈到如何为移民家庭提供健康保健服务，减少他们对现有社区管理者的怀疑，打消他们的疑虑，为他们提供切实可用的实际方案，这些都是为了打造immigrant-friendly的社区环境。虽然文中没有直接提及，但四个选项中"打造移民友好的社区""帮助移民使用现成的服务""评估现有医保体系""帮助护理人员理解移民家庭的影响"，只有A和B与原文相关，而A包含B的内容，故本题最佳答案为A。

Passage Four

76. C。细节题。第一段中谈到今年是西班牙大流感的一百周年，并提醒尽管科学技术在过去的一个世纪里取得了巨大进步，但流行病的危险仍然存在。因此C选项是正确答案。A选项"提醒全球防范即将到来的流感大流行"中，流感与原文中的influenza-like virus有区别，是混淆项。

77. D。细节题。第二段中说："But these urgent undertakings are not sufficient. If the World is to tackle many factors that raise our risk of a devastating pandemic, the medical community may have to…publicly engage with controversial issues that some observers would consider nonmedical." 即走出医院，参与有争议性的、非医学类的议题。因此D为原文的正确改写。

78. B。细节题。第三段讲到，高收入国家，尤其是美国和欧洲，总想着把自己和世界隔离开来。认为将自己与世界隔离开可以防止疾病传播的想法是不合理的，言外之意即需要保持开放的心态。

79. D。细节题。第四段讲到，低收入国家抵制疫苗是一个永恒的挑战，高收入国家对疫苗的抵制也日益高涨，且只是冰山一角。一旦疫情袭来，毫无抵抗之力。由此可推断出，D为正确选项。文中并未提及高收入国家是否应该向低收入国家学习，事实上，情况都很不乐观。

80. D。推理题。最后一段讲到最根本的一点，医学专家可以进入公共领域，需要他们的声音来面对这些问题（公共领域的非医学问题）。因此D为正确答案。C选项是混淆项：越来越多的医学专家参与有争议性的问题，are involved in表明是当下的状态，与原文中的prefer to avoid的现实状况不吻合。

Passage Five

81. D。细节题。第一段中讲到the words history and physical almost always appear together in that order，即先问病史，再做检查，这是惯常的顺序。D选项是正确的改写。A选项的意思是"检查在先，记录病史在后"，be preceded by意为"被……领先"，是混淆项。

82. D。细节题。第二段中讲到我们在解剖实验室工作，彻底地检查，然后我们自己编写患者的病史，即在为尸体做检查的基础上编写病史，与D选项的内容是一致的。

83. C。推理题。创建讣告写作计划是为了更好地理解尸体捐赠者的生平，而非为了提升学生的写作水平（A选项），也并非为了激发学生对解剖学的兴趣和训练他们检查身体的技能，更多是为了建立和解剖对象之间的合作伙伴关系。因此C选项是最佳答案。

84. C。细节题。Dr. Carol Kennedy在小镇农场长大，是Georgetown医学院1972级的学生，她去世后想继续为Georgetown医学院的学生（就像作者一样）服务。由此可判断C是正确答案。

85. A。主旨题。本文主要讲如何培养医学生与被解剖对象之间的伙伴关系，如何在解剖前去还原他的病历，并列举了Dr. Carol Kennedy的例子来说明这个过程。因此A选项是最佳答案。

Passage Six

86. B。主旨题。题干问的是第一段的主旨大意。由第二段第一句That's close to how a cancer vaccine works（与癌症疫苗的工作原理类似）可知，第一段讲的是疫苗的工作原理。

87. A。细节题。根据第二段中的Most experts see cancer vaccines as a hybrid of treatment and prevention可知，A选项（既是治疗性的，也是预防性的）是正确答案。

88. A。细节题。第三段中讲到在非病毒性癌症的情况下，所谓的"暴露"是基因和环境以及一系列其他未知因素的组合，这些因素可能因人而异。因此，用疫苗来做非病毒癌症的预防是比较困难的。

89. A。推理题。该段主题句为首句，大意是：使用疫苗来预防无病患者的非病毒性癌症大不相同。一方面，确定一个人患上特定类型癌症的机会比确定暴露于流感病毒或水痘病毒而患病的可能性要困难得多。虽说是"暴露"（在某种可能性或者病毒下），但实际是多种因素的组合。言下之意即"暴露"在非病毒疫苗和"暴露"在其他因素下是不同的。因此A选项是正确总结。

90. C。细节题。最后一段讲到：癌症疫苗最适用于已经通过手术、化学疗法或放射疗法诊断和治疗疾病的患者。然后他们将接受免疫接种，以防止癌症复发和扩散。因此C为正确选项。全文都在讲癌症疫苗很难用来防范正常人的非病毒性癌症患病的可能性，更无法代替传统的治疗方案，因此A，B，D都是错误选项。

武汉大学 2022 年博士研究生入学考试英语试题
（阅读部分）

Passage One

When Georgian judo champion David Khakaleshvili boarded a bus to go to his weigh-in at the Atlanta Games, he didn't expect the driver would get lost. By the time the defending gold medalist made it to the right venue, his Olympics were over. The competition at the 1996 Games may have been outstanding, but its transport system was not. Athletes and spectators missed events or were stranded for hours by a dysfunctional bus network, overcrowded trains and grid-locked city streets. The snafus received scathing notices in the international media. Sydney's Olympic organizers, on a fact-finding visit to the Games, came away convinced that the best transport network is the kind nobody talks about.

The task of coordinating the movement of people to and from venues during the 2000 Games falls to the Olympic Roads and Traffic Authority. Its "No. 1 priority is obviously the athletes", says corporate affairs director Paul Willoughby. "But there's no question that the media are a very important client group." While senior Games officials and V.I.P.s will get the limousine treatment, extra 3,800 buses have been organized to transport team and technical officials, sponsors, 10,200 athletes and 17,600 journalists.

Spectators and visitors to the city may find it tougher to get around. Transport is traditionally not Sydney's strong point: a sprawling city of 4 million people, it lacks a comprehensive subway system, time-saving ring roads or an easy-to-navigate street network. Homebush Bay, where competition in more than half of the 28 Olympic sports will take place, is 18km from the city center, and the remaining Games venues are dotted all over Sydney. For limousines and buses, ORTA is setting up a network of marked Olympic road routes, clear-ways and dedicated transit lanes. But with spectator parking outlawed at venues, and surrounding streets accessible only to local residents and Games officials, trains will be the main form of public transport for ticket holders. And they are already plagued by frequent breakdowns and delays. Says rail commuter Giselle Mawer: "It's going to be total bedlam. The system's barely coping now. It took my daughter two hours to get home from school last night, and it's only a few kilometers away."

With 31 million commuter trips—more than two and a half times the usual number—expected on Sydney's railways during the Games, ORTA cannot guarantee that there won't be problems or accidents, concedes Willoughby, "but we have a whole range of contingency plans in place if things go wrong," he says. Olympic Park Station, designed to handle 50,000 passengers an hour, has successfully coped with large-scale test events. But even if Sydney's Olympic transport network functions to plan, with up to 500,000 spectators expected at Homebush Bay on the busiest days of competition, 90-min waiting times at that station will be the norm, notes Willoughby.

Organizers are counting on the cooperation of Sydney-siders not attending the Games. In a frank message to residents while in town in April, I.O.C. vice-president and transport working group member Anta De Frantz urged them "not to use the transport system or the roads while the Games are on". While some locals would rather be anywhere else in September, few will be content to just sit at home. "That's never been ORTA's intention," says Willoughby. But if ORTA's plans go off the rails, the best view of the Olympics could be the one on a television screen.

16. ORTA is responsible for _____.

    A. making schedule of games

    B. building arenas for the Olympic sports

    C. picking up athletes from other cities to Sydney

    D. transporting people to and from places of Olympic competition

17. Which of the following details are NOT mentioned in the passage?

    A. 17,600 journalists will come to report the Games.

    B. Homebush Bay is 18km away from the city center.

    C. Limousines will be provided for some Games officials.

    D. There will be 10,200 athletes, technical officials and sponsors.

18. We may infer from Willoughby's words that he _____.

    A. is confident that the Sydney's Olympic Games will be a success

    B. is afraid that there might be commuting problems for the Games

C. cannot find solutions to the unexpected problems that might occur

D. wants Sydney residents to stay at home to watch games on TV

19. The underlined expression "go off the rails" means "_____".

    A. get off the train

    B. go to the wrong side of the tracks

    C. move away from the intended goal

    D. proceed smoothly as planned

20. The passage mainly aims at _____.

    A. criticizing ORTA's preparation work for the Olympic Games

    B. introducing public transportation system in Sydney

    C. revealing the problems concerning transport for the Olympic Games

    D. persuading local people not to use trains when the Games are on

Passage Two

I promised to work, but still bet that Jerry couldn't teach me to draw. I wanted very much to learn to draw, for a reason that I kept to myself: I wanted to convey an emotion I have about the beauty of the world. It's difficult to describe because it's an emotion. It's analogous to the feeling one has in religion that has to do with a god that controls everything in the universe: there's a generality aspect that you feel when you think about how things that appear so different and behave so differently are all run "behind the scenes" by the same organization, the same physical laws. It's an appreciation of the mathematical beauty of nature, of how she works inside; a realization that the phenomena we see result from the complexity of the inner workings between atoms; a feeling of how dramatic and wonderful it is. It's a feeling of awe—of scientific awe—which I felt could be communicated through a drawing to someone who had also had this emotion. It could remind him, for a moment, of this feeling about the glories of the universe.

Jerry turned out to be a very good teacher. He told me first to go home and draw anything. So I tried to draw a shoe; then I tried to draw a flower in a pot. It was a mess!

The next time we met I showed him my attempts. "Oh, look!" he said. "You see, around in back here, the line of the flower pot doesn't touch the leaf." (I had meant the line to come up to the leaf.) "That's very good. It's a way of showing depth. That's very clever of you."

"And the fact that you don't make all the lines the same thickness (which I didn't mean to do) is good. A drawing with all the lines the same thickness is dull." It continued like that: Everything that I thought was a mistake, he used to teach me something in a positive way. He never said it was wrong; he never put me down. So I kept trying, and I gradually got a little bit better, but I was never satisfied.

21. The underlined word "organization" in Paragraph 1 most nearly means "_____".

    A. corporation

    B. rules of physics

    C. social group

    D. arrangements of objects

22. Which of the following experiences is closest to what the author describes as "dramatic and wonderful"?

    A. Proving a physical law.

    B. Creating a beautiful sculpture.

    C. Seeing a masterful painting for the first time.

    D. Appreciating the power of physical laws in nature.

23. What assumption does the author make about the appreciation of art?

    A. It is rather difficult for a scientist.

    B. It comes only through the experience of creating art.

    C. It is not as important as the appreciation of science.

    D. It is enhanced by having experiences similar to those that inspired the artist.

24. The author suggests that the "way of showing depth" is actually _____.

    A. unintentional   B. unattractive

    C. impossible   D. easy to accomplish

25. In what way was the author "never satisfied"?

    A. He was never able to fully appreciate great art.

    B. He was unable to convey fully his feelings about the beauty of the world.

    C. He was not able to replicate his teacher's talent for appreciating his students.

    D. He was never able to draw a realistic flower pot.

Passage Three

The discovery of dinosaurs in the 19th century provided, or so it appeared, a quintessential case for the negative correlation of size and smarts. With their pea brains and giant bodies, dinosaurs became a symbol of lumbering stupidity. Their extinct seemed only to confirm their flawed design.

Dinosaurs were not even granted the usual solace of a giant—great physical prowess. Dinosaurs have usually been reconstructed as slow and clumsy. In the standard illustration, Brontosaurus wades in a murky pond because he cannot hold up his own weight on land.

Dinosaurs have been making a strong comeback, in this age of "I'm OK; You're OK." Most paleontologists are now willing to view them as energetic, active, and capable animals. The Brontosaurus that wallowed in its pond a generation ago is now running on land, while pairs of males have been seen twinning their necks about each other in elaborate sexual combat for access to females (much like the neck wrestling of giraffes). Modern anatomical reconstructions indicate strength and agility, and many paleontologists now believe that dinosaurs were warm-blooded.

The idea of warm-blooded dinosaurs has captured the public imagination and received a torrent of press coverage. Yet another vindication of dinosaurian capability has received very little attention, although I regard it as equally significant. I refer to the issue of stupidity and its correlation with size. The revisionist interpretation, which I support in this column, does not enshrine dinosaurs as paragons of intellect, but it does maintain that they were not small-brained after all. They had the "right-sized" brains for reptiles of their body size.

I don't wish to deny that the flattened, minuscule head of large-bodied Stegosaurus houses little brain from our subjective, top-heavy perspective, but I do wish to assert that we should not expect more of the beast. First of all, large animals have relatively smaller brains than related, small animals. The correlation of brain size with body size among kindred animals (all reptiles, all mammals for example) is remarkably regular. As we move from small to large animals, from mice to elephants or small lizards to Komodo dragons, brain size increases, but not so fast as body size. In other words, bodies grow faster than brains, and large animals have low ratios of brain weight to body weight. In fact, brains grow only about two-thirds as fast as bodies. Since we have no reason to believe that large animals are consistently stupider than their smaller relatives, we must conclude that large animals require relatively less brain to do as well as smaller animals. If we do not recognize this relationship, we are likely to underestimate the mental power of very large animals, dinosaurs in particular.

If behavioral complexity is one consequence of mental power, then we might expect to uncover among dinosaurs some signs of social behavior that demand coordination, cohesiveness and recognition. Indeed we do, and it cannot be accidental that these signs were overlooked when dinosaurs labored under the burden of a falsely imposed obtuseness. Multiple trackways have been uncovered, with evidence for more than twenty animals travelling together in parallel movement. Did some dinosaurs live in herds? At the Davenport Ranch sauropod trackway, smaller footprints lie in the center and larger ones at the periphery. Could it be that some dinosaurs travelled much as some advanced herbivorous mammals do today, with large adults at the borders sheltering juveniles in the center?

But the best illustration of dinosaurian capability may well be the fact most often cited against them — their demise.

The remarkable thing about dinosaurs is not that they became extinct, but that they dominated the earth for so long. Dinosaurs held sway for 100 million years while mammals, all the while, lived as small animals in the interstices of their world. After 70 million years on top, we mammals have an excellent track record and good prospects for the future, but we have yet to display the staying power of dinosaur.

People, on this criterion, are scarcely worth mentioning — 5 million years perhaps since Australopithecus, a mere 50,000 for our own species, Homo sapiens. Try the ultimate test within our system of values: Do you know anyone who would wager a substantial sum even at favorable odds on the proposition that Homo sapiens will last longer than Brontosaurus?

26. In the context of the passage as a whole, it is reasonable to infer that the underlined phrase in Paragraph 3 means that _____.

   A. the Brontosaurus evolved from living in the water to living on land

   B. scientists' understanding of the Brontosaurus's lifestyle has changed within the last generation

   C. standard illustrations of dinosaurs still inaccurately depict their lifestyles

   D. the Brontosaurus eventually learned to hold up its own weight on land

27. The passage suggests that some fossil evidence about dinosaur behavior has been overlooked in the past because scientists _____.

   A. had preconceived ideas about the intelligence of dinosaurs

   B. believed that mammals were not capable of social formations

C. did not have the current data about the dinosaur's brain size

D. did not have the necessary equipment to discover the social patterns of dinosaurs

28. What does the passage offer as evidence that dinosaurs may have exhibited complex behaviors?

A. Modern anatomical reconstructions indicating strength and agility.

B. Fossils revealing that dinosaurs labored under severe burdens.

C. Footprints of varying sizes indicating that dinosaurs travelled with advanced herbivorous mammals.

D. Multiple trackways in which footprint size and location indicate social order.

29. What does the author mean when he states in the last paragraph that "people...are scarcely worth mentioning"?

A. Compared to the complex social behavior of dinosaurs, human behavior seems simple.

B. Compared to the longevity of dinosaurs, humans have been on earth a very short time.

C. Compared to the size of dinosaurs, humans seem incredibly small.

D. Compared to the amount of study done on dinosaurs, study of human behavior is severely lacking.

30. According to the passage, what is the revisionist interpretation concerning the relationship between intelligence and physical size?

A. Dinosaurs actually had relatively large brains.

B. Dinosaurs were paragons of intellect.

C. Dinosaurs were relatively small-brained.

D. Dinosaurs' brains were appropriately sized.

31. What does the author suggest in Paragraph 5 when he states that Stegosaurus has a small brain from "our subjective, top-heavy perspective"?

A. Humans are unusually smart in their judgement of other species.

B. The human physical construction is deformed by the largeness of the scull.

C. It is unfair to judge other species by human standards.

D. Not all species have a brain as small relative to body weight as do humans.

32. The passage states that the ratio of brain weight to body weight in larger animals, as compared to smaller animals, is _____.

    A. higher   B. lower

    C. the same   D. overestimated

33. According to the passage, which of the following correctly stated the relationship of brain size to body size?

    A. The brain grows at two-thirds the rate of body growth.

    B. At maturity, the brain weighs an average of one-third of body weight.

    C. Large animals are not consistently less intelligent than smaller animals.

    D. Brain size is independent of body size.

34. The author states that the best illustration of dinosaurs' capability is their dominance of the earth for _____.

    A. 100,000 years   B. 5 million years

    C. 70 million years   D. 100 million years

35. As it is used in the last paragraph, the term Australopithecus most nearly means _____.

    A. the last of the dinosaurs, which became extinct 5 million years ago

    B. the first Homo sapiens, who appeared on earth 50,000 years ago

    C. an early version of humankind, but a different species

    D. a physically larger species of human with a much smaller brain

武汉大学2022年博士研究生入学考试英语试题 （阅读部分）答案与解析

Passage One

16. D。细节题。信息出现在文章第二段首句：在 2000 年奥运会期间，协调人员进出场馆的任务落在了奥林匹克道路交通管理局（ORTA）的肩上。选项 D"运送人员往返奥运比赛场地"与原文意思相符。故答案为 D。

17. D。推理题。选项 A，B，C 的信息分别与第二段中的 "While senior Games officials and V.I.P.s will get the limousine treatment, extra 3,800 buses have been organized to transport team and technical officials, sponsors, 10,200 athletes and 17,600 journalists." 和第三段中的 "Homebush Bay, where competition in more than half of the 28 Olympic sports will take place, is 18km from the city center…" 对应。由此可知，选项 D 中的数字 10,200 仅仅是运动员（athletes）的人数，而不是包含运动员、技术人员和赞助商的总人数，此项与原文不符。故答案为 D。

18. B。推理题。根据题干中的关键词 Willoughby 定位至第四段。第四段中提及："威洛比指出，但即使悉尼的奥运交通网络按计划运行，在比赛最繁忙的日子里，霍姆布什湾 (Homebush Bay) 预计将有多达 50 万名观众，在那个车站等待 90 分钟将是常态。" 由此可知，Willoughby 担心奥运会期间因人流太大带来的交通问题。选项 B 符合文意。故答案为 B。

19. C。词义题。画线词组出现的语境是文章最后一段最后一句话。最后一段提出国际奥委会副主席号召人们在比赛期间不要占用交通系统，但是当地居民不会只待在家中。因此，文章最后提及如果 ORTA's plans go off the rails，导致的结果是观看奥运会的最佳视角可能是电视屏幕，言外之意是人们只能待在家里观看奥运会的比赛。由此可推知，这里所说的意外情况是 "ORTA 的计划偏离预期"。结合选项可知，选项 C "偏离预期目标" 符合文意。故答案为 C。

20. C。主旨题。文章首段提及亚特兰大奥运会很出色，但城市的交通系统却并非如此。（The competition at the 1996 Games may have been outstanding, but its transport system was not.）随后进一步说明悉尼为 2000 年奥运会期间顺利运送运动员往返比赛场地制订的计划（ORTA's plan），随后指出该计划可能存在的问题。由此可知，本文主要是关于奥运会的交通问题。选项 C 与文意相符。故答案为 C。

Passage Two

21. B。词义题。画线单词出现的语境为：…there's a generality aspect that you feel…by the same organization, the same physical laws. 句意：当你思考看似不同、行为迥异的事物都由同一个组织、同一套物理法则 "幕后" 运作时，你会感受到一种普遍性。分析句子可知，the same physical laws 是对 organization 的解释，选项 B 为同义替换，故答案为 B。

22. D。推理题。dramatic and wonderful 出现的语境为：It's an appreciation of the mathematical beauty of nature…a feeling of how dramatic and wonderful it is. 分析句子可知，句子的前面部分是对 a feeling of how dramatic and wonderful it is 的解释。句意：这是对大自然数学之美的欣赏，是对它内在运作方式的欣赏；我们所看到的现象是由原子间内部运作

的复杂性引起的，你会感到它是多么戏剧化和美妙。选项 D"欣赏自然界物理规律的力量"与文意相符，作者在感叹和赞美大自然的规律和力量。故答案为 D。

23．B。推理题。作者在第一段主要说明了他对自然科学力量和运行规则的赞美，并在段末说明了可以通过绘画传递这种情感。第二段提及老师 Jerry 建议他回家先画出来，之后作者尝试着去绘画。由此可推知，作者认为对艺术的欣赏源于创造艺术的体验，选项 B 与文意相符。故答案为 B。

24．A。推理题。文中第三段提及：Jerry 评价作者的画时说"花盆的线条没有碰到叶子"，并称赞这是一种显示深度的方式，但实际上作者本来是要把线条延伸到叶子上的。由此可知，这种表示深度的方式实际上是作者的无意之举。可知选项 A 符合文意。故答案为 A。

25．B。推理题。文章第一段说作者想要通过绘画表现对大自然的赞美之情，并且说自己之后一直在努力，但从不满足，由此可推知，作者不满足的是没有充分表达赞美之情。选项 B 符合文意。故答案为 B。

Passage Three

26．B。推理题。画线部分语境为：大多数古生物学家现在都愿意将它们视为精力充沛、活跃的动物和有能力的动物。一代前被认为在池塘里打滚的雷龙现在在陆地上奔跑。由此可推知，古生物学家关于恐龙生活方式的理解在过去一代中发生了变化。选项 B 与文意相符。故答案为 B。

27．A。推理题。根据题干信息定位至第六段。段首提及：If behavioral complexity is one consequence of mental power, then we might expect to uncover among dinosaurs some signs of social behavior that demand coordination, cohesiveness and recognition. Indeed we do, and it cannot be accidental that these signs were overlooked when dinosaurs labored under the burden of a falsely imposed obtuseness. 句意：如果行为复杂性是脑力的一个结果，那么我们可能希望在恐龙群体中发现一些需要协调、凝聚力和认可的社会行为迹象。事实上，我们确实发现了，当恐龙在错误强加的迟钝负担下活动时，这些迹象被忽视并不是偶然的。根据此处信息可知，这些迹象被忽略的原因在于 when dinosaurs labored under the burden of a falsely imposed obtuseness，也就是说，人们误认为那些需要协调、凝聚力的社会行为迹象是恐龙身材庞大却头脑愚笨的结果。文章第五段末也指出了这一观点：由于我们没有理由相信大型动物总是比它们的小型亲属更笨，我们必须得出结论，大型动物需要较少的大脑就能做得和小型动物一样好。如果我们没有认识到这种关系，我们很可能会低估非常大的动物（特别是恐龙）的脑力。根据以上信息可以推断出，过去，一些关于恐龙行为的化石证据被忽视了，这是因为科学家们对恐龙的智力有先入为主的想法。选项 A 符合文意。故答案为 A。

28. D。细节题。根据题干关键词 complex behaviors 定位至第六段。第六段段首说明恐龙的一些社会行为恰恰说明了恐龙的智慧。之后又进一步举例说明。已经发现了多处行迹，有证据表明有 20 多只动物在平行移动。有些恐龙是群居的吗？在达文波特牧场蜥脚类恐龙行迹中，较小的足迹位于中心，较大的足迹位于外围。是否有些恐龙像今天的一些高级食草哺乳动物一样活动，大型成年恐龙在边缘保护中间的幼崽？选项 D 与文意相符。故答案为 D。

29. B。推理题。根据题干定位至最后一段。很明显，此段段首是将人类与恐龙对比。在上一段中，作者提及，恐龙统治了地球一亿年，而哺乳动物则一直以小型动物的身份生活在世界的缝隙中。之后末段提及，按照这个标准，人类几乎不值得一提——也许从南方古猿开始算起距今才 500 万年，我们自己的物种——智人距今只有 5 万年。由此可知，作者是在将人类的短暂历史与恐龙的漫长历史做比较。故答案为 B。

30. D。细节题。根据题干定位至第四段。此段中对 revisionist interpretation 做了解释：The revisionist interpretation, which I support in this column, does not enshrine dinosaurs as paragons of intellect, but it does maintain that they were not small-brained after all. They had the "right-sized" brains for reptiles of their body size. 由此可知，恐龙的大脑 "大小合适"，是适合它们的身型的。选项 D 符合文意。故答案为 D。

31. C。推理题。根据题干定位至第五段：I don't wish to deny that the flattened, minuscule head of large-bodied Stegosaurus houses little brain from our subjective, top-heavy perspective, but I do wish to assert that we should not expect more of the beast. 由此可知，作者不想否认，从我们主观的、头重脚轻的角度来看，大型剑龙扁平的小脑袋里几乎没有大脑，但作者确实想断言，我们不应该对这种动物期望过高。由此可推知，作者认为用人类的标准来评判其他物种是不公平的。故答案为 C。

32. B。细节题。第五段提出 large animals have low ratios of brain weight to body weight（大型动物的大脑重量与体重的比率较低）。由此可知，与小型动物相比，大型动物的大脑重量与体重之比要低一些。故答案为 B。

33. A。细节题。文章第五段提及：In fact, brains grow only about two-thirds as fast as bodies. 由此可知，选项 A 与原文信息一致。

34. D。细节题。本题主要考查数字。根据题干和数字选项定位至倒数第二段。此段中提及 Dinosaurs held sway for 100 million years。故答案为 D。

35. C。推理题。根据题干定位至最后一段。此段中提及人类起源于500万年前的南方古猿（Australopithecus），由此可知，南方古猿是早期人类的一支。随后又提及我们现代人人种——智人（Homo sapiens）—— 仅有5万年的历史。由此推知，南方古猿（Australopithecus）是不同于我们现代人人种的人类物种。选项C符合文意。故答案为C。

武汉大学2019年博士研究生入学考试英语试题（阅读部分）

Passage One

One of the most intriguing stories of the Russian Revolution concerns the identity of Anastasia, the youngest daughter of Czar Nicholas II. During his reign over Russia, the Czar had planned to revoke many of the harsh laws established by previous czars. Some workers and peasants, however, clamored for more rapid social reform. In 1918, a group of these people known as Bolsheviks overthrew the government. On July 17 or 18, they murdered the Czar and what was thought to be his entire family.

Although witnesses vouched that all the members of the Czar's family had been executed, there were rumors suggesting that Anastasia had survived. Over the years, a number of women claimed to be Grand Duchess Anastasia. Perhaps the most famous claimant was Anastasia Tschaikovsky, who was also known as Anna Anderson.

In 1920, 18 months after the Czar's execution, this terrified young woman was rescued from drowning in a Berlin river. She spent two years in a hospital, where she attempted to reclaim her health and shattered mind. The doctors and nurses thought that she resembled Anastasia and questioned her about her background. She disclaimed any connection with the Czar's family. Eight years later, however, she claimed that she was Anastasia. She said that she had been rescued by two Russian soldiers after the czar and the rest of her family had been killed. Two brothers named Tschaikovsky had carried her into Romania. She had married one of the brothers, who had taken her to Berlin and left her there, penniless and without a vocation. Unable to invoke the aid of her mother's family in Germany, she had tried to drown herself.

During the next few years, scores of the czar's relatives, ex-servants, and acquaintances interviewed her. Many of these people said that her looks and mannerisms were evocative of the Anastasia that they had known. Her grandmother and other relatives denied that she was the real Anastasia, however.

Tired of being accused of fraud, Anastasia immigrated to the United States in 1928 and took the name Anna Anderson. She still wished to prove that she was Anastasia, though, and returned to Germany in 1933 to bring suit against her mother's family. There she declaimed to the court, asserting that she was indeed Anastasia and deserved her inheritance.

In 1957, the court decided that it could neither confirm nor deny Anastasia's identity. Although it will probably never be known whether this woman was the Grand Duchess Anastasia, her search to establish her identity has been the subject of numerous books, plays, and movies.

1. Some Russian peasants and workers _____ for social reform.

   A. longed   B. cried out

   C. begged   D. hoped

2. Witnesses _____ that all members of the czar's family had been executed.

   A. gave assurance   B. thought

   C. hoped   D. convinced some

3. Tschaikovsky initially _____ any connection with the czar's family.

   A. denied   B. stopped

   C. noted   D. justified

4. In court she _____ maintaining that she was Anastasia and deserved her inheritance.

   A. finally appeared   B. spoke forcefully

   C. gave testimony   D. gave evidence

Passage Two

The victory of the small Greek democracy of Athens over the mighty Persian empire in 490 B. C. is one of the most famous events in history. Darius, king of the Persian Empire, was furious because Athens had interceded for the other Greek city-states in revolt against Persian domination. In anger the king sent an enormous army to defeat Athens. He thought it would take drastic steps to pacify the rebellious part of the empire.

Persia was ruled by one man. In Athens, however, all citizens helped to rule. Ennobled by this participation, Athenians were prepared to die for their city-state. Perhaps this was the secret of the remarkable victory at Marathon, which freed them from Persian rule. On their way to Marathon, the Persians tried to fool some Greek city-states by claiming to have come in peace. The frightened citizens of Delos refused to believe this. Not wanting to abet the conquest of Greece, they fled from their city and did not return until the Persians had left. They were wise, for the Persians next conquered the city of Eritrea and captured its people.

Tiny Athens stood alone against Persia. The Athenian people went to their sanctuaries. There they prayed for deliverance. They asked their gods to expedite their victory. The Athenians refurbished their weapons and moved to the plain of Marathon, where their little band would meet the Persians. At the last moment, soldiers from Plataea reinforced the Athenian troops.

The Athenian army attacked, and Greek citizens fought bravely. The power of the mighty Persians was offset by the love that the Athenians had for their city. Athenians defeated the Persians in both archery and hand combat. Greek soldiers seized Persian ships and burned them, and the Persians fled in terror, Herodotus, a famous historian, reports that 6,400 Persians died, compared with only 192 Athenians.

5. Athens had _____ the other Greek city-states against the Persians.

    A. refused help to   B. intervened on behalf of

    C. wanted to fight   D. defeated

6. Darius took drastic steps to _____ the rebellious Athenians.

    A. weaken   B. destroy   C. calm   D. irritate

7. The people of Delos did not want to _____ the conquest of Greece.

    A. end   B. encourage

    C. think about   D. daydream about

8. The Athenians were _____ by some soldiers who arrived from Plataea.

    A. welcomed   B. strengthened   C. held   D. captured

Passage Three

Conflict had existed between Spain and England since the 1570s. England wanted a share of the wealth that Spain had been taking from the lands it had claimed in the Americas.

Elizabeth I, Queen of England, encouraged her staunch admiral of the navy, Sir Francis Drake, to raid Spanish ships and towns. Though these raids were on a small scale, Drake achieved dramatic success, adding gold and silver to England's treasury and diminishing Spain's supremacy.

Religious differences also caused conflict between the two countries. Whereas Spain was Roman Catholic, most of England had become Protestant, King Philip II of Spain wanted to claim the throne and make England a Catholic country again. To satisfy his ambition and also to retaliate against England's theft of his gold and silver, King Philip began to build his fleet of warships, the Spanish Armada, in January 1586.

Philip intended his fleet to be indestructible. In addition to building new warships, he marshaled 130 sailing vessels of all types and recruited more than 19,000 robust soldiers and 8,000 sailors. Although some of his ships lacked guns and others lacked ammunition, Philip was convinced that his Armada could withstand any battle with England.

The martial Armada set sail from Lisbon, Portugal, on May 9, 1588, but bad weather forced it back to port. The voyage resumed on July 22 after the weather became more stable.

The Spanish fleet met the smaller, faster, and more maneuverable English ships in battle off the coast of Plymouth, England, first on July 31 and again on August 2. The two battles left Spain vulnerable, having lost several ships and with its ammunition depleted. On August 7, while the Armada lay at anchor on the French side of the Strait of Dover. England sent eight burning ships into the midst of the Spanish fleet to set it on fire. Blocked on one side, the Spanish ships could only drift away, their crews in panic and disorder. Before the Armada could regroup, the English attacked again on August 8.

Although the Spaniards made a valiant effort to fight back, the fleet suffered extensive damage. During the eight hours of battle, the Armada drifted perilously close to the rocky coastline. At the moment when it seemed that the Spanish ships would be driven onto the English shore, the wind shifted, and the Armada drifted out into the North Sea. The Spaniards recognized the superiority of the English fleet and returned home, defeated.

9. Sir Francis Drake added wealth to the treasury and diminished Spain's _____.

    A. unlimited power   B. unrestricted growth

    C. territory   D. treaties

10. King Philip recruited many _____ soldiers and sailors.

    A. warlike   B. strong

    C. accomplished   D. timid

11. The two battles left the Spanish fleet _____.

    A. open to change   B. triumphant

C. open to attack   D. defeated

12. The Armada was _____ on one side.

A. closed off   B. damaged

C. alone   D. circled

Passage Four

Mount Vesuvius, a volcano located between the ancient Italian cities of Pompeii and Herculaneum, has received much attention because of its frequent and destructive eruptions. The most famous of these eruptions occurred in A.D. 79.

The volcano had been inactive for centuries. There was little warning of the coming eruption, although one account unearthed by archaeologists says that a hard rain and a strong wind had disturbed the celestial calm during the preceding night. Early the next morning, the volcano poured a huge river of molten rock down upon Herculaneum, completely burying the city and filling the harbor with coagulated lava.

Meanwhile, on the other side of the mountain, cinders, stones and ashes rained down on Pompeii. Sparks from the burning ash ignited the combustible rooftops quickly. Large portions of the city were destroyed in the conflagration. Fire, however, was not the only cause of destruction. Poisonous sulphuric gases saturated the air. These heavy gases were not buoyant in the atmosphere and therefore sank toward the earth and suffocated people.

Over the years, excavations of Pompeii and Herculaneum have revealed a great deal about the behavior of the volcano. By analyzing data, much as a zoologist dissects an animal specimen, scientists have concluded that the eruption changed large portions of the area's geography. For instance, it turned the Sarno River from its course and raised the level of the beach along the Bay of Naples. Meteorologists studying these events have also concluded that Vesuvius caused a huge tidal wave that affected the world's climate.

In addition to making these investigations, archaeologists have been able to study the skeletons of victims by using distilled water to wash away the volcanic ash. By strengthening the brittle bones with acrylic paint, scientists have been able to examine the skeletons and draw conclusions about the diet and habits of the residents. Finally, the excavations at both Pompeii and Herculaneum have yielded many examples of classical art, such as jewelry made of bronze, which is an alloy of copper and tin. The eruption of Mount Vesuvius and its tragic consequences have provided everyone with a wealth of data about the effects that volcanoes can have on the surrounding area. Today volcanologists can locate and predict eruptions, saving lives and preventing the destruction of other cities and cultures.

13. Herculaneum and its harbor were buried under _____ lava.

    A. liquid   B. solid

    C. flowing   D. gas

14. The poisonous gases were not _____ in the air.

    A. able to float   B. visible

    C. able to evaporate   D. invisible

15. Scientists analyzed data about Vesuvius in the same way that a zoologist _____ a specimen.

    A. describes in detail

    B. studies by cutting apart

    C. photographs

    D. charts

16. _____ have concluded that the volcanic eruption caused a tidal wave.

    A. Scientists who study oceans

    B. Scientists who study atmospheric conditions

    C. Scientists who study ash

    D. Scientists who study animal behavior

Passage Five

Normally a student must attend a certain number of courses in order to graduate, and each course which he attends gives him a credit which he may count towards a degree. In many American universities the total work for a degree consists of thirty-six courses each lasting for one semester. A typical course consists of three classes per week for fifteen weeks; while attending a university a student will probably attend four or five courses during each semester. Normally a student would expect to take four years attending two semesters each year. It is possible to spread the period of work for the degree over a longer period. It is also possible for a student to move between one university and another during his degree course, though this is not in fact done as a regular practice.

For every course that he follows a student is given a grade, which is recorded, and the record is available for the student to show to prospective employers. All this imposes a constant pressure and strain of work, but in spite of this some students still find time for great activity in student affairs. Elections to position in student organizations arouse much enthusiasm. The effective work of main-training discipline is usually performed by students who advise the academic authorities. Any student who is thought to have broken the rules, for example, by cheating has to appear before a student court. With the enormous number of students, the operation of the system does involve a certain amount of activity. A student who has held one of these positions of authority is much respected and it will be of benefit to him later in his career.

17. According to the first paragraph an American student is allowed _____.

    A. to live in a different university

    B. to take a particular course in a different university

    C. to live at home and drive to classes

    D. to get two degrees from two different universities

18. American university students are usually under pressure of work because _____.

    A. their academic performance will affect their future careers

    B. they are heavily involved in student affairs

    C. they have to observe university discipline

    D. they want to run for positions of authority

19. Some students are enthusiastic for positions in student organizations probably because _____.

    A. they hate the constant pressure and strain of their study

    B. they will then be able to stay longer in the university

    C. such positions help them get better jobs

    D. such positions are usually well paid

20. The student organizations seem to be effective in _____.

    A. dealing with the academic affairs of the university

    B. ensuring that the students observe university regulations

    C. evaluating students' performance by bringing them before a court

    D. keeping up the students' enthusiasm for social activities

武汉大学2019年博士研究生入学考试英语试题
（阅读部分）答案与解析

Passage One

1. A。事实细节题。文中首段第三句提及："Some workers and peasants，however，clamored for more rapid social reform." 即但有些工农群众要求加快社会改革。选项A中的longed是文中clamored的同义替换。故答案为A。

2. B。事实细节题。文章第一段末句 "On July 17 or 18，they murdered the czar and what was thought to be his entire family." 提及，布尔什维克的人杀死了沙皇以及他们认为的沙皇全家人。第二段首句也提到："Although witnesses vouched that all the members of the czar's family had been executed，there were rumors suggesting that Anastasia had survived." 即尽管目击者证明沙皇家族的所有成员都已被处决，但有传闻称，阿纳斯塔西娅（Anastasia）幸免于难，由此可知，目击者只是自己认为沙皇全家已经被杀死了。故答案为B。

3. A。事实细节题。文章第三段 "The doctors and nurses thought that she resembled Anastasia and questioned her about her background. She disclaimed any connection with the czar's family." 提及，医生和护士认为她长得很像阿纳斯塔西娅（Anastasia），于是询问她的背景。但是她否认与沙皇家族有任何联系。denied "否认" 与文中disclaimed "拒绝承认" 为同义转换。故答案为A。

4. B。事实细节题。文章倒数第二段 "There she declaimed to the court，asserting that she was indeed Anastasia and deserved her inheritance." 中的asserting "明确肯定；断言" 与spoke forcefully为同义转换。故答案为B。

Passage Two

5. B。事实细节题。文章首段 "Darius，king of the Persian Empire，was furious because Athens had interceded for the other Greek city-states in revolt against Persian domination." 中提及波斯帝国的国王大流士非常愤怒，因为雅典为那些反抗波斯统治的其他希腊城邦求情。文中interceded for与选项B中的intervened on behalf of为同义转换。故答案为B。

6. C。事实细节题。见文章第一段最后一句，"He thought it would take drastic steps

to pacify the rebellious part of the empire." 即他认为需要采取激烈的措施来平息帝国内部的叛乱。文中pacify意为"在（有战争的地区、国家等）实现和平"，选项中只有calm与文意相符。故答案为C。

7. B。事实细节题。第二段"Not wanting to abet the conquest of Greece, they fled from their city and did not return until the Persians had left."中abet意为"教唆；唆使；煽动；怂恿"，其英文释义为：to help or encourage sb. to do sth. wrong，B选项encourage符合词义。故答案为B。

8. B。事实细节题。第三段"At the last moment, soldiers from Plataea reinforced the Athenian troops."中reinforced意为"加强；给……加强力量（或装备）；使更强大"，与strengthened意思相同，故答案为B。

Passage Three

9. A。事实细节题。第二段末句"Drake achieved dramatic success, adding gold and silver to England's treasury and diminishing Spain's supremacy."中supremacy表示"霸权"，四个选项中只有A选项unlimited power与supremacy意思相近，其他选项，unrestricted growth"无限制增长"、territory"领土，版图"和treaties"条约，协定"均不符合原文词义。故答案为A。

10. B。事实细节题。第四段"he marshaled 130 sailing vessels of all types and recruited more than 19,000 robust soldiers and 8,000 sailors"中提及King Philip征募了1万9千多名精壮的士兵和8千多名水手。文中robust"强健的；强壮的；结实的"与strong意思一致。故答案为B。

11. C。事实细节题。第六段"The two battles left Spain vulnerable, having lost several ships and with its ammunition depleted."中vulnerable表示"易受……伤害的"。本句意为：这两场战役让西班牙变得不堪一击，损失了几艘船，弹药也耗尽了。选项中open to attack表示"易受攻击的"，符合文意。故答案为C。

12. A。事实细节题。信息出现在第六段"Blocked on one side, the Spanish ships could only drift away, their crews in panic and disorder."中，句中提及西班牙战舰（Armada号）被封锁（blocked）在一边，与blocked意思相近的是closed off"堵塞（路口等）"。故答案为A。

Passage Four

13. A。信息推断题。第二段末句"Early the next morning, the volcano poured a huge

river of molten rock...filling the harbor with coagulated lava." 提及，第二天清晨，火山喷发出一条巨大的熔岩河，将赫库兰尼姆这座城市完全掩埋，凝固的熔岩填满了港口。由句中的a huge river of molten rock可知，赫库兰尼姆和港口被熔岩掩埋，选项中liquid "液体" 与文中的river信息对应。故答案为A。

14．A。事实细节题。第三段末句 "These heavy gases were not buoyant in the atmosphere and therefore sank toward the earth and suffocated people." 中提及，重气体（heavy gases）、不易浮（not buoyant）。able to float "能够飘浮的" 符合文意。故答案为A。

15．B。信息推断题。第四段 "By analyzing data...scientists have concluded that the eruption changed large portions of the area's geography." 中提及，科学家们分析数据就像动物学家解剖动物标本一样。根据常识，animal specimen "动物标本" 就是将动物切片研究，选项B "切分研究" 与文意相符。故答案为B。

16．B。事实细节题。由第四段末句 "Meteorologists studying these events have also concluded that Vesuvius caused a huge tidal wave that affected the world's climate." 可知，研究这些事件的气象学家还得出结论，维苏威火山喷发引起了巨大的潮汐波，影响了世界气候。根据文中关键词tidal wave和climate可知，meteorologists指的是 "气象学家"，选项B "研究气候现象的科学家" 与文意相符。故答案为B。

Passage Five

17．B。事实细节题。文章首段最后一句 "It is also possible for a student to move between one university and another... as a regular practice." 提到，学生在攻读学位期间可以在两所不同的学校上课，选项B "在一所不同的学校学习一门特殊的课程" 与文意相符。选项A和C在原文中未提及，选项D中提到获得两个学位（two degrees），而原文只是说在不同的学校上课，并非在不同的学校都获得学位。故答案为B。

18．A。事实细节题。文章第二段第二句中的all this指的是前一句提到的学生所修的每一门课的成绩都会被记录下来，给未来的雇主看，即这将影响他们将来的就业（For every course that he follows a student is given a grade, which is recorded, and the record is available for the student to show to prospective employers.），选项A与文意相符。选项B "积极参与学生事务"、选项C "遵守校方纪律" 均与题干问题无关；选项D文中并未提及。故答案为A。

19．C。信息推断题。文章最后一段末句 "A student who has held one of these positions of authority is much respected and it will be of benefit to him later in his career." 指出，担任过领导职位的学生很受人尊敬，对他将来的职业生涯也很有利。由此可知，担任过领导职位的学生将来会找到更好的工作，选项C与文意相符。故答案为C。

20．B。信息推断题。文章第二段 "The effective work of main-training discipline is usually performed by students... involve a certain amount of activity." 中提及维持纪律的有效工作通常由向学术当局提供建议的学生来完成。任何被认为违反规定的学生，例如作弊，都必须出庭受审。由于学生人数众多，系统的运行确实涉及一定的活动。由此可知，学生组织在维持学校纪律方面起到了一定的作用。选项B中的observe university regulations "遵守学校规定" 与文中的maintain discipline信息对应。故答案为B。

复旦大学2018年博士研究生入学考试英语试题（阅读部分）

Passage One

Child prodigies evoke awe, wonder and sometimes jealousy: how can such young children display the kinds of musical or mathematical talents that most adults will never master, even with years of dedicated practice? Lucky for these despairing types, the prevailing wisdom suggests that such comparisons are unfair—prodigies are born, not made (mostly). Practice alone isn't going to turn out the next 6-year-old Mozart.

So finds a recent study of eight young prodigies, which sought to shed some light on the roots of their talent. The prodigies included in the study are all famous, having achieved acclaim and professional status in their fields by the ripe age of 10. All of the prodigies had stories of remarkable early abilities.

The study found a few key characteristics these youngsters had in common. For one, they all had exceptional working memories—the system that holds information active in the mind, keeping it available for further processing. Working memory isn't just the ability to remember long strings of numbers. It is the ability to hold and process quantities of information, both verbal and non-verbal—such as, say, memorizing a musical score and rewriting it in your head. All the children in the study scored off the charts when tested on measures of working memory: they placed in at least the 99th percentile, with most in the 99.9th percentile.

Surprisingly, however, the study found that not all of the prodigies had high IQs. Indeed, while they had higher-than-average intelligence, some didn't have IQs that were as elevated as their performance and early achievements would suggest. One child had an IQ of just 108, at the high end of normal.

There was something else striking too. The authors found that prodigies scored high in autistic traits, most notably in their ferocious attention to detail. They scored even higher on this trait than did people diagnosed with Asperger's syndrome, a high-functioning form of autism that typically includes obsession with details. Three of the eight prodigies had a diagnosed autism spectrum disorder themselves. What's more, four of the eight families included in the study reported autism diagnoses in first- or second-degree relatives, and three of these families reported a total of 11 close relatives with autism. In the general population, by contrast, about 1 in 88 people have either autism or Asperger's.

Yet, despite the obvious similarities, very little research has been done on the connection between autism and extreme talent. One previous study, published in 2007, did find that close relatives of prodigies—like close relatives of people with autism—tended to score higher on autistic traits, particularly in problems with social skills, difficulty switching attention and intense attention to detail. Other than that, however, the issue hasn't been studied systematically, beyond the observation that autism is often seen in savants, or people with exceptional abilities who have other simultaneous impairments.

Prodigies, in contrast, appear to benefit from certain autistic tendencies while avoiding the shortfalls of others. On a standard assessment of traits associated with autism, the prodigies in the current study scored higher than a control group on all measures, including attention to detail and problems with social skills or communication. Comparing these children with those who have full-blown autism or Asperger's could therefore potentially help pinpoint what goes wrong in those who develop disabling forms of autism and what goes right in others with similar traits who simply benefit from enhanced abilities.

The current study is a small one, and much more research needs to be done to elucidate the connections between highly gifted children and those with autism spectrum conditions. But the findings strongly suggest that such connections exist.

1. According to Paragraph 1, what is the common idea towards child prodigies?

    A. They are not created.

    B. Practice can create child prodigies.

    C. They must be created.

    D. Musical child prodigies are created within several years.

2. Which of the following is TRUE according to the recent study?

   A. All the child prodigies don't have high IQs.

   B. All the child prodigies don't have IQs.

   C. All the child prodigies have autism at the same time.

   D. Child prodigies come into being after a good education.

3. What can we learn from Paragraph 5?

   A. All these eight prodigies are diagnosed with autism.

   B. Prodigies are more likely to suffer from autism than the ordinary people.

   C. Children diagnosed with autism are likely to become a prodigy.

   D. Child prodigies are those with autism having something in common.

4. What is the main idea of the passage?

   A. What do talent and autism have in common?

   B. What are the characteristics of talent?

   C. What are the findings about a mental disease called autism?

   D. What is autism?

5. Such a passage is most likely to be found in _____.

   A. a business magazine

   B. a newspaper

   C. a sports program on TV

   D. the science column of a magazine

Passage Two

Whenever you see an old film, even one made as little as ten years ago, you cannot help being struck by the appearance of the women taking part. Their hair-styles and make-up look outdated; their skirts look either too long or too short; their general appearance is, in fact, slightly **ludicrous**. The men taking part in the film, on the other hand, are clearly recognizable. There is nothing about their appearance to suggest that they belong to an entirely different age.

This illusion is created by changing fashions. Over the year, the great majority of men have successfully resisted all attempts to make them change their style of dress. The same cannot be said for women. Each year a few so-called top designers in Paris or London lay down the law and women the whole world over rush to obey. The decrees of the designers are unpredictable and dictatorial. This year, they decide in their arbitrary fashion, skirts will be short and waists will be high; zips are in and buttons are out. Next year the law is reversed and far from taking exception, no one is even mildly surprised.

If women are mercilessly exploited year after year, they have only themselves to blame. Because they shudder at the thought of being seen in public in clothes that are out of fashion, they are annually black-mailed by the designers and the big stores. Clothes, which have been worn, only a few times have to be discarded because of the dictates of fashion. When you come to think of it, only a woman is capable of standing in front of a wardrobe packed full of clothes and announcing sadly that she has nothing to wear.

Changing fashions are nothing more than the deliberate creation of waste. Many women squander vast sums of money each year to replace clothes that have hardly been worn. Women, who cannot afford to discard clothing in this way, waste hours of their time altering the dresses they have. Hem-lines are taken up or let down; waist-lines are taken in or let out; neck-lines are lowered or raised, and so on.

No one can claim that the fashion industry contributes anything really important to society. Fashion designers are rarely concerned with vital things like warmth, comfort and durability. They are only interested in outward appearance and they take advantage of the fact that women will put up with any amount of discomfort, providing they look right. There can hardly be a man who hasn't at some time in his life smiled at the sight of a woman shivering in a flimsy dress on a wintry day, or delicately picking her way through deep snow in dainty shoes.

When comparing men and women in the matter of fashion, the conclusions to be drawn are obvious. Do the constantly changing fashions of women's clothes, one wonders, reflect basic qualities of fickleness and instability? Men are too sensible to let themselves be bullied by fashion designers. Do their unchanging styles of dress reflect basic qualities of stability and reliability? That is for you to decide.

6. The main idea of this passage is that _____.

    A. new fashions in clothes reflect the qualities of women

    B. new fashions in clothing are created solely for commercial exploitation of women

    C. the top designers seem to have the right to create new fashions

D. men have the basic quality of reliability

7. What does "ludicrous" mean in Paragraph 1?

   A. Fashionable.   B. Glamorous.

   C. Absurd.   D. Charming.

8. Why does the general appearance of actresses look ludicrous?

   A. Because they want their appearance in the fashion.

   B. Because the top designers want them to follow the fashion.

   C. Because the top designers want them to make fashion.

   D. Because the top designers want them to lead the fashion.

9. Why are women mercilessly exploited by the fashion designers?

   A. They love new fashion.   B. They love new clothes.

   C. They want to look beautiful.   D. They are too vain.

10. What are fashion designers interested in?

   A. Outward appearance.   B. Comfort.

   C. Beauty.   D. Durability.

Passage Three

In her novel of "Reunion, American Style", Rona Jaffe suggests that a class reunion "is more than a sentimental journey. It is also a way of answering the question that lies at the back of nearly all our minds. Did they do better than I?"

Jaffe's observation may be misplaced but not completely lost. According to a study conducted by social psychologist Jack Sparacino, the overwhelming majority who attend reunions aren't there invidiously to compare their recent accomplishments with those of their former classmates. Instead, they hope, primarily, to relive their earlier successes.

Certainly, a few return to show their former classmates how well they have done; others enjoy observing the changes that have occurred in their classmates (not always in themselves, of course). But the majority who attend their class reunions do so to relive the good times they remember having when they were younger. In his study, Sparacino found that, as high school students, attendees had been more popular, more often regarded as attractive, and more involved in extracurricular activities than those classmates who chose not to attend. For those who turned up at their reunions, then, the old times were also the good times!

It would appear that Americans have a special fondness for reunions, judging by their prevalence. Major league baseball players, fraternity members, veterans groups, high school and college graduates, and former Boy Scouts all hold reunions on a regular basis. In addition, family reunions frequently attract blood relatives from faraway places who spend considerable money and time to reunite.

Actually, in their affection for reuniting with friends, family or colleagues, Americans are probably no different from any other people, except that Americans have created a mind-boggling number and variety of institutionalized forms of gatherings to facilitate the satisfaction of this desire. Indeed, reunions have increasingly become formal events that are organized on a regular basis and, in the process, they have also become big business.

Shell Norris of Class Reunion, Inc., says that Chicago alone has 1,500 high school reunions each year. A conservative estimate on the national level would be 10,000 annually. At one time, all high school reunions were organized by volunteers, usually female homemakers. In the last few years, however, as more and more women have entered the labor force, alumni reunions are increasingly being planned by specialized companies rather than by part-time volunteers.

The first college reunion was held by the alumni of Yale University in 1792. Graduates of Pennsylvania, Princeton, Stanford, and Brown followed suit. And by the end of the 19th century, most 4-year institutions were holding alumni reunions.

The variety of college reunions is impressive. At Princeton, alumni parade through the town wearing their class uniforms and singing their alma mater. At Marietta College, they gather for a dinner-dance on a steamship cruising the Ohio River.

Clearly, the thought of cruising on a steamship or marching through the streets is usually not, by itself, sufficient reason for large numbers of alumni to return to campus. Alumni who decide to attend their reunions share a common identity based on the years they spent together as undergraduates. For this reason, universities that somehow establish a common bond—for example, because they are relatively small or especially prestigious—tend to draw substantial numbers of their alumni to reunions. In an effort to enhance this common identity, larger colleges and universities frequently build their class reunions on participation in smaller units, such as departments or schools. Or they encourage "affinity reunions" for groups of former cheerleaders, editors, fraternity members, musicians, members of military organizations on campus, and the like.

Of course, not every alumnus is fond of his or her alma mater. Students who graduated during the late 1960s may be especially reluctant to get involved in alumni events. They were part of the generation that conducted sit-ins and teach-ins directed at university administrators, protested military recruitment on campus and marched against "establishment politics". If this generation has a common identity, it may fall outside of their university ties—or even be hostile to them. Even as they enter their middle years, alumni who continue to hold unpleasant memories of college during this period may not wish to attend class reunions.

11. According to the passage, Sparacino's study _____.

    A. provided strong evidence for Jaffe's statement

    B. showed that attendees tended to excel in high school study

    C. found that interest in reunions was linked with school experience

    D. found evidence for attendees' intense desire for showing off success

12. Which of the following is NOT mentioned as a distinct feature of U.S. class reunions?

    A. U.S. class reunions are usually occasions to show off one's recent success.

    B. Reunions are regular and formal events organized by professional agencies.

    C. Class reunions have become a profitable business.

    D. Class reunions have brought about a variety of activities.

13. What mainly attracts many people to return to campus for reunion?

    A. The variety of activities for class reunion.

    B. The special status their university enjoys.

    C. Shared experience beyond the campus.

    D. Shared undergraduate experience on campus.

14. The rhetorical function of the first paragraph is to _____.

    A. introduce Rona Jeffe's novel

    B. present the author's counterargument

    C. serve as prelude to the author's argument

    D. bring into focus on contrasting opinions

15. What is the passage mainly about?

    A. Reasons for popularity and attendance for alumni reunions.

    B. A historical perspective for alumni reunions in the United States.

C. Alumni reunions and American university traditions.

D. Alumni reunion and its social and economic implications.

Passage Four

It is becoming acceptable again to talk of computers performing human tasks such as problem-solving and pattern-recognition.

After years in the wilderness, the term "artificial intelligence" (AI) seems poised to make a comeback. AI was big in the 1980s but vanished in the 1990s. It re-entered public consciousness with the release of AI, a movie about a robot boy. This has ignited public debate about AI, but the term is also being used once more within the computer industry. Researchers, executives and marketing people are now using the expression without irony or inverted commas. And it is not always hype. The term is being applied, with some justification, to products that depend on technology that was originally developed by AI researchers. Admittedly, the rehabilitation of the term has a long way to go, and some firms still prefer to avoid using it. But the fact that others are starting to use it again suggests that AI has moved on from being seen as an over-ambitious and under-achieving field of research.

The field was launched, and the term "artificial intelligence" coined, at a conference in 1956 by a group of researchers that included Marvin Minsky, John McCarthy, Herbert Simon and Alan Newell, all of whom went on to become leading figures in the field. The expression provided an attractive but informative name for a research programme that encompassed such previously disparate fields as operations research, cybernetics, logic and computer science. The goal they shared was an attempt to capture or mimic human abilities using machines. That said, different groups of researchers attacked different problems, from speech recognition to chess playing, in different ways; AI unified the field in name only. But it was a term that captured the public imagination.

Most researchers agree that AI peaked around 1985. A public reared on science-fiction movies and excited by the growing power of computers had high expectations. For years, AI researchers had implied that a breakthrough was just around the corner. Marvin Minsky said in 1967 that within a generation the problem of creating "artificial intelligence" would be substantially solved. Prototypes of medical-diagnosis programs and speech recognition appeared to be making progress. It proved to be a false dawn. Thinking computers and household robots failed to materialize, and a backlash ensued. "There was undue optimism in the early 1980s", says David Leake, a researcher at Indiana University. "Then when people realized these were hard problems, there was retrenchment. By the late 1980s, the term AI was being avoided by many researchers, who opted instead to align themselves with specific sub-disciplines such as neural networks, agent technology, case-based reasoning, and so on."

Ironically, in some ways AI was a victim of its own success. Whenever an apparently mundane problem was solved, such as building a system that could land an aircraft unattended, the problem was deemed not to have been AI in the first place. "If it works, it can't be AI" as Dr Leake characterizes it. The effect of repeatedly moving the goal-posts in this way was that AI came to refer to "blue-sky" research that was still years away from commercialization. Researchers joked that AI stood for "almost implemented". Meanwhile, the technologies that made it onto the market, such as speech recognition, language translation and decision-support software, were no longer regarded as AI. Yet all three once fell well within the umbrella of AI research.

But the tide may now be turning, according to Dr Leake. HNC Software of San Diego, backed by a government agency, reckon that their new approach to artificial intelligence is the most powerful and promising approach ever discovered. HNC claim that their system, based on a cluster of 30 processors, could be used to spot camouflaged vehicles on a battlefield or extract a voice signal from a noisy background-tasks humans can do well, but computers cannot. "Whether or not their technology lives up to the claims made for it, the fact that HNC are emphasizing the use of AI is itself an interesting development" says Dr Leake.

Another factor that may boost the prospects for AI in the near future is that investors are now looking for firms using clever technology, rather than just a clever business model, to differentiate themselves. In particular, the problem of information overload, exacerbated by the growth of e-mail and the explosion in the number of web pages, means there are plenty of opportunities for new technologies to help filter and categorize information-classic AI problems. That may mean that more artificial intelligence companies will start to emerge to meet this challenge.

The 1969 film, *2001: A Space Odyssey*, featured an intelligent computer called HAL 9000. As well as understanding and speaking English, HAL could play chess and even learned to lip read. HAL thus encapsulated the optimism of the 1960s that intelligent computers would be widespread by 2001. But 2001 has been and gone, and there is still no sign of a HAL-like computer. Individual systems can play chess or transcribe speech, but a general theory of machine intelligence still remains elusive. It may be, however, that the comparison with HAL no longer seems quite so important, and AI can now be judged by what it can do, rather than by how well it matches up to a 30-year-old science-fiction film. "People are beginning to realize that there are impressive things that these systems can do," says Dr Leake hopefully.

16. According to the researchers, in the late 1980s, there was a feeling that _____.

    A. a general theory of AI would never be developed

    B. original expectations of AI may not have been justified

    C. a wide range of applications was close to fruition

    D. more powerful computers were the key to further progress

17. In Dr. Leake's opinion, the reputation of AI suffered as a result of _____.

    A. changing perceptions

    B. premature implementation

    C. poorly planned projects

    D. commercial pressures

18. The prospects for AI may benefit from _____.

    A. existing AI applications

    B. new business models

    C. orders from Internet-only companies.

    D. new investment priorities.

19. What does the irony in Paragraph 5 function?

    A. To point out the wrong opinion before.

    B. To introduce the contrary statement.

    C. To highlight why AI failed in 1980s.

    D. To elucidate AI's development history.

20. What is the author's attitude to the prospect of AI?

    A. Optimistic.   B. Negative.

    C. Opposing.   D. Struggling.

复旦大学2018年博士研究生入学考试英语试题
（阅读部分）答案与解析

Passage One

1. A。细节题。通过第一段中的 "prodigies are born, not made (mostly)" 可知，大家普遍认为，神童是天生的，不是造就的，故A选项是正确答案。

2. A。细节题。通过第四段中的 "Surprisingly, however, the study found that not all of the prodigies had high IQs. Indeed, while they had higher-than-average intelligence" 可知，不是所有的神童都有高智商，故A选项是正确的。要注意，A选项中all...not是部分否定的表达方式。

3. B。推理题。定位到第五段，该段讲到8个神童中有3个被诊断患有自闭症谱系障碍。此外，研究中的8个家庭中有4个家庭报告了一级或二级亲属的自闭症诊断，其中3个家庭报告共有11名近亲患有自闭症。相比之下，在普通人群中，大约88人中只有1人患有自闭症或阿斯伯格综合征。由此可以推理，神童比起普通人更容易患自闭症。

4. B。主旨题。本文从描述神童开始，逐步过渡到神童研究中的发现：智商普遍很高、患自闭症的可能性比普通人更大，这些都是神童的一些共存的特点，因此本文主旨并非在寻找神童与自闭症之间的关系，而是放大来看这个特殊群体中存在的一些共同特点。故本题答案为B。

5. D。推理题。这是一篇有关神经科学、心理学、社会学等跨学科研究的文章，以神童为研究对象，涉及自闭症等神经科学研究、家庭教育研究，可知出现在杂志的科研专栏的可能性最大。故本题答案为D。

Passage Two

6. B。推断题。创制新时装就是对女性的商业性剥削。答案遍及全文。也有几段突出描述。如：第二段第四句"每年，巴黎或伦敦的一些所谓高级设计师制定出条条框框，全世界的女性争先恐后地遵守服从。设计师的条令难以预测，说一不二。"第三段"要说女性年年被无情地剥削之事，只能怪她们自己。由于她们一想起在公共场所穿着过时的衣服就会发抖，所以她们每年都被设计师和大商店讹诈(勒索)……"第四段"许多女性(每年)浪费大笔钱财来置换她们几乎从未穿过的服装，不断变化的时尚就是故意创造浪费。"选项A"时装反映女性的秉性"这句话在最后一段结论中提及，但不是中心思想。选项D"男人具有可靠的基本素质"明显不对。选项C"高级设计师似乎有权创造新款式"这是作者在批评设计者，并不是文章主旨。

7．C。语义题。看似词汇题，实则语义走向题。该词的上文讲到老电影中的女性发型和妆容过时，裙子不是太长就是太短，整体看上去就很ludicrous，这里需要选择一个和outdated, too long或者too short一致的贬义走向的词，只有absurd满足这个要求。

8．D。推断题。因为高级设计师请她们领导时装潮流。这是常识，设计师推出新颖服装，首先是让演员试装——等于时装模特的效用，掀起可以领导时装的新潮流。故D选项正确。选项A"她们要打扮入时"，这只是演员的一方面。选项B"随大流"、选项C"做做样子"都是不对的。

9．D。推断题。这在文章的好几段内都提到了。如第一题中提及的第二、三、四段。如第三段后半部分"只穿了几次的衣服就因为时尚的要求而弃之一边。当你想到只有女性能站在堆满衣服的衣柜前，悲哀地诉说她没有衣服穿。"第四段的后半段"花不起大笔钱财买衣服的女性会花上好几个小时把已有的衣服改来改去"。第五段后半部分"男人一生中经常可以看到大冬天妇女穿着薄薄的衣衫瑟瑟发抖，或者穿着精致的鞋在雪地上小心翼翼地行走，这都令他们发笑"。最后一段结论，画龙点睛地点明"女性服装的时尚不断变化，人们不禁要问，这是不是反映了女性轻浮和易变的基本素质(秉性)？"选项A"她们爱新时尚"、选项B"她们爱新衣服"、选项C"她们想看上去美"这三项只是虚荣的部分组成。

10．A。细节题。外观。答案在第五段："没有人认为时装工业为社会做过真正的贡献。时装设计师很少关心保暖、舒服和耐穿这类紧要的事，他们只是对外观感兴趣，他们利用了女性的心理：只要看着美，她们能忍受一切(痛苦)不舒服……"选项B"舒适"、选项C"美"、选项D"耐穿"这三项均不正确。

Passage Three

11．C。细节题。通过人名定位到文中第二段"According to a study conducted by social psychologist Jack Sparacino...Instead, they hope, primarily, to relive their earlier successes."即他们参加聚会不是为了进行成就攀比（compare accomplishment），而是为了回忆早时的成功。earlier success肯定是上学时的共同时光，即school experience。因此本题答案为C。

12．A。细节题。第五段中讲到"...reunions have increasingly become formal events that are organized on a regular basis and, in the process, they have also become big business.（聚会越来越成为定期组织的正式活动，而且已经成了一门不错的生意。）"，第六段中的"alumni reunions are increasingly being planned by specialized companies（都是由专业公司组织）"，倒数第三段中的"The variety of college reunions is impressive.（各式各样的聚会真是让人大开眼界。）"，这些信息分别对应B，C，D选项。只有A选项（炫富）没有提及。

13. D。细节题。倒数第二段中讲道："Alumni who decide to attend their reunions share a common identity...somehow establish a common bond"，即校友们愿意参加校友会的主要原因是基于大学共度时光中建立的共同身份，由此缔结了一种共同纽带。因此D选项是该句的正确改写，为正确答案。

14. D。推断题。第一段讲到Rona Jaffe的新书，暗指大学校友会更多在攀比（Did they do better than I？），第二段首句则否定了这个观点（misplaced），并提出另一个研究，该研究中指出校友会更多地不是为了炫富，而是为了寻找共同经历和身份。因此第一段的主要功能是为了引入并关注不同的新观点。故D选项为正确答案。

15. A。主旨题。全文从第二段引入校友会或者其他聚会的观点后，就开始分析校友会的历史、参加校友会的人群，以及当下校友会的组织方式，B，C，D都是文中的几个分论点，也是校友们重聚的原因。对全文主旨总结最好的是A选项。

Passage Four

16. B。细节题。根据late 1980s可定位到原文第四段"By the late 1980s, the term AI was being avoided by many researchers, who opted instead to align themselves with specific sub-disciplines such as neural networks, agent technology, case-based reasoning, and so on."即20世纪80年代后期，AI研究者避免使用这个术语，而是开创了很多二级学科，比如神经网络、代理人科技、案例演绎等。这么做的原因是以前的研究都没有取得成果（false dawn）。

17. D。细节题。直到文中第三段，作者一直在讲AI是如何蓬勃发展，并在1985年达到了顶峰。后来因为Thinking computers and household robots failed to materialize...Then when people realized these were hard problems, there was retrenchment，会思考的电脑和做家务的机器人未能实现，接着就发生了各种偏移。人们突然就意识到前途艰难，投资紧跟着就变少。因此AI受损于观念改变，不再有undue optimism。

18. D。细节题。从倒数第二段中的"Another factor that may boost the prospects for AI in the near future is that investors are now looking for firms using clever technology... That may mean that more artificial intelligence companies will start to emerge to meet this

challenge." 可知，影响AI未来的因素是投资者们不仅仅将其作为生意来看，更多的是在寻找如何使用这项聪明技术的商业体。因此，AI的前景会从观念的改变上受益。

19. C。推断题。该段讲到AI一度遭遇与实际问题解决划清界限的尴尬局面。第五段中讲到AI被定义为blue-sky research（天马行空的研究），即AI太不接地气，使得AI被研究者们避之不及。当然在历史上，AI也因激发了公众的想象力而声名大噪。因此，这个irony主要在强调AI失败的原因。

20. A。态度题。文中谈到AI的历史发展过程，虽然历经数十年的跌宕起伏，但由最后一句话 "'People are beginning to realize that there are impressive things that these systems can do,' says Dr Leake hopefully." 可知，他对AI的未来是充满希望的。因此态度词选择optimistic是合理的。

四川大学2018年博士研究生入学考试英语试题（阅读部分）

Passage One

Guns. Everywhere guns.

Let me start this discussion by pointing out that I am not anti-gun. I'm pro-knife. Consider the merits of the knife.

In the first place, you have to catch up with someone to stab him. A general substitution of knives for guns would promote physical fitness. We'd turn into a whole nation of great runners. Plus, knives don't discharge themselves. And people are seldom killed while cleaning their knives.

As a civil libertarian, I of course support the *Second Amendment*. And I believe it means exactly what it says: "A well-regulated militia being necessary to the security of a free state, the right of the people to keep and bear arms shall not be infringed." Fourteen-year-old boys are not part of a well-regulated militia. Members of wacky religious cult are not part of a well-regulated militia. Permitting unregulated citizens to have guns is destroying the security of this free state.

I am intrigued by the arguments of those who claim to follow the judicial doctrine of original intent. How do they know it was the dearest wish of Thomas Jefferson's heart that teenage drug dealers should cruise the cities of this nation perforating their fellow citizens with assault rifles? Channeling?

There is more hooey spread about the *Second Amendment*. It says quite clearly that guns are for those who form part of a well-regulated militia, i.e., the armed forces including the National Guard. The reasons for keep them away from everyone else get clearer by the day.

The comparison most often used is that of the automobile, another lethal object that is regularly used to wreak great casualty. Obviously, this society is full of people who haven't got enough common sense to sue an automobile properly. But we don't want to outlaw cars.

We do, however, license them and their owners, restrict their use to presumably sane and sober adults and keep track of who sells them to whom. At a minimum, we should do the same with guns.

In truth, there is no rational argument for guns in this society. This is no longer a frontier nation in which people hunt their own food. It is a crowded, overwhelmingly urban country in which letting people have access to guns is a continuing disaster. Those who want guns — whether for target shooting, hunting, or potting rattlesnakes（get a hoe）— should be subjected to the same restrictions placed on gun owners in England, a nation in which liberty has survived nicely without an armed populace.

The argument that "guns don't kill people" is patent nonsense. Anyone who has ever worked in a cop shop knows how many family arguments ended in murder because there was a gun in the house. Did the gun kill someone? No. But if there had been no gun, no one would have died, at least not without a good foot face first. Guns do kill. Unlike cars, that is all they do.

Michael Crichton makes an interesting argument about technology in his thriller *Jurassic Park*. He points out that power without discipline is making this society into disasters. By the time someone who studies the martial arts becomes a master — literally able to kill with bare hands — that person has also undergone years of training and discipline. But any fool can pick up a gun and kill with it.

"A well-regulated militia" surely implies both long training and long discipline. That is the least, the very least, that should be required of those who are permitted to have guns, because a gun is literally the power to kill. For years, I used to enjoy making fun of my gun-nuts friends about their psychosexual hang-ups — always in a spirit of a good cheer, you understand. But letting the noisy minority in the National Rifle Association force us to allow this casualty to continue is just plain insane.

I do not think gun nuts have a power hang-up. I don't know what is missing in their psyches that they need to feel they have the power to kill. But no sane society would allow this to continue.

Ban the damn things. Ban them all. You want protection? Get a dog.

1. The author claims that he is "*pro-knife*", because he believes that _____.

    A. knives are weapons more efficient than guns

    B. knives force people to take part in physical sports

    C. fewer lives might be lost if knives are used as weapons

    D. a man who is anti-gun should use knives to kill

2. Most likely, a civil libertarian such as the author would believe that _____.

    A. guns should not be banned even if the only thing they do is to kill

    B. every citizen in the country should possess guns according to the law

    C. only the psychologically normal should be allowed to own guns

    D. religious believers and school children should be allowed to own guns

3. Which of the following statements is not true according to the passage?

    A. Thomas Jefferson didn't want drug-dealers to own guns.

    B. Automobiles can be as dangerous as guns in claiming lives.

    C. Freedom can be guaranteed even if the population is not armed.

    D. Rigid discipline may reduce casualty from gun-shooting.

4. Most likely, the author's "*gun-nuts friends*" are _____.

    A. hard nuts to crack   B. anti-gun activists

    C. gun-crazy people   D. disciplined militia

5. The general tone of this passage is _____.

    A. pungent   B. desperate   C. menacing   D. humorous

Passage Two

According to Sybil Evans, a conflict-resolution expert in New York City, there are three components to blame for our societal bad behaviors: time, technology and tension.

What is eating up our time? To begin with, Americans work longer hours and are rewarded with less vacation time than people in any other industrial society. Over an average year, for example, most British employees work 250 hours less than most Americans; most Germans work a full 500 hours less. And most Europeans are given four to six weeks' vacation every year, compared to the average American's two weeks. To make matters worse, many Americans face long stressful commutes at the beginning and end of each long workday.

Once we Americans finally get home from work, our busy day is rarely done. We are involved in community activities; our children participate in sports, school programs, and extracurricular activities; and our houses, yards and cars cry out for maintenance. To make matters worse, we are reluctant to use the little bit of leisure time we do have to catch up on our sleep. Compared with Americans of the nineteenth and nearly twentieth centuries, most of us are chronically sleep deprived. While our ancestors typically slept nine-and-a-half hours a night, many of us feel lucky to get seven. We're critical of "lazy" people who sleep longer, and we associate naps with toddlerhood. (In doing so, we ignore the example pf successful people including Winston Churchill, Albert Einstein, and Napoleon, all of who were devoted to their afternoon naps.)

The bottom line: we are time-challenged and just plain tired — and tired people are cranky people. We're ready to blow — to snap at the slow-moving cashier, to tap the bumper of the slowpoke ahead of us, or to do something far worse.

Technology is also to blame for the bad behavior so widespread in our culture. Amazing gadgets were supposed to make our lives easier — but have they? Sure, technology has its positive aspects. It is a blessing, for instance, to have a cell phone on hand when your car breaks down far from home or to be able to "instant message" a friend on the other side of the globe. But the downsides are many. Cell phones, pagers, fax machines, handheld computers, and the like have robbed many of us what was once valuable downtime. Now we're always available to take that urgent call or act on that last-minute demand. Then there is the endless pressure of feeling we need to keep up with our gadgets' latest technological developments. For example, it's not sufficient to use your cell phone for phone calls. Now you must learn to use the phone for text-messaging and downloading games. It's not enough to take still photos with your digital camera. You should know how to shoot ultra high-speed fast-action clips. It's not enough to have an enviable CD collection. You should be downloading new songs in MP3 format. The computers in your house should be connected by a wireless router, and online via high-speed DSL service. In other words, if it's been more than ten minutes since you've updated your technology, you're probably behind.

In fact, you're not only behind; you're a stupid loser. At least, that's how most of us end up feeling as we're confronted with more and more unexpected technologies: do-it-yourself checkout at the supermarket, the telephone "help center" that offers a record of series of messages, but no human help. And feeling like losers makes us frustrated and, you guessed it, angry. "It's not any one thing but lots of little things that make people feel like they don't have control of their lives," says Jane Middleton-Moz, an author and therapist. "A sense of helplessness is what riggers rage. It's why people end up licking ATM machines."

Her example is not far-fetched. According to a survey of computer users in Great Britain, a quarter of those under age 25 admitted to having kicked or punched their computers on at least one occasion. Others confessed to yanking out cables in a rage, forcing the computer to crash. On this side of the Atlantic, a Wisconsin man, after repeated attempts to get his daughter's malfunctioning computer repaired, took it to the store where he had bought it, placed it in the foyer, and attacked it with a sledgehammer. Arrested and awaiting a court appearance, he told local reporters, "It feels good, in a way." He had put into action a fantasy many of us have had — that of taking out our feelings of rage on the machines that so frustrate us.

Tension, the third major culprit behind our epidemic of anger, is intimately connected with our lack of time and the pressures of technology. Merely our chronic exhaustion and our frustration in the face of a bewildering array of technologies would be enough to cause our stress levels to skyrocket, but we are dealing with much more. Our tension is often fueled by a reserve of anger that might be the result of a critical boss, marital discord, or (something that many of today's men and women experience, if few will admit it) a general sense of being stupid and inadequate in the face of the demands of modern life. And along with the challenges of everyday life, we now live with a widespread fear of such horrors as terrorist acts, global warming, and antibiotic-resistant diseases. Our sense of dread may be out of proportion to actual threads because of technology's ability to bombard us so constantly with worrisome information. Twenty-four hours a day news stations bring a stream of horror into our living rooms. As we work on our computers, headlines and graphic images are never more than a mouse-click away.

6. Most likely the author of this passage is a _____.

    A. psychological advisor   B. government official

    C. medical doctor   D. magazine columnist

7. Which of the following is a true inference from the passage?

    A. Taking a nap every day is associative for young children.

B. All people who hit ATMs do so because they are helpless.

C. Reducing tension may help making people more peaceful.

D. Lazy people keep the American tradition of previous centuries.

8. All of the following phrases describe the negative influences of modern technology on Americans EXCEPT "_____".

　　A. more irritable　　　　　　　　　B. desperate in updating skills

　　C. helpless in controlling　　　　　D. more critical of news report

9. In the last paragraph, the word "epidemic" is closest in meaning with "_____".

　　A. expression　　　B. syndrome　　　C. celebrity　　　D. horror

10. Most appropriately, this passage can be entitled "_____".

　　A. Rage and Its Causes in Modern America

　　B. Modern Technology and Its Unwanted Results

　　C. Sleeping Circle among Modern Americans

　　D. Factors that lead to Bad Behavior on American Roads

Passage Three

Our brains' very different makeup leads to our very different methods of interacting with the world around us. Simon Baron-Cohen, author of *the Essential Difference: Men, Women, and the Extreme Male Brain*, has labeled the classic female mental process as "empathizing". He defines empathizing as "the drive to identify another person's emotional and thoughts, and to respond to these with and appropriate emotion." Empathizers are constantly measuring and responding to the surrounding emotional temperature. They are concerned about showing sensitivity to the people around them. This empathetic quality can be observed in virtually all aspects of women's life from the choice of typically female-dominated careers (nursing, elementary school teaching, social work) to reading matter popular mainly with women (romantic fiction, articles about relationships, advice columns about how people can get along better) and to women's interaction family, and sympathy for each other's concerns. So powerful is the empathizing mindset that it even affects how the typical female memory works. Ask a woman when a particular event happened, and she often pinpoints it in terms of an occurrence that had emotional content: "That was the summer my sister broke her leg," or "That was around the time Gene and Mary got into such an awful argument."

Likewise, she is likely to bring her empathetic mind to bear on geography. She'll remember a particular address not as 11th on Market Streets but being "near the restaurant where we went on our anniversary", or "around the corner from Liz's old apartment".

In contrast, Baron-Cohen calls the typical male mindset "systemizing", which he defines as "the drive to analyze and explore a system, to extract underlying rules that govern the behavior of a system." A systemizer is less interested in how people feel than in how things work. Again, the systematic brain influences virtually all aspects of the typical man's life. Male-dominated professions (such as engineering, computer-programming, auto repair, and mathematics) rely heavily on systems, formulas, and patterns, and very little on the ability to intuit another person's thoughts or emotions. Reading materials most popular with men includes science fiction and history, as well as factual "how-to" magazines on such topics as computers, photography, home repair, and woodworking. When they get together with male friends, men are far less likely to engage in intimate conversation than they are to share an activity: watching or playing sports, working on a car, bowling, golfing, or fishing. Men's conversation is peppered with dates and addresses, illustrating their comfort with systems: "back in 1996 when I was living in Boston…" or "The best way to the new stadium is to go all the way out Walnut Street to 33rd and then get on the bypass…"

One final way that men and women differ is in their typical responses to problem-solving. Ironically, it may be this very activity — intended on both sides to eliminate problems — that creates the most conflict between partners of the opposite sex. To a woman, the process of solving a problem is all-important. Talking about a problem is a means of deepening the intimacy between her and her partner. The very anatomy of her brain, as well as her accompanying empathetic mindset, makes her want to consider all sides of a question and to explore various possible solutions. To have a partner who is willing to explore a problem with her is deeply satisfying. She interprets that willingness as an expression of the other's love and concern.

But men have an almost completely opposite approach when it comes to dealing with a problem. Everything in their mental makeup tells them to focus narrowly on the issue, solve it, and get it out of the way. The ability to fix a problem quickly and efficiently is, to them, a demonstration of their power and competence. When a man hears his female partner begin to describe a problem, his strongest impulse is to listen briefly and then tell her what to do about it. From his perspective, he has made a helpful and loving gesture; from hers, he's short-circuited conversation that could have deepened and strengthened their relationship.

The challenge that confronts men and women is to put aside ideas of "better" and "worse" when it comes to their many differences. Our diverse brain development, our ways of interacting with the world and our modes of dealing with problems all have their strong points. In some circumstances, a typically feminine approach may be more effective; in others, a classically masculine mode may have the advantage. Our differences aren't going to disappear; my daughter, now a middle-schooler, regularly tells me she loves me, while her teenage brothers express their affection by grabbing me in a headlock. Learning to understand and appreciate one another's gender-specific qualities is the key to more rich and rewarding lives together.

11. The word "*empathizing*" in the first paragraph can best be replaced by "_____".

 A. changing oneself to be like another

 B. stepping into another's space

 C. taking oneself for another

 D. putting oneself on another's position

12. An empathetic person is likely to do all of the following except _____.

 A. criticizing graduate students

 B. enjoying socialization

 C. understanding others' feelings

 D. reading love stories

13. Which of the following is not something that men would like to do?

 A. Empathizing and systemizing are two directly hostile predispositions.

 B. Different mindsets between sexes are not necessarily incompatible.

 C. No purpose is served as men focus on results but women on process.

 D. Data analysis has been more masculine than feminine as a tradition.

14. Which of the following is not something that men would like to do?

 A. Carpentering.　　　　B. Hunting preys.

 C. Reading romantics.　　D. Competitive sports.

15. A "rewarding life" in the last paragraph means one that _____.

 A. brings about good payment　　B. is fruitful

 C. pays back a lot in cash　　D. wins an award

Passage Four

If animals could talk, what wonderful stories they would tell. The eagle could already see that the earth was round when men were still afraid of falling off its edge. The whale could have warned Columbus about a barrier between Europe and India and saved that explorer a lot of anxiety. Justice would be more properly served if animals could give **testimony**. There would probably be a reduction in crime and quite possibly an increase in the divorce rate. All of us would have to alter our behavior in some way or another, for our environment would be considerably changed.

The idea of talking animal is as old and as widespread among human societies as language itself. No culture lacks a legend on which some animal plays a speaking role. All over West African, children listen to folk tales in which a "spider-man" is the hero. And there is hardly an animal who does not figure in Aesop's famous fables. Many authors have exploited the idea successfully, among them Hugh Lofting, the creator of the famous Doctor Dolittle. The good doctor's forte was animal communication, and he is no doubt fiction's most prodigious language learner. Still Doctor Dolittle and his adventures are fantasies for children, and the idea of communicating with our fellow animal tenants of this globe as we communicate with our fellow human tenants is absurd. Or is it?

Whether language is the exclusive property of the human species is an interesting question. The answer depends on what properties of human language are considered. If language is viewed only as a system of communication, then obviously many species communicate. Humans also use systems other than their language to relate to each other and to send "messages." To understand human language, one needs to see what, if anything, is special and unique to language. If we find that there are no such special properties, then we will have to conclude that language, as we have been discussing it, is not, as claimed, uniquely human.

Most humans who acquire language utilize speech sounds to express meanings, but such sounds are not a necessary aspect of language, as was shown in the case of sign languages. The use of speech sounds is therefore not a basic property of human language and it is possible that the chirping of birds, the squeaking of dolphins, and the dancing of bees, and the manipulation of plastic chips by chimpanzees represent systems similar to human language. If animal communication systems are not similar to human languages, it will not because they fail to have speech sounds.

Conversely, if animals vocally imitate human utterances, this does not mean they possess language. We have already seen that language is a system which relates sounds and meanings (or gestures and meanings). "Talking" birds such as parrots and mynah birds are capable of faithfully reproducing words and phrases of human language. The birds imitate what they have heard. But when a parrot says "Polly wants a cracker" she may really want a ham sandwich or a drink of water or nothing at all. A bird that has leaned to say "hello" or "good-bye" is as likely to use one as the other, regardless of whether people are arriving or departing. The bird's "utterances" carry no meaning. They are speaking neither English nor their own language when they sound like us.

Talking birds do not dissect the sounds of their imitation into discrete units. *Polly and Molly* do not "rhyme" for a parrot. They are as different as "hello" and "good-bye" (or as similar). One property of all human languages is the "discreteness" of the speech or gestural units, which are ordered and reordered, combined and split apart. A parrot says what it is taught, or what it hears, and no more. If Polly learns "Polly wants a cracker" and "Polly wants a doughnut" and also learns to imitate the single words "whisky" and "bagel", she will not spontaneously produce, as children do, "Polly wants whisky" or "Polly wants a bagel". If she learns *cat* and *cats* and *dog* and *dogs* and then learns *parrot*, she will be unable to "form the plural" *parrots* (as in *cats*).

A parrot does not take speech to pieces, nor can it form an unlimited set of utterances from a finite set of units. Thus, the ability to produce sounds similar to those used in human language cannot be equated with the ability to learn a human language in the seventeenth century, the philosopher and mathematician Rene Descartes pointed out what we have been discussing here: that the ability to use language is not based on the physiological abilities to produce speech or speech-like sounds. He concluded:

It is not the want of organs that [prevents animals from making] …known their thoughts… for it is evident that magpies and parrots are able to utter words just like ourselves, and yet they cannot speak as we do, that is , so as to give evidence that they think of what they say. On the other hand, men who, being born deaf and dumb, are in the same degree, or even more than the brutes, **destitute of** *the organs which serve the others for talking, are in the habit of themselves inventing certain signs by which they make themselves understood.*

16. Which of the following statements is true according to the passage?

    A. Animals do have their own languages that human beings cannot understand.

    B. Human beings came to believe that the earth was round later than animals did.

C. The meaning of animal utterance is not based on the meanings of its component units.

D. Columbus would have discovered India instead of America, warned by whales.

17. The word "*testimony*" in the first paragraph means "_____".

    A. participating in a test   B. drafting a testament

    C. producing evidence to a fact   D. providing an ultimate truth

18. According to the author, no animal communication can be a language because _____.

    A. the design features special to human language are not found therein

    B. animals do not have the same pronunciation system as that of humans

    C. the "messages" sent by them are only a part of human communication

    D. the definition of animal language differs from that of human language

19. Which of the following is not a property of animals' vocal imitation of human speech?

    A. There is no phonetic structure composed of units.

    B. The words in an utterance do not have definite references.

    C. The connection of expression and thoughts is not established.

    D. The sounds in an utterance are not sufficiently identifiable.

20. In the last paragraph, the phrase "*destitute of*" can best be replaced by "_____".

    A. divorced from   B. depriving of

    C. for lack of   D. in presence of

Passage Five

Emphasizing commonalities is not just a matter of a scientific taste. The design of any adaptive biological system — the explanation of how it works — is almost certain to be uniform across individuals in a sexually reproducing species, because sexual recombination would fatally scramble the blueprints for qualitatively different designs. There is, to be sure, a great deal of genetic diversity among individuals; each person is biochemically unique. But natural selection is a process that feeds on that variation, and (aside from functionally equivalent varieties of molecules) when natural selection creates adaptive designs, it does so by using the variation up: the variant genes that specify more poorly designed organs disappear when their owners starve, get eaten, or die mateless. To the extent that mental modules are complex products of natural selection, genetic variation will be limited to quantitative variation, not differences in basic design. Genetic differences among people, no matter how fascinating they are to us in love, biography, personnel, gossip, and politics, are of minor interest to us when we appreciate what makes minds intelligent at all.

Similarly, an interest in mind design puts possible innate differences between sexes and races in a new light. With the exception of the maleness-determining gene on the Y-chromosome, every functioning gene in a man's body is also found in a woman's and vice versa. The maleness gene is a developmental switch that can activate some suites of genes and deactivate others, but the same blueprints are in both kinds of bodies, and the default condition is identity of design. There is some evidence that the sexes depart from this default in the case of the psychology of reproduction and the adaptive problems directly and indirectly related to it, which is not surprising; it seems unlikely that peripherals as different as the male and female reproductive systems would come with the same software. But the sexes face essentially similar demands for most the rest of cognition, including language, and I would be surprised if there were differences in design between them.

21. Which of the following is the best paraphrase of the first sentence in the first paragraph?

    A. Scientists have a taste different from common people.

    B. Science has more interest than just commonalities.

    C. Universality is not restricted to scientific pursuit.

    D. Commonality is not the only emphasis of science.

22. By "natural selection is a process that feeds on that variation" the author means that _____.

    A. such variation gives feedback to natural selection

    B. natural selection is a process of variation of feedings

    C. variations are functional modules of natural process

    D. natural selection could not work without that variation

23. Which of the following statements is true according to the author?

    A. Individual differences are only variations in amount

B. Differences in essence result from sexual reproduction

C. Both qualitative and quantitative differences are equally important

D. Phenomena are composed of commonalities

24. The author of this passage hopes to make it clear that _____.

A. default designs are different from males to females in their bodies

B. men and women are the same in genetic makeup save in reproduction systems

C. psychology of reproduction determines the male and female genetic designs

D. the behaviors of men and women can be changed by changing the software

25. Obviously, the author is a(n) _____ in his standpoint concerning what science is.

A. rationalist   B. empiricist

C. phenomenologist   D. naturalist

Passage Six

Syntax is complex, but the complexity is there for a reason. For our thought are surely even more complex, and we are limited by a mouth that can pronounce a single word at a time. Science has begun to crack the beautifully designed code that our brains used to convey complex thought as words and their orderings.

The workings of syntax are important for another reason. Grammar offers a clear refutation of the empiricist doctrine that there is nothing in the mind that was not first in the senses. Traces, cases, NPs, and the other *paraphernalia* of syntax are colorless, odorless, and tasteless, but hey, or something like them, must be a part of our unconscious mental life. This should not be surprising to a thoughtful computer scientist. There is no way one can write a halfway intelligent program without defining variables and data structures that do not directly correspond to anything in the input or output. For example, a graphics program that had to store an image of a triangle inside a circle would not store the actual keystrokes that the user typed to draw the shapes, because the same shapes could have been drawn in a different order or with a different device like a mouse of a light pen. Nor would it store the list of dots that have to be lit up to display the circle around and leave the triangle in place, or make the circle bigger or smaller, and one long list of dots would not allow the program to know which dots belong to the circle and which to the triangle. Instead, the shapes would be stored in some more abstract format (like the coordinates of a few defining points for each shape), a format that mirrors neither the inputs nor the outputs to the program but that can be translated to and from them when the need arises.

Grammar, a form of mental software must have evolved under similar design specifications. Though psychologists under the influence of empiricism often suggest that grammar mirrors commands to the speech muscles, melodies in speech sounds, or mental scripts for the ways that people and things tend to interact, I think all these suggestions miss the mark. Grammar is a protocol that has to interconnect the ear, the mouth and the mind, three very different kinds of machine. It cannot be tailored to any of them but must have an abstract logic of its own.

26. According to the first paragraph, the author would agree that _____.

    A. whatever complex concept or thought can all be expressed by one sentence

    B. words organized according to a syntactic rule make a sentence meaningful

    C. it is science that provides the beautiful design to a language

    D. syntax is necessary because pronunciation is limited

27. The word "*paraphernalia*" in the second paragraph means most probably "_____".

    A. devices   B. paragraphs

    C. chemicals   D. words

28. According to this essay, grammar is _____.

    A. an empirical test   B. a system of rules

    C. a reflection of interaction   D. a machine of logic

29. Which of the following sums up best the main idea of this essay?

    A. A thoughtful computer scientist is one who is familiar with linguistic theories.

    B. Everything one sees, hears, or feels constitutes the reliable data for sciences.

    C. What science should do is to understand the mechanism behind phenomena.

    D. Language is the same as programming because the output depends on the input.

30. The author of this essay is most likely a _____.

    A. teacher of English   B. computer scientist

    C. linguist   D. psychologist

四川大学2018年博士研究生入学考试英语试题（阅读部分）答案与解析

Passage One

1. C。推理题。由第三段中的"In the first place, you have to catch up with someone to stab him"与倒数第五段中的"No. But if there had been no gun, no one would have died, at least not without a good foot race first. Guns do kill. Unlike cars, that is all they do."可知，作者想表达的是，如果用刀来作为杀人武器，会比枪费劲得多，故C选项"如果刀被用作武器，那么死亡人数可能会减少"是正确答案。

2. C。推理题。由第八段中的"We do, however, license them and their owner, restrict their use to presumably sane and sober adults and keep track of who sells them to who. At a minimum, we should do the same with guns."可知，C选项"只有心理正常的人才可以获准拥有枪支"正确。

3. A。推理题。由第五段中的"How do they know it was the dearest wish of Thomas Jefferson's heart that teenage drug dealers should cruise the cities of this nation perforating their fellow citizens with assault rifles?"可知，文中并未明确指出Thomas Jefferson是否同意毒贩拥有枪支，而是用尖刻的诙谐口吻来讽刺那些想用美国立法精神来捍卫枪支使用自由的人，"他们怎么知道这是Thomas Jefferson当初最真的想法，想让十来岁的贩毒青少年端着冲锋枪横扫大街上的同胞呢"，而Thomas Jefferson是否同意，文中并未给出明确答案，故A选项不符合文意。从文中第七段和第八段可知B选项正确，从倒数第五段最后两句"Guns do kill. Unlike cars, that is all they do."可知C选项符合文意，从倒数第三段可知D选项符合文意。因此本题正确答案为A。

4. C。推理题。由倒数第二段中的"I do not think gun nuts have a power hang-up. I don't know what is missing in their psyches that they need to feel they have the power to kill."可知，nut与psyche意思相关，是对某事或者某物心态很奇特的人。A"难以打开的坚果"，B"反对枪支的积极分子"，C"对枪狂热的人"，D"遵守纪律的人"，可知C是正确选项。

5. A。推理题。由第三段中的"A general substitution of knives for guns should promote physical fitness. We'd turn into a whole nation of great runners.（用刀代替枪的普

遍做法会促进身体健康。我们会变成一个伟大的跑步者的国家。）"与最后一段中的"Ban the damn things. Ban them all. You want protection? Get a dog."可知，作者的语气更多的是尖刻，故A选项正确。这里要注意humorous（幽默的）和pungent（尖刻的）之间的区别，幽默往往让人愉悦，尖刻更多带有讽刺。

Passage Two

6. D。推理题。本文首段提到 "According to Sybil Evans, a conflict-resolution expert in New York City, there are three components to blame for our societal bad behaviors: time, technology and tension.（纽约冲突解决专家Sybil Evans认为，有三种因素导致社会性不良行为：时间、科技和紧张关系。）"这是文章的主题。作者在后文长篇大论地分析三种因素与不良行为的细致关系。心理咨询师、政府官员以及医生的角色都不如"杂志专栏作家"合适。

7. C。推理题。由第二段中的 "What is eating up our time…industrial society." 和最后一段中的 "Tension, the third major culprit behind our epidemic of anger…pressures of technologies…" 可知，C选项"缓解紧张可能有助于使人们更加平静"是正确答案。

8. D。推理题。由第五段中的 "Then there is the endless pressure of feeling we need to keep up with our gadgets' latest technological developments.（此外，我们还会有无尽的压力，觉得自己需要跟上电子产品的最新技术发展。）"与该段最后一句 "…in other words, if it's been more than ten minutes since you've updated your technology, you've probably behind.（换句话说，如果你已经超过十分钟仍未再次升级，你可能就落后了。）"可推知，A "更加急躁"和B "极度渴望更新技能"在文中有提及；由第六段中的 "At least, that's how most of us end up feeling as we're confronted with more…they don't have control of their lives…（当我们面对越来越多意想不到的技术时……让人们觉得他们无法控制自己的生活……）"可知，C "无法控制"在文中亦有提及。故D选项为正确答案。

9. B。词汇题。最后一段中的 "Tension, the third major culprit behind our epidemic of anger, is intimately connected with our lack of time and the pressures of technologies would be enough to cause our stress levels to skyrocket, but we dealing with much more.（紧张是我们传染性的愤怒现象背后的第三大原因，它与我们缺乏时间和技术带给我们的压力密切相关。）"，epidemic表示anger的程度，是一种社会性症候，因此B选项（综合症状）是正确答案。

10. A。推理题。由第一段中的 "there are three components" 及最后一段可知，本文

主题为愤怒这种社会传染病背后的原因分析，因此A选项（愤怒及其在现代美国的起因）是正确答案。B，C，D均为该主题下不同层次的细节问题。

Passage Three

11．D。推理题。由第一段中的"Simon Baron-Cohen…has labels the classis female mental process as 'empathizing'. He defines empathizing as…"可知，Simon将"移情"定义为"识别他人情绪和想法的动力，并以适当的情绪回应这些情绪和想法"，本题正确答案为D（设身处地为别人着想）。

12．A。推理题。由第一段中的"Empathizers are constantly measuring and responding to the surrounding emotional temperature… to the people around them."可知，移情者不断估量和回应周围的情绪温度，他们在意对周围的人表现出体恤。由此可推知，"批评毕业生"与原文不符合。

13．D。推理题。由第二段中的"Male-dominated professions… rely heavily on systems, formulas, and patterns, and very little on the ability to intuit another person's thoughts or emotions."可知，男性主导的职业很大程度上依赖于系统、公式和模式，很少依赖于直觉感知他人想法和情感的能力，由此可推知D选项（作为一种传统，数据分析更男性化，而非女性化）正确。

14．C。推理题。由第二段中的"Reading materials most popular with men includes science fiction and history, as well as factual 'how-to' magazines on such topics as computers, photography，home repair, and woodworking."可知，"阅读爱情故事"不是男性喜欢做的事情，故C为正确答案。

15．B。推理题。由最后一段中的"Our diverse brain development…all have their strong points."可知，我们多种多样的大脑开发，我们与世界互动的方式和处理问题的方式都有其优点。"Learning to understand and appreciate one another's gender-specific qualities…rich and rewarding lives together."意为："学会理解和欣赏彼此的性别特质对一起获得更加丰富和更有收获的生活非常重要。"由此可知，B选项"有收获的"是正确答案。

Passage Four

16．B。推理题。由第一段中的"The eagle could already see that the earth was round when men were still afraid of falling off its edge."可知，B选项是正确答案（对地球是圆的

这个认知，人类晚于动物）。

17．C。词汇题。由第一段中的"Justice would be more properly served if animals could give testimony.（如果动物能作证，那么正义将得到更好的伸张。）"可知，testimony为"证据"的意思，故C选项为正确答案。

18．A。推理题。由第三段中的"If we find that there are no such special properties, then we will have to conclude that language, as we have been discussing it, is not, as claimed, uniquely human.（如果我们发现没有这种特性，那么我们将不得不得出这样的结论：正如我们一直所讨论的那样，语言并非我们所声称的人类特有的。）"可知，A选项（在那里没有发现人类语言特定的结构特点）是正确答案。

19．D。推理题。由倒数第二段中的"Thus, the ability to produce sounds similar to those used in human language cannot be equated with the ability to learn a human language.（产生与人类语言相似的声音的这种能力不能等同于学习人类语言的能力。）"可知，"动物话语中的声音不能被充分识别"与原文内容不符，故D选项为正确答案。

20．B。推理题。由最后一段中的"On the other hand, men who, being born deaf and dumb, are in the same degree, or even more than the brutes, destitute of the organs… inventing certain signs by which then make themselves understood."可知，这里的destitute of the organ与前面的born deaf and dumb相对，即"缺失相应的器官"。因此本题正确答案为B选项。

Passage Five

21．C。推理题。由第一段中的"Emphasizing commonalities is not just a matter of a scientific taste.（强调共性不仅仅是科学品位的问题。）"可知，C选项"共性并不局限于科学追求"正确。

22．D。推理题。由第一段中的"…when natural selection creates adaptive designs, it does so… when their owners starve, get eaten, or die mateless.（当自然选择创造出适应性设计时，它是通过利用变异来实现的，即设计较差的器官的变种基因会随着其所有者饿死、被吃掉或是在没有配偶的情况下死亡而消失。）"可知，D选项"自然选择在没有变异的情况下不能运作"是正确答案。

23．D。推理题。由第一段中的"There is, to be sure, a great deal of genetic diversity among individuals; each person is biochemically unique."可知，个体差异不仅仅是数量上的差异，在生物化学角度上都是独一无二的，可判断A选项与原文不符；由第一段中的"The design of any adaptive biological system…because sexual recombination would fatally scramble the blueprints for qualitatively different design. （任何适应性生物系统的设计——对其工作原理的解释——在有性繁殖的物种中几乎可以肯定个体间是一致的，因为有性生殖的遗传因子重组会打乱本质上有差异的设计）"可知，差异就是本质的，而不是由有性生殖造成的，故B选项与原文不符；由第一段中的"Genetic differences among people... when we appreciate what makes minds intelligent at all"可知，"人与人之间的基因差异——无论在爱情、经历、人事、八卦或是政治上对我们多么奇妙——在我们判断是什么让智商不同时就都不值一提了"，本质才是最重要的。因此C选项与原文不符合。本题正确答案为D选项。

24．B。推理题。由最后一段中的"With the exception of the maleness-determining gene on the Y-chromosome, every functioning gene in a man's body is also found in a woman's and vice versa. （除了生殖系统，男性体内的每一个起作用的基因都存在于女性体内，反之亦然。）"可知，B选项"除了生殖系统，男女基因构成都是一样的"正确。

25．C。推理题。由第一段中的"Emphasizing commonalities is not just a matter of a scientific taste... blueprints for qualitatively different designs."可知，强调共性不只是一个科学体验的问题，任何适应性生物系统的设计——对其工作原理的解释——在有性繁殖的物种中几乎可以肯定个体间是一致的，因为有性生殖的遗传因子重组会打乱本质上有差异的设计蓝图。故C选项（现象学家）是正确答案。

Passage Six

26．B。推理题。由第一段中的"Science has begun to crack the...as words and their orderings. （科学已经开始破解这个设计精妙的密码，大脑使用文字及各种组合来传达复杂的思想。）"可推知B选项"根据语法规则的单词使句子有意义"是正确答案。

27．A。词汇题。由第二段中的"Traces, cases, NPs and the other paraphernalia of syntax ...or something like them, must be a part of our unconscious mental life."可知，paraphernalia 与traces，cases是同等性质的东西，本句意为"痕迹、（语法）格、名词短语和其他的语法工具是无色、没有气味、没有味道的，但与它们类似的东西肯定是我们无意识的心理活动的一部分。"可推知，paraphernalia有"设备，工具"的意思，故device是正确答案。

28．B。推理题。由最后一段中的"Grammar is a protocol that has to interconnect the ear, the mouth and the mind, three every different kinds of machine. （语法是一种规约，它必须使耳朵、嘴巴和大脑这三种非常不同的设备相互联系。）"可知，B选项"一个规则体系"是正确答案。

29. C。主旨题。由第一段和第二段的内容可知，语法的工作原理之所以重要还有另外一个原因。语法对经验主义的学说提出了明确的驳斥，该学说认为，头脑中没有什么不是首先在感觉中出现的。故C选项"科学应该做的是理解现象背后的机制"是正确答案。A选项"一位有思想的计算机科学家是一个熟悉语言理论的人"，B选项"一个人的所见所闻所感构成了科学的可靠数据"，D选项"语言和编程是一样的，因为输出依赖于输入"，此三项均不正确。

30. C。推理题。由最后一段中的"I think all these suggestions miss the mark. Grammar is a protocol that has to interconnect the ear, the mouth and the mind, three very different kinds of machine."可知，C选项"语言学家"是正确答案，因为文中提到，语法是一种规约，它需要耳朵、嘴巴和大脑这三种不同的工具相互联系。

上海交通大学2018年博士研究生入学考试英语试题（阅读部分）

Passage One

Over the years, biologists have suggested two main pathways by which sexual selection may have shaped the evolution of male birdsong. In the first, male competition and intrasexual selection produce relatively short, simple songs used mainly in territorial behavior. In the second, female choice and intersexual selection produce longer, more complicated songs used mainly in mate attraction; like such visual ornamentation as the **peacock's tail**, elaborate vocal characteristics increase the male's chances of being chosen as a mate, and he thus enjoys more reproductive success than his less ostentatious rivals. The two pathways are not mutually exclusive, and we can expect to find examples that reflect their interaction. Teasing them apart has been an important challenge to evolutionary biologists.

Early research confirmed the role of intrasexual selection. In a variety of experiments in the field, males responded aggressively to recorded songs by exhibiting territorial behavior near the speakers. The breakthrough for research into intersexual selection came in the development of a new technique for investigating female response in the laboratory. When female cowbirds raised in isolation in sound-proof chambers were exposed to recordings of male song, they responded by exhibiting mating behavior. By quantifying the responses, researchers were able to determine what particular features of the song were most important. In further experiments on song sparrows, researchers found that when exposed to a single song type repeated several times or to a repertoire of different song types, females responded more to the latter. The beauty of the experimental design is that it effectively rules out confounding variables; acoustic isolation assures that the female can respond only to the song structure itself.

If intersexual selection operates as theorized, males with more complicated songs should not only attract females more readily but should also enjoy greater reproductive success. At first, however, researchers doing fieldwork with song sparrows found no correlation between larger repertoires and early mating, which has been shown to be one indicator of reproductive success; further, common measures of male quality used to predict reproductive success, such as weight, size, age, and territory, also failed to correlate with song complexity.

The confirmation researchers had been seeking was finally achieved in studies involving two varieties of warblers. Unlike the song sparrow, which repeats one of its several song types in bouts before switching to another, the warbler continuously composes much longer and more variable songs without repetition. For the first time, researchers found a significant correlation between repertoire size and early mating, and they discovered further that repertoire size had a more significant effect than any other measure of male quality on the number of young produced. The evidence suggests that warblers use their extremely elaborate songs primarily to attract females, clearly confirming the effect of intersexual selection on the evolution of birdsong.

1. The passage is primarily concerned with _____.

    A. showing that intrasexual selection has a greater effect on birdsong than does intersexual selection

    B. contrasting the role of song complexity in several species of birds

    C. describing research confirming the suspected relationship between intersexual selection and the complexity of birdsong

    D. demonstrating the superiority of laboratory work over field studies in evolutionary biology

2. The author mentions the peacock's tail in Paragraph 1 most probably in order to _____.

    A. cite an exception to the theory of the relationship between intrasexual selection and male competition

    B. illustrate the importance of both of the pathways that shaped the evolution of birdsong

    C. draw a distinction between competing theories of intersexual selection

    D. give an example of a feature that may have evolved through intersexual selection by female choice

3. According to the passage, which of the following is specifically related to intrasexual selection?

    A. Female choice.   B. Territorial behavior.

    C. Complex song types.   D. Large song repertoires.

4. Which of the following, if true, would most clearly demonstrate the interaction mentioned in beginning of the second paragraph?

    A. Female larks respond similarly both to short, simple songs and to longer, more complicated songs.

    B. Male canaries use visual ornamentation as well as elaborate song repertoires for mate attraction.

    C. Both male and female blackbirds develop elaborate visual and vocal characteristics.

    D. Male jays use songs to compete among themselves and to attract females.

5. The passage indicates that researchers raised female cowbirds in acoustic isolation in order to _____.

    A. eliminate confounding variables

    B. approximate field conditions

    C. measure reproductive success

    D. quantify repertoire complexity

6. According to the passage, the song sparrow is unlike the warbler in that the song sparrow _____.

    A. uses songs mainly in territorial behavior

B. continuously composes long and complex songs

C. has a much larger song repertoire

D. repeats one song type before switching to another

Passage Two

"Deep reading"— as opposed to the often superficial reading we do on the Web — is an endangered practice, one we ought to take steps to preserve as we would a historic building or a significant work of art. Its disappearance would jeopardize the intellectual and emotional development of generations growing up online, as well as the preservation of a critical part of our culture: the novels, poems and other kinds of literature that can be appreciated only by readers whose brains, quite literally, have been trained to understand them.

Recent research in cognitive science and psychology has demonstrated that deep reading—slow, immersive, rich in sensory detail and emotional and moral complexity—is a distinctive experience, different in kind from the mere decoding of words. Although deep reading does not, strictly speaking, require a conventional book, the built-in limits of the printed page are uniquely helpful to the deep reading experience. A book's lack of hyperlinks (超链接), for example, frees the reader from making decisions — should I click on this link or not? —allowing her to remain fully immersed in the narrative.

That immersion is supported by the way the brain handles language rich in detail, indirect reference and figures of speech: by creating a mental representation that draws on the same brain regions that would be active if the scene were unfolding in real life. The emotional situations and moral dilemmas that are the stuff of literature are also vigorous exercise for the brain, propelling us inside the heads of fictional characters and even, studies suggest, increasing our real-life capacity for empathy（认同）.

None of this is likely to happen when we're browsing through a website. Although we call the activity by the same name, the deep reading of books and the information-driven reading we do on the Web are very different, both in the experience they produce and in the capacities they develop. A growing body of evidence suggests that online reading may be less engaging and less satisfying, even for the "digital natives" to whom it is so familiar. Last month, for example, Britain's National Literacy Trust released the results of a study of 34,910 young people aged 8 to 16. Researchers reported that 39% of children and teens read daily using electronic devices, but only 28% read printed materials every day. Those who read only onscreen were three times less likely to say they enjoy reading very much and a third less likely to have a favorite book. The study also found that young people who read daily only onscreen were nearly two times less likely to be above-average readers than those who read daily in print or both in print and onscreen.

7. What does the author say about "deep reading"?

    A. It serves as a complement to online reading.

    B. It should be preserved before it is too late.

    C. It is mainly suitable for reading literature.

    D. It is an indispensable part of education.

8. Why does the author advocate the reading of literature?

    A. It helps promote readers' intellectual and emotional growth.

    B. It enables readers to appreciate the complexity of language.

    C. It helps readers build up immersive reading habits.

    D. It is quickly becoming an endangered practice.

9. In what way does printed-page reading differ from online reading?

    A. It ensures the reader's cognitive growth.

    B. It enables the reader to be fully engaged.

    C. It activates a different region of the brain.

    D. It helps the reader learn rhetorical devices.

10. What do the studies show about online reading?

    A. It gradually impairs one's eyesight.

    B. It keeps arousing readers' curiosity.

    C. It provides up-to-date information.

    D. It renders reading less enjoyable.

11. What do we learn from the study released by Britain's National Literacy Trust?

    A. Onscreen readers may be less competent readers.

    B. Those who do reading in print are less informed.

    C. Young people find reading onscreen more enjoyable.

    D. It is now easier to find a favorite book online to read.

Passage Three

Nothing succeeds in business books like the study of success. The current business-book boom was launched in 1982 by Tom Peters and Robert Waterman with "In Search of Excellence". It has been kept going ever since by a succession of gurus and would-be gurus who promise to distil the essence of excellence into three (or five or seven) simple rules.

"The Three Rules" is a self-conscious contribution to this type; it even includes a bibliography of "success studies". Messrs Raynor and Mumtaz Ahmed work for a consultancy, Deloitte, that is determined to turn itself into more of a thought-leader and less a corporate repairman. They employ all the tricks of the success genre. They insist that their conclusions are "measurable and actionable" — guide to behavior rather than analysis for its own sake. Success authors usually serve up vivid stories about how exceptional businesspeople stamped their personalities on a company or rescued it from a life-threatening crisis. Messrs Raynor and Ahmed are happier chewing the numbers: they provide detailed appendices on "calculating the elements of advantage" and "detailed analysis".

The authors spent five years studying the behaviour of their 344 "exceptional companies", only to come up at first with nothing. Every hunch（直觉）led to a blind alley and every hypothesis to a dead end. It was only when they shifted their attention from how companies behave to how they think that they began to make sense of their voluminous material.

Management is all about making difficult trade-offs in conditions that are always uncertain and ever-changing. But exceptional companies approach these trade-offs with two simple rules in mind, sometimes consciously, sometimes unconsciously. First: better before cheaper. Companies are more likely to succeed in the long run if they compete on quality or performance than on price. Second: revenue before cost. Companies have more to gain in the long run from driving up revenue than by driving down costs.

Most success studies suffer from two faults. There is "the halo（光环）effect", whereby good performance leads commentators to attribute all manner of virtues to anything and everything the company does. These virtues then suddenly become vices when the company fails. Messrs Raynor and Ahmed work hard to avoid these mistakes by studying large bodies of data over several decades. But they end up embracing a different error: stating the obvious. Most businesspeople will not be surprised to learn that it is better to find a profitable niche（缝隙市场）and focus on boosting your revenues than to compete on price and cut your way to success. The difficult question is how to find that profitable niche and protect it.

There, "The Three Rules" is less useful.

12. What kind of business books are most likely to sell well?

    A. Books on excellence.   B. Guides to management.

    C. Books on business rules.   D. Analyses of market trends.

13. What does the author imply about books on success so far?

    A. They help businessmen one way or another.

    B. They are written by well-recognised experts.

    C. They more or less fall into the same stereotype.

    D. They are based on analyses of corporate leaders.

14. How does "The Three Rules" different from other success books according to the passage?

    A. It focuses on the behavior of exceptional businessmen.

    B. It bases its detailed analysis on large amount of data.

    C. It offers practicable advice to businessmen.

    D. It draws conclusion from vivid examples.

15. What does the passage say contributes to the success of exceptional companies?

    A. Focus on quality and revenue.

    B. Management and sales promotion.

    C. Lower production costs and competitive prices.

    D. Emphasis on after-sale service and maintenance.

16. What is the author's comment on "The Three Rules"?

    A. It can help to locate profitable niches.

    B. It has little to offer to businesspeople.

    C. It is noted for its detailed data analysis.

    D. It fails to identify the keys to success.

Passage Four

Antarctica has actually become a kind of space station — a unique observation post for detecting important changes in the world's environment. Remote from major sources of pollution and the complex geological and ecological systems that prevail elsewhere,

Antarctica makes possible scientific measurements that are often sharper and easier to interpret than those made in other parts of the world.

Growing numbers of scientists therefore see Antarctica as a distant-early-warning sensor, where potentially dangerous global trends may be spotted before they show up to the north. One promising field of investigation is glaciology. Scholars from the United States, Switzerland, and France are pursuing seven separate but related projects that reflect their concern for the health of the West Antarctic Ice Sheet — a concern they believe the world at large should share.

The Transantarctic Mountains, some of them more than 14,000 feet high, divide the continent into two very different regions. The part of the continent to the "east" of the mountains is a high plateau covered by an ice sheet nearly two miles thick. "West" of the mountain, the half of the continent south of the Americas is also covered by an ice sheet, but there the ice rests on rock that is mostly well below sea level. If the West Antarctic Ice Sheet disappeared, the western part of the continent would be reduced to a sparse cluster of islands.

While ice and snow are obviously central to many environmental experiments, others focus on the mysterious "dry valley" of Antarctica, valleys that contain little ice or snow even in the depths of winter. Slashed through the mountains of southern Victoria Land, these valleys once held enormous glaciers that descended 9,000 feet from the polar plateau to the Ross Sea. Now the glaciers are gone, perhaps a casualty of the global warming trend during the 10,000 years since the ice age. Even the snow that falls in the dry valleys is blasted out by vicious winds that roars down from the polar plateau to the sea. Left bare are spectacular gorges, rippled fields of sand dunes, clusters of boulders sculptured into fantastic shapes by 100-mile-an-hour winds, and an aura of extraterrestrial desolation.

Despite the unearthly aspect of the dry valleys, some scientists believe they may carry a message of hope of the verdant parts of the earth. Some scientists believe that in some cases the dry valleys may soak up pollutants faster than pollutants enter them.

17. What is the best title for this passage?

    A. Antarctica and Environmental Problems

    B. Antarctica: Earth's Early-Warning Station

    C. Antarctica: a Unique Observation Post

    D. Antarctica: a Mysterious Place

18. What would the result be if the West Antarctic Ice Sheet disappeared?

    A. The western part of the continent would be disappeared.

    B. The western part of the continent would be reduced.

    C. The western part of the continent would become scattered islands.

    D. The western part of the continent would be reduced to a cluster of islands.

19. Why are the Dry Valleys left bare?

    A. Vicious wind blasts the snow away.

    B. It rarely snows.

    C. Because of the global warming trend and fierce wind.

    D. Because of sand dunes.

20. Which of the following is true?

    A. The "Dry Valleys" have nothing left inside.

    B. The "Dry Valleys" never held glaciers.

    C. The "Dry Valleys" may carry a message of hope for the verdant.

    D. The "Dry Valleys" are useless to scientists.

21. What is the meaning of "an aura of extraterrestrial desolation"?

    A. Aliens' footprints after they arrived there.

    B. A bleak atmosphere isolated from the earth.

    C. A mysterious existence left by other planets.

    D. Some lights never seen by the people on earth.

Passage Five

Mass transportation revised the social and economic fabric of the American city in three fundamental ways. It catalyzed physical expansion, it sorted out people and land uses, and it accelerated the inherent instability of urban life. By opening vast areas of unoccupied land for residential expansion, the omnibuses, horse railways, commuter trains, and electric trolleys pulled settled regions outward two to four times more distant from city centers than they were in the premodern era. In 1850, for example, the borders of Boston lay scarcely two miles from the old business district; by the turn of the century the radius extended ten miles. Now those who could afford it could live far removed from the old city center and still commute there for work, shopping, and entertainment. The new accessibility of land around the periphery of almost every major city sparked an explosion of real estate development and fueled what we now know as urban sprawl. Between 1890 and 1920, for example, some 250,000 new residential lots were recorded within the borders of Chicago, most of them located in outlying areas. Over the same period, another 550,000 were plotted outside the city limits but within the metropolitan area. Anxious to take advantage of the possibilities of commuting, real estate developers added 800,000 potential building sites to the Chicago region in just thirty years — lots that could have housed five to six million people.

Of course, many were never occupied; there was always a huge surplus of subdivided, but vacant, land around Chicago and other cities. These excesses underscore a feature of residential expansion related to the growth of mass transportation: urban sprawl was essentially unplanned. It was carried out by thousands of small investors who paid little heed to coordinated land use or to future land users. Those who purchased and prepared land for residential purposes, particularly land near or outside city borders where transit lines and middle-class inhabitants were anticipated, did so to create demand as much as to respond to it. Chicago is a prime example of this process. Real estate subdivision there proceeded much faster than population growth.

22. With which of the following subjects is the passage mainly concerned?

    A. Types of mass transportation.

    B. Instability of urban life.

    C. How supply and demand determine land use.

    D. The effect of mass transportation on urban expansion.

23. Why does the author mention both Boston and Chicago?

    A. To demonstrate positive and negative effects of growth.

    B. To exemplify cities with and without mass transportation.

    C. To show mass transportation changed many cities.

    D. To contrast their rate of growth.

24. According to the passage, what was one disadvantage of residential expansion?

    A. It was expensive.

    B. It happened too slowly.

    C. It was unplanned.

D. It created a demand for public transportation.

25. The author mentions Chicago in the second paragraph as an example of a city, _____.

    A. that is large

    B. that is used as a model for land development

    C. where the development of land exceeded population growth

    D. with an excellent mass transportation system

上海交通大学2018年博士研究生入学考试英语试题（阅读部分）答案与解析

Passage One

1. C。主旨题。本文开篇就讲了文章大意：two main pathways by which sexual selection may have shaped the evolution of male birdsong，即性间选择和性内选择对雄性鸟叫的形成作用，因此主题词最完整的是C选项。

2. D。目的题。答案就在该定位处的前后：like such visual ornamentation as the peacock's tail, … enjoys more reproductive success than his less ostentatious rivals。这里是个类比：如果雄性孔雀尾巴不够鲜艳，被雌性选择成配偶的概率就低；如果雄性孔雀的声音不够精致，成功的概率也会低于它们更花哨的对手。因此，提及孔雀尾巴是为了例证被雌性动物性间选择的重点，故选项D为正确答案。

3. B。细节题。通过定位intrasexual selection和命题顺序定位到第二段：Early research confirmed the role of intrasexual selection … by exhibiting territorial behavior near the speakers，早期研究证实了性内选择的角色，雄性鸟类会通过展示领地行为来做出强有力的反应。第一句是论点，第二句是论点的扩展，这是典型的例证题。故选项B正确。

4. D。推断题。第二段开头是一个对比：Early research confirmed the role of intrasexual selection …The breakthrough for research into intersexual selection came in the development of a new technique for investigating female response in the laboratory.早期研究证实了性内选择的作用，对性间选择研究的突破来自实验室里调查雌性反应的新技术。这是论点，能证明该论点的论据选项中，只有D选项（雄性松鸦用歌声来相互竞争并吸引雌

性）最完整。A选项没有涉及intrasexual selection和inters exualselection，B偏离了bird song 的主题，C选项没有涉及性选择。

5. A。推断题。在无声环境中饲养雌性牛鸟，然后将其置于声音环境下，看它们的反应。该段末尾有一句总结：The beauty of the experimental design is that … the female can respond only to the song structure itself，即实验设计的美妙之处在于它有效地排除了混杂的变量；声音隔离确保了雌性只能对歌曲结构本身做出反应。不难判断本题答案为A。

6. D。细节题。关于song sparrow和warbler的区别，可定位在最后一段Unlike the song sparrow … the warbler continuously composes much longer and more variable songs without repetition，这里要分清问的是song sparrow还是warbler，原文中定语从句which指代的是song sparrow，说它是先重复一种歌再换成其他的种类，可知与D选项一致。

Passage Two

7. B。细节题。通过命题顺序从第一段开始找答案，大意是"深度阅读应该像历史古迹或艺术作品一样被保护起来"，说明深度阅读已经濒临灭绝了。因此B选项（在为时未晚之前保护深度阅读）是正确答案。

8. A。推断题。从第二段的首句Recent research in cognitive science and psychology has demonstrated that deep reading—slow, immersive, rich in sensory detail and emotional and moral complexity…可知，深度阅读实际是缓慢的、沉浸式的阅读，是对丰富的感性细节、情绪及道德的复杂程度的体验，即它可以帮助读者发展智力和情感成长。故A选项正确。B选项"使读者能欣赏语言的复杂性"不是深度阅读的目的，而是深度阅读的对象；C选项"帮助读者建立沉浸式阅读习惯"是同义重复，即深度阅读就是沉浸式阅读，D选项"很快变成濒危行为"与本题无关。故A选项为正确答案。

9. B。细节题。用printed-page reading定位到第二段the built-in limits of the printed page are uniquely helpful to the deep reading experience … allowing her to remain fully immersed in the narrative，即阅读纸质版的书会让读者完全沉浸在叙事中。故B选项为正确答案。

10. D。细节题。通过online reading 定位到最后一段中的A growing body of evidence suggests that online reading may be less engaging and less satisfying可知，在线阅读会减少阅读的黏性，难以让人满意。因此正确答案为D。

11. A。细节题。通过Britain's National Literacy Trust定位到最后一段的最后一句：The study also found that young people who read daily only onscreen … in print or both in print and onscreen，即屏幕阅读者成为中等偏上的阅读者的概率比纸媒或者纸媒加屏幕阅读者少两倍。故A选项为正确答案。

Passage Three

12．A。推断题。题干问题为："以下哪种商业图书最可能大卖？"根据关键词 business books 定位到第一段中的"Nothing succeeds in business books like the study of success."即商业图书中最成功的就是对成功的研究。如今商业图书的繁荣始于1982年的一本名为《追求卓越》的书。从那以后，一系列大师将这种繁荣持续了下来，他们承诺提取卓越的本质并把它简化成3（5或7）个简单的规则。由此可知，A选项"研究卓越的书"为正确答案。

13．C。推断题。由第二段可知，他们使用了成功学图书的所有诡计。他们坚持说他们的结论是可衡量的和可执行的——引导行为而不是分析。成功学作者们经常准备好了一些生动的关于卓越的商人是怎样把自己的个性刻画于自己的公司之中，或怎样把公司从致命危机中拯救出来的故事。文中的usually暗示，成功学作者们经常这样做，可知C选项"他们或多或少陷入了同样的思维定式"为正确答案。

14．B。推断题。题干问题为：作者认为《三大规则》这本书与其他成功学图书有何不同？根据关键词大写的*Three Rules*定位，发现剩下的文章内容几乎都是在说这本书。于是动用顺序原则优先看第三段大意就是：他们前五年对344家优秀公司进行的研究毫无成果。直到他们把注意力从卓越公司做了什么转移到总结卓越公司的思考方式，他们浩瀚的研究素材才有成果。由此可知他们的重点是站在卓越公司的角度思考动因以分析成功，所以选项B"此书详细的分析是基于海量的数据。"为正确答案。

15。A。细节题。题干问题为：文章认为卓越公司的成功是依靠以下哪个选项？根据关键词exceptional companies 定位到第四段。大意就是：卓越公司有两大原则：第一，打质量仗而不是价格仗；第二，开源而不是节流。由此可知选项A"专注于质量和收入。"为正确答案。

16．D。推断题。题干问题为：作者对《三大规则》这本书有何评价？根据关键词 *Three Rules*和comment，并按照顺序原则定位到最后一段最后两句。大意是：此书犯了另一个错误，就是忽视了商人们的难题是获得盈利并保持领先。在这个方面，此书没那么有用。由此得出作者对此书并不是完全认可，所以选项D"它未能指出成功的关键。"为正确答案。

Passage Four

17．A。推断题。选项B"南极洲：地球的预警站。"选项C"南极洲：独一无二的观测站。"选项D"南极洲：神秘的地方。"三个选项都是文章的组成部分，而A选项是其他选项的归纳概括，故为正确答案。

18．D。细节题。第三段"横断南极的山脉，有的高达一万四千多英尺，把这块大陆分成情况各异的两个地区。山脉以东的大陆部分是由差不多两英里厚的冰层覆盖的高原；山脉以西，即美洲以南的半个大陆也为冰层所覆盖。可是，这里冰层覆盖在大大低于海平面的岩石上。如果西南极洲冰层消失，那南极大陆西部将成为稀疏的岛群。"可知选项D正确。

19．C。推断题。在第四段："……这些干谷甚至在寒冬季节也很少有冰雪。它们插在南维多利亚陆地的山脉中，一度曾有从极地高原到罗斯海的深度为9 000英尺的冰河。现在冰河已不存在，很可能是冰河时代之后一万年间地球变暖的结果。即使落入干谷的雪也被从极地高原咆哮入海的邪恶狂风吹散了。留下来的是光秃秃的壮观的峡谷，起伏的沙丘，被时速100英里的大风雕刻成奇形怪状的巨石群，以及外星荒凉的景象。"综合原文不难看出，全球变暖，狂风劲吹，干谷只能变成光秃秃的了。本题是因果逻辑关系题，A，B，D选项都是现象。

20．C。细节题。答案是第五段第一句"尽管干谷具有神秘的一面，科学家却相信它们可能为地球上葱绿的地方带来了希望的信息"。故选项C正确。

21．B。推断题。此处大意是：即使是落在干谷中的雪也被从极地高原咆哮入海的邪恶狂风吹散了。留下来的是光秃秃的壮观的峡谷、起伏的沙丘、被时速100英里的大风雕刻成奇形怪状的巨石群，以及外星荒凉的景象。根据上下文，此处应该选择B，并非指真正出现了外星球或者星际之间的神秘事件，而是一种荒凉的气氛。

Passage Five

22．D。推断题。文章开门见山提出这一点"公共交通运输从三个根本方面改变了美国城市的社会和经济结构"。后面文章内容就是这三个方面的具体化。选项A"公共交通运输类型。"选项B"城市生活的不稳定性。"选项C"供需如何决定土地利用。"这三项文中作为具体问题提到了，但并不是文章涉及的主题。故选项D"公共交通运输对城市扩展的影响。"为正确答案。

23．C。推断题。答案见第一段第四句"举例说，1850年，波士顿的边界离老的商业地区几乎不到2英里，到了这个世纪末，其半径扩至10英里。现在有支付能力的人可以在远离老的城市中心的地方居住，仍然可以通勤到市中心工作、购物和娱乐"。第七句"在1890年至1920年间，芝加哥境内记录了约25万个新住宅地块，其中大部分位于郊区。在同一时期，另有55万人在城市范围外但在大都市区内被计划安置。由于急于利用通勤的可能性，房地产开发商在短短30年内为芝加哥地区增加了80万个潜在建筑用地——这些用地原本可以容纳500万至600万人。"选项A"表示成长的正反两方面效果。"选项B"列举有和无公共交通运输的城市为例。"选项D"对比两者成长率。"这三项都不是本文中列举两城市例子的目的。只有选项C"说明公共交通改变了许多城市。"正确。

24．C。细节题。见第二段第二、三句"城市扩张蔓延根本无计划，几千个小的投资商进行扩展，毫不考虑相互协调配合利用土地，也不考虑未来土地利用"。故选项C"没有计划。"正确。

25．C。答案详见第二段"那些出于居住目的购买和准备土地的人，尤其是在城市边界附近或之外的土地上，预计会有公交线路和中产阶级居民，这样做是为了创造需求，也是为了应对需求。芝加哥就是这一过程的典型例子。那里的房地产细分比人口增长快得多。"选项A"城市大"，选项B"用作土地开发的样板"，选项D"具有优越的公共交通系统，都没有讲到土地开发和人口之间的关系"只有选项C"土地开发超过人口增长速度"正确。

南京大学2015年博士研究生入学考试英语试题
（阅读部分）

Passage One

According to sociologists, there are several different ways in which a person may become recognized as the leader of a social group in the United States. In the family, traditional cultural patterns confer leadership on one or both of the parents. In other cases, such as friendship groups, one or more persons may gradually emerge as leaders, although there is no formal process of selection. In larger groups, leaders are usually chosen formally through election or recruitment.

Although leaders are often thought to be people with unusual personal ability, decades of research have failed to produce consistent evidence that there is any category of "natural leaders". It seems that there is no set of personal qualities that all leaders have in common; rather, virtually any person may be recognized as a leader if the person has qualities that meet the needs of that particular group.

Furthermore, although it is commonly supposed that social groups have a single leader, research suggests that there are typically two different leadership roles that are held by different individuals. Instrumental leadership is leadership that emphasizes the completion of tasks by a social group. Group members look to instrumental leaders to "get things done". Expressive leadership, on the other hand, is leadership that emphasizes the collective well-being of a social group's member. Expressive leaders are less concerned with the overall goals of the group than with providing emotional support to group members and attempting to minimize tension and conflict among them. Group members expect expressive leaders to maintain stable relationships within the group and provide support to individual members.

Instrumental leaders are likely to have a rather secondary relationship to other group members. They give orders and may discipline group members who inhibit attainment of the group's goals. Expressive leaders cultivate a more personal or primary relationship to others in the group. They offer sympathy when someone experiences difficulties or is subjected to discipline, are quick to lighten a serious moment with humor, and try to resolve issues that threaten to divide the group. As the differences in these two roles suggest, expressive leaders generally receive more personal affection from group members; instrumental leaders, if they are successful in promoting group goals, may enjoy a more distant respect.

36. What does the passage mainly discuss?

    A. The problems faced by leaders.

    B. How leadership differs in small and large groups.

    C. How social groups determine who will lead them.

    D. The role of leaders in social groups.

37. The passage mentions all of the following ways by which people can become leaders EXCEPT _____.

    A. recruitment

    B. formal election process

    C. specific leadership training

    D. traditional cultural patterns

38. In mentioning "natural leaders" in Paragraph 2, the author is making the point that _____.

    A. few people qualify as "natural leaders"

    B. there is no proof that "natural leaders" exist

    C. "natural leaders" are easily accepted by the members of a social group

D. "natural leaders" share a similar set of characteristics

39. Which of the following statements about leadership can be inferred from Paragraph 2?

    A. A person who is an effective leader of a particular group may not be an effective leader of another group.

    B. Few people succeed in sharing a leadership role with another person.

    C. A person can best learn how to be an effective leader by studying research on leadership.

    D. Most people desire to be leaders but can produce little evidence of their qualifications.

40. The passage indicates that instrumental leaders generally focus on _____.

    A. ensuring harmonious relationship

    B. sharing responsibility with group members

    C. identifying new leaders

    D. achieving a goal

Passage Two

The word hospice is hundreds of years old. It comes to us from the time called the Middle Ages in Europe. Religious groups then provided hospice as a place where travellers could stay. Sometimes the groups also offered a place for the sick and the dying. Today the word hospice means more than a place. It means a way of caring for the dying. In the modern sense of the word, it means that, if possible, dying people can receive care at home during their last days; and the healthcare workers do not try to lengthen the lives of the dying with modern medical equipment. Instead, care-givers make every effort to control or stop the patients' pain. It also means that patients get help for their emotional needs in addition to their physical needs.

A British woman Cicely Saunders was the first major activist for hospice care in modern times. Cicely Saunders worked as a nurse in a hospital right after World War II, where she met a man who was dying of cancer. Together they found ideas about the best possible treatment for people who would never get well again. They talked about treatments that would permit patients to discuss their feelings and to take part in activities meaningful to them. They planned a system that would allow dying people to be surrounded by the people and things they loved most. The dying man gave Cicely Saunders enough money to study to become a doctor. By 1967 Dr. Saunders had organized and opened St. Christopher's Hospice in London.

In 1974, after the America's first hospice started in New Haven, others followed suit in cities throughout the country. Organizers had a difficult job. They had to teach the public about the idea of hospice. They had to get money from companies, religious groups and citizens. And they had to negotiate with local governments to use public money to care for the dying. Thanks to their unyielding determination and painstaking efforts, hospice has grown in America. Dr. Jo Magno, the President of the National Hospice Organization, said that working with the dying occasionally made her sad. Yet she remembers the words of Dr. Cicely Saunders — "We cannot add days to life, but we can add life to days."

41. What is the original meaning of the word "hospice" ?

A. It was a place where the homeless old people were taken care of.

B. It was a place where religious people lived.

C. It was a place offered by churches for the travellers.

D. It was a place where doctors treated patients.

42. In the modern sense of the word, hospice includes all of the following EXCEPT _____.

A. a priest is invited to pray for the dying

B. a dying patient is taken care of at his home

C. efforts are made to reduce the pain of the dying people

D. the psychological needs of the dying are considered and cared for

43. What did Cicely and the man talk about?

A. How to advise the hospital to treat the dying patients.

B. How to make arrangement for the patients who had no hope of recovery.

C. The meaningful activities for all patients to take part in.

D. The kind of people that are allowed to visit the patients.

44. How did Cicely Saunders complete her study?

A. By working part-time.

B. By obtaining a fellowship.

C. With the help of a man's money.

D. Through her management of St. Christopher's Hospice.

45. Which is a correct statement about the early American hospice?

A. It was an immediate success as a result of the effort by Dr. Cicely.

B. It was probably not easy to persuade companies to provide financial support.

C. Many people readily accepted the new idea.

D. Local governments forbade what they did.

Passage Three

What we today call American folk art was, indeed, art of, by, and for ordinary, everyday "folks" who, with increasing prosperity and leisure, created a market for art of all kinds, and especially for portraits. Citizens of prosperous, essentially middle-class republics—whether ancient Romans, seventeenth century Dutch burghers, or nineteenth century Americans—have always shown a marked taste for portraiture. Starting in the late eighteenth century, the United States contained increasing numbers of such people, and of the artists who could meet their demands.

The earliest American folk art portraits come, not surprisingly, from New England—especially Connecticut and Massachusetts—for this was a wealthy and populous region and the center of a strong craft tradition. Within a few decades after the signing of the *Declaration of Independence* in 1776, the population was pushing westward, and portrait painters could be found at work in western New York, Ohio, Kentucky, Illinois, and Missouri. Midway through its first century as a nation, the United States' population had increased roughly five times, and eleven new states had been added to the original thirteen. During these years the demand for portraits grew and grew, eventually to be satisfied by camera. In 1839 the daguerreotype was introduced to America, ushering in the age of photograph, and within a generation the new invention put an end to the popularity of painted portraits. Once again an original portrait became a luxury, commissioned by the wealthy and executed by the professional.

But in the heyday of portrait painting—from the late eighteenth century until the 1850's—anyone with a modicum of artistic ability could become a limner, as such a portraitist was called. Local craftspeople—sign, coach, and house painters—began to paint portraits as a profitable sideline; sometimes a talented man or woman who began by sketching family members gained a local reputation and was besieged with requests for portraits; artists found it worth their while to pack their paints, canvases, and brushes and to travel the countryside, often combining house decorating with portrait painting.

46. In Lines 3–5 the author mentions seventeenth century Dutch burghers as an example of a group that _____.

    A. consisted mainly of self-taught artists

    B. appreciated portraits

    C. influenced American folk art

    D. had little time for the arts

47. According to the passage, where were many of the first American folk art portraits painted?

    A. In western New York.

    B. In Illinois and Missouri.

    C. In Connecticut and Massachusetts.

    D. In Ohio.

48. The word "this" in Line 9 refers to _____.

    A. a strong craft tradition

    B. American folk art

    C. New England

    D. western New York

49. The phrase "ushering in" in Line 16 is closest in meaning to "_____".

    A. beginning

    B. demanding

    C. publishing

    D. increasing

50. According to the passage, which of the following contributed to a decline in the demand for paint portraits?

    A. The lack of a strong craft tradition.

    B. The westward migration of many painters.

    C. The growing preference for landscape paintings.

D. The invention of the camera.

Passage Four

What percentage of the population in a modern technological society is, like myself, in the fortunate position of being workers? At a guess I would say sixteen percent, and I do not think that figure is likely to get bigger in the future.

Technology and the division of labor have done two things: by eliminating in many fields the need for special strength or skill, they have made a very large number of paid occupations which formerly were enjoyable work into boring labor, and by increasing productivity they have reduced the number of necessary laboring hours. It is already possible to imagine a society in which the majority of the population, that is to say, its laborers, will have almost as much leisure as in earlier times was enjoyed by the aristocracy. When one recalls how aristocracies in the past actually behaved, the prospect is not cheerful. Indeed, the problem of dealing with boredom may be even more difficult for such a future mass society than it was for aristocracies. The latter, for example, ritualized their time; there was a season to shoot grouse, a season to spend in town, etc. The masses are more likely to replace an unchanging ritual by fashion which changes as often as possible in the economic interest of certain people. Again, the masses cannot go in for hunting, for very soon there would be no animals left to hunt. For other aristocratic amusements like gambling, dueling, and warfare, it may be only too easy to find equivalents in dangerous driving, drug-taking, and senseless acts of violence. Workers seldom commit acts of violence, because they can put their aggression into their work, be it physical like the work of a smith, or mental like the work of a scientist or an artist. The role of aggression in mental work is aptly expressed by the phrase "getting one's teeth into a problem".

51. According to the passage, the writer believes the majority of the population _____.

A. are unhappy with what they do

B. will get bigger in their number in the future

C. agree with him on his classification

D. are in the fortunate position of being workers

52. According to the passage, technology and the division of labor have done all the following EXCEPT _____.

   A. increasing the joy of the paid occupations

   B. making skill and special strength unnecessary in work

   C. causing jobs to be dull labor

   D. decreasing working hours

53. What can be inferred from the passage about special strength and skill?

   A. Special strength and skill must be abandoned if people want to enjoy their work.

   B. Special strength and skill are necessary for people to find their work enjoyable.

   C. Special strength or skill causes work to be boring.

   D. Special strength or skill reduces the number of necessary laboring hours.

54. According to the passage, aristocracy dealt with boredom by _____.

   A. enjoying more leisure

   B. working with laborers

   C. demanding difficult work for the masses

   D. ritualizing their time

55. Which of the following is one of the amusements of the masses?

   A. Hunting.   B. Gambling.

   C. Foolish acts of violence.   D. Doing scientific research.

南京大学2015年博士研究生入学考试英语试题
（阅读部分）答案与解析

Passage One

36. D。主旨题。首段第一句提到，在美国，一个人有可能通过很多不同的方式成为一个社会团体的领导。之后的段落着重说明社会团体中两种不同的领导：建设性的领导和富于表现力的领导。由此可知，文章主要说明在社会团体中不同领导的角色。故答案为 D。

37. C。细节题。根据题干可定位至首段第二、三、四句。句中提及在家庭中的 traditional cultural patterns 对应选项 D 的内容；在较大团体中的 formal process of election or recruitment 分别对应选项 B 和选项 A 的内容。选项 C 在文中未提及。故答案为 C。

38. B。推理题。第二段中的 decades of research have failed to produce consistent evidence that there is any category of "natural leaders" 指出，几十年的研究未能提供一致的证据表明存在 "天生的领导" 这一类别。之后进一步说明 there is no set of personal qualities that all leaders have in common，即没有所有领导共有的所谓 "领导品质" 的证据。以上信息与选项 B 中提及的 no proof that "natural leaders" exist 一致。故答案为 B。

39. A。推理题。第二段中指出 there is no set of personal qualities that all leaders have in common，即没有所有领导共有的所谓 "领导品质"。此段最后一句指出 any person may be recognized as a leader if the person has qualities that meet the needs of that particular group，即几乎任何一个人只要拥有符合特定团体需要的品质，都有可能被认定为领导者。而 particular group（特定团体）的设定说明一个团体的领导并不一定能够胜任另外一个团体的领导角色，与选项 A 信息一致。故答案为 A。

40. D。细节题。根据题干定位至第三段中的 "Instrumental leadership is leadership that emphasizes the completion of tasks by a social group." 此句指出建设型领导是那种强调社会团体完成任务型的领导，而随后对 expressive leadership 进行了说明，指出富于表现力的领导较少关注团队的整体目标（less concerned with the overall goals of the group），显然，这点与建设型领导是不同的。由此可知，instrumental leadership 更加关注达成目标。故答案为 D。

Passage Two

41. C。细节题。题干中问的是 "hospice" 最初的意思（original meaning），根据题干定位至文章首段第二句中的 Religious groups then provided hospice as a place where travellers could stay。故答案为 C。

42. A。细节题。根据题干定位至文章首段中的 "Today the word hospice means more than a place." 之后的信息。句中的 dying people can receive care at home during their last days 与选项 B 对应；care-givers make every effort to control or stop the patients' pain 与选项 C 对应；patients get help for their emotional needs in addition to their physical needs 与选项 D 对应，只有选项 A 的内容在文中未提及。故答案为 A。

43. B。推理题。文中第二段提及 Cicely 与一位将死的癌症患者讨论对于那些无法治愈的患者的最佳治疗方法。同时，他们计划了一项能够让那些将死之人所最热爱的人和物陪伴在他们身边的医疗体系。由此可知，Cicely 和癌症患者讨论的是如何安排那些无法治愈的患者的治疗，故答案为 B。

44. C。细节题。根据题干定位至第二段倒数第二句话 The dying man gave Cicely Saunders enough money to study，由此可知，Cicely Saunders 完成学业的钱来自这位濒临死亡的男士的资助。故答案为 C。

45. B。推理题。根据题干定位至文章最后一段。根据此段中的 "Organizers had a difficult job." 可知，组织者遇到了一系列的困难。由此可知，选项 A 中提及的 immediate success 与文意不符。文中提及 "They had to teach the public about the idea of hospice." 可知公众对终极关怀的理念是不太理解的，选项 C 与此信息不符；根据 they had to negotiate with local governments to use public money to care for the dying 可知，当地政府并不是禁止（forbid）该机构，而是不愿意使用公共资金来照顾濒死之人，选项 D 也不正确。根据文中的 They had to get money from companies 可知组织者们不得不努力从企业获得资金支持，与选项 B 内容一致。故答案为 B。

Passage Three

46. B。细节题。题干中提及 seventeenth century Dutch burghers，作者以此为例是为了说明文章首段首句提出的观点，即美国民间艺术是由普通百姓所拥有、创造并享受的艺术。随着财富和闲暇与日俱增，他们创造了各种艺术的市场，特别是肖像绘画。由此可知，答案为 B。

47. C。细节题。根据题干定位至第二段中的 The earliest American folk art portraits come, not surprisingly, from New England—especially Connecticut and Massachusetts，由此可知美国最早的民间艺术画像来自新英格兰地区——特别是康涅狄格州和马萨诸塞州。故答案为 C。

48. C。指代题。this 之前提及美国最早的民间艺术画像来自新英格兰地区（New England），之后解释了原因：该地区富裕、人口稠密，而且是浓厚艺术传统的中心。由此可知，this 指代的是前面提及的 New England。故答案为 C。

49. A。词义题。根据第二段中的 the demand for portraits grew and grew, eventually to be satisfied by camera 可知，美国独立后的 50 年间，肖像绘画的需求不断增长，直到有了照相机才算得到满足。之后提及 In 1839 the daguerreotype was introduced to America，即银版照相法于 1839 年传入美国。Camera（相机），Daguerreotype（银版照相法）与 ushering in the age of photography 中的 photography（摄影）说明的内容一致。由此可知，随着银版照相法于 1839 年传入美国，摄影时代到来了，故 ushering in 的意思应为 "到来，

开始"，故答案为 A。

50．D。细节题。第二段提及摄影时代的到来致使在不超过一代人的时间内，手工画像就不再风靡了。根据 within a generation the new invention put an end to the popularity of painted portraits 可知，手工画像需求的减少源自相机的发明，故答案为 D。

Passage Four

51．A。推理题。作者在文章首段提及在一个现代化的技术社会里，总人口中有多大比例的人能够像自己一样有幸成为工作者呢（in the fortunate position of being workers），作者在这里使用了 fortunate，但实际上劳动者并不幸运。因为在之后的段落中，作者提及技术和劳动分工在许多领域取消了对特别才能和技术的需求，将大量原本令人愉快的工作变成了乏味的劳动（enjoyable work into boring labor）；劳动者有了更多的闲暇时间。但是对劳动者来说，在未来这样一个大众社会里，要解决"无聊"这个问题，也许比过去的贵族们要困难得多（the problem of dealing with boredom may be even more difficult for such a future mass society than it was for aristocracies）。由此可知，对大多数人来说，他们对于所做的事情并没有感到快乐。故答案为 A。

52．A。细节题。根据题干定位至第二段：by eliminating in many fields the need for special strength or skill 与选项 B 对应；made a very large number of paid occupations which formerly were enjoyable work into bring labor 与选项 C 对应；reduced the number of necessary laboring hours 与选项 D 对应。选项 A 中提及 increasing the joy of the paid occupations 与 the prospect is not cheerful 意义相悖，由此可知答案为 A。

53．B。推理题。文中第二段首句提及技术和劳动分工通过在许多领域取消了对特别才能和技术的需求，将大量原本令人愉快的工作变成了乏味的劳动，言外之意是：那些需要特殊才能和技术的工作可以给劳动者带来快乐，故答案为 B。

54．D。细节题。根据题干定位至文章第二段中的 the latter, for example, ritualized their time，由此可知答案为 D。

55．C。细节题。the masses 在文中指的是第二段中的 the majority of the population，即 its laborers，也就是下文提到的 the masses，与 workers 相对；根据第二段最后三句可知，senseless acts of violence 是他们的一种消遣方式，与选项 C 一致，故答案为 C。

山东大学2015年博士研究生入学考试英语试题
（阅读部分）

Passage One

I've been writing for most of my life. The book *Writing Without Teachers* introduced me to one distinction（区别）and one practice that has helped my writing processes tremendously. The distinction is between the creative mind and the critical mind. While you need to employ both to get to a finished result, they cannot work in parallel no matter how much we might like to think so.

Trying to criticize writing on the fly is possibly the single greatest barrier to writing that most of us encounter. If you are listening to that 5th grade English teacher who corrects your grammar while you are trying to capture a fleeting（稍纵即逝的）thought, the thought will die. If you capture the fleeting thought and simply share it with the world in raw form, no one is likely to understand. You must learn to create first and then criticize if you want to make writing the tool for thinking that it is.

The practice that can help you past your learned bad habits of trying to edit as you write is what Elbow calls "free writing". In free writing, the objective is to get words down on paper non-stop, usually for 15-20 minutes. No stopping, no going back, no criticizing. The goal is to get the words flowing. As the words begin to flow, the ideas will come from the shadows and let themselves be captured on your notepad or your screen.

Now you have raw materials that you can begin to work with using the critical mind that you've persuaded to sit on the side and watch quietly. Most likely, you will believe that this will take more time than you actually have and you will end up staring blankly at the pages as the deadline draws near.

Instead of staring at a blank, start filling it with words no matter how bad. Halfway through your available time, stop and rework your raw writing into something closer to finished products. Move back and forth until you run out of time and the final result will most likely be far better than your current practices.

1. When the author says the creative mind and the critical mind "cannot work in parallel" in the writing process, he means _____.

    A. one cannot use them at the same time

    B. they cannot be regarded as equally important

    C. they are in constant conflict with each other

    D. no one can be both creative and critical

2. What prevents people from writing on is _____.

    A. putting their ideas in raw form

    B. ignoring grammatical soundness

    C. attempting to edit as they write

    D. trying to capture fleeting thoughts

3. What is the chief objective of the first stage of writing?

    A. To organize one's thoughts logically.

    B. To get one's ideas down.

    C. To choose an appropriate topic.

    D. To collect raw materials.

4. One common concern of writers about "free writing" is that _____.

    A. it overstresses the role of the creative mind

    B. it does not help them to think clearly

    C. it may bring about too much criticism

    D. it takes too much time to edit afterwards

5. In what way does the critical mind help the writer in the writing process?

    A. It allows him to sit on the side and observe.

    B. It helps him to come up with new ideas.

    C. It saves the writing time available to him.

    D. It improves his writing into better shape.

Passage Two

"The world's environment is surprisingly healthy. Discuss." If that were an examination topic, most students would tear it apart, offering a long list of complaints: from local smog（烟

雾）to global climate change, from the felling（砍伐）of forests to the extinction of species. The list would largely be accurate, the concern legitimate. Yet the students who should be given the highest marks would actually be those who agreed with the statement. The surprise is how good things are, not how bad.

After all, the world's population has more than tripled during this century, and world output has risen hugely, so you would expect the earth itself to have been affected. Indeed, if people lived, consumed and produced things in the same way as they did in 1900 (or 1950, or indeed 1980), the world by now would be a pretty disgusting place: smelly, dirty, toxic and dangerous.

But they don't. The reasons why they don't, and why the environment has not been mined, have to do with prices, technological innovation, social change and government regulation in response to popular pressure. That is why, today's environmental problems in the poor countries ought, in principle, to be solvable.

Raw materials have not run out, and show no sign of doing so. Logically, one day they must: the planet is a finite place. Yet it is also very big, and man is very ingenious. What has happened is that every time a material seems to be running short, the price has risen and, in response, people have looked for new sources of supply, tried to find ways to use less of the material, or looked for a new substitute. For this reason prices for energy and for minerals have fallen in real terms during the century. The same is true for food. Prices fluctuate, in response to harvests, natural disasters and political instability; and when they rise, it takes some time before new sources of supply become available. But they always do, assisted by new farming and crop technology. The long-term trend has been downwards.

It is where prices and markets do not operate properly that this benign（良性的）trend begins to stumble, and the genuine problems arise. Markets cannot always keep the environment healthy. If no one owns the resource concerned, no one has an interest in conserving it or fostering it: fish is the best example of this.

6. According to the author, most students _____.

   A. believe the world's environment is in an undesirable condition

   B. agree that the environment of the world is not as bad as it is thought to be

   C. get high marks for their good knowledge of the world's environment

   D. appear somewhat unconcerned about the state of the world's environment

7. The huge increase in world production and population _____.

   A. has made the world a worse place to live in

B. has had a positive influence on the environment

C. has not significantly affected the environment

D. has made the world a dangerous place to live in

8. One of the reasons why the long-term trend of prices has been downwards is that _____.

   A. technological innovation can promote social stability

   B. political instability will cause consumption to drop

   C. new farming and crop technology can lead to overproduction

   D. new sources are always becoming available

9. Fish resources are diminishing because _____.

   A. no new substitutes can be found in large quantities

   B. they are not owned by any particular entity

   C. improper methods of fishing have mined the fishing grounds

   D. water pollution is extremely serious

10. The primary solution to environmental problems is _____.

   A. to allow market forces to operate properly

   B. to curb consumption of natural resources

   C. to limit the growth of the world population

   D. to avoid fluctuations in prices

Passage Three

Low-level slash-and-burn farming doesn't harm rainforest. On the contrary, it helps farmers and improves forest soils. This is the unorthodox view of a German soil scientist who has shown that burnt clearings in the Amazon, dating back more than 1,000 years, helped creates patches of rich, fertile soil that farmers still benefit from today.

Most rainforest soils are thin and poor because they lack minerals and because the heat and heavy rainfall destroy most organic matter in the soils within four years of it reaching the forest floor. This means topsoil contains few of the ingredients needed for long-term successful farming. But Bruno Glaser, a soil scientist of the University of Bayreuth, has studied unexpected patches of fertile soils in the central Amazon. These soils contain lots of organic matter.

Glaser has shown that most of this fertile organic matter comes from "black carbon" — the organic particles from camp fires and charred（烧成炭的）wood left over from thousands of years of slash-and-burn farming. "The soils, known as Terra Preta, contained up to 70 times more black carbon than the surrounding soils," says Glaser.

Unburnt vegetation rots quickly, but black carbon persists in the soil for many centuries. Radiocarbon dating shows that the charred wood in Terra Preta soils is typically more than 1,000 years old.

"Slash-and-burn farming can be good for soils provided it doesn't completely burn all the vegetation, and leaves behind charred wood," says Glaser. "It can be better than manure （粪 肥）." Burning the forest just once can leave behind enough black carbon to keep the soil fertile for thousands of years. And rainforests easily regrow after small-scale clearing. Contrary to the conventional view that human activities damage the environment, Glaser says: "Black carbon combines with human wastes is responsible for the richness of Terra Preta soils."

Terra Preta soils turn up in large patches all over the Amazon, where they are highly prized by farmers. All the patches fall within 500 square kilometers in the central Amazon. Glaser says the widespread presence of pottery（陶器）confirms the soil's human origins.

The findings add weight to the theory that large areas of the Amazon have recovered so well from past periods of agricultural use that the regrowth has been mistaken by generations of biologists for "virgin" forest.

During the past decade, researchers have discovered hundreds of large earth works deep in the jungle. They are up to 20 meters high and cover up to a square kilometer. Glaser claims that these earth works, built between AD 400 and 1400, were at the heart of urban civilizations managed to feed themselves.

11. We learn from the passage that the traditional view of slash-and-burn farming is that _____.

    A. it does no harm to the topsoil of the rainforest

    B. it destroys rainforest soils

    C. it helps improve rainforest soils

    D. it diminishes the organic matter in rainforest soils

12. Most rainforest soils are thin and poor because _____.

    A. the composition of the topsoil is rather unstable

    B. black carbon is washed away by heavy rains

    C. organic matter is quickly lost due to heat and rain

D. long-term farming has exhausted the ingredients essential to plant growth

13. Glaser made his discovery by _____.

    A. studying patches of fertile soils in the central Amazon

    B. examining pottery left over by ancient civilizations

    C. test-burning patches of trees in the central Amazon

    D. radiocarbon-dating ingredients contained in forest soils

14. What does Glaser say about the regrowth of rainforest?

    A. They take centuries to regrow after being burnt.

    B. They cannot recover unless the vegetation is burnt completely.

    C. Their regrowth will be hampered by human habitation.

    D. They can recover easily after slash-and-burn farming

15. From the passage it can be inferred that _____.

    A. human activities will do grave damage to rainforests

    B. Amazon rainforest soils used to be the richest in the world

    C. farming is responsible for the destruction of the Amazon rainforests

    D. there once existed an urban civilization in the Amazon rainforests

Passage Four

In a purely biological sense, fear begins with the body's system for reacting to things that can harm us — the **so-called fight-or-flight response**. "An animal that can't detect danger can't stay alive," says Joseph LeDoux. Like animals, humans evolved with an elaborate mechanism for processing information about potential threats. At its core is a cluster of neurons（神经元）deep in the brain known as the amygdala（扁桃核）.

LeDoux studies the way animals and humans respond to threats to understand how we form memories of significant events in our lives. The amygdala receives input from many parts of the brain, including regions responsible for retrieving memories. Using this information, the amygdala appraised a situation — I think this charging dog wants to bite me — and triggers a response by radiating nerve signals throughout the body. These signals produce the familiar signs of distress: trembling, perspiration and fast-moving feet, just to name three.

This fear mechanism is critical to the survival of all animals, but no one can say for sure whether beasts other than humans know they're afraid. That is, as LeDoux says, "if you put that system into a brain that has consciousness, then you get the feeling of fear."

Humans, says Edward M. Hallowell, have the ability to call up images of bad things that happened in the past and to anticipate future events. Combine these higher thought processes with our hardwired danger-detection systems, and you get a near-universal human phenomenon: worry.

That's not necessarily a bad thing, says Hallowell. "When used properly, worry is an incredible device," he says. After all, a little healthy worrying is okay if it leads to constructive action — like having a doctor look at that weird spot on your back.

Hallowell insists, though, that there's a right way to worry. "Never do it alone, get the facts and then make a plan," he says. Most of us have survived a recession, so we're familiar with the belt-tightening strategies needed to survive a slump.

Unfortunately, few of us have much experience dealing with the threat of terrorism, so it's been difficult to get facts about how we should respond. That's why Hallowell believes it was okay for people to indulge some extreme worries last fall by asking doctors for Cipro and buying gas masks.

16. The "so-called fight-or-flight response" (Line 2, Para. 1) refers to "_____".

    A. the biological process in which human beings' sense of self-defense evolves

    B. the instinctive fear human beings feel when faced with potential danger

    C. the act of evaluating a dangerous situation and making a quick decision

    D. the elaborate mechanism in the human brain for retrieving information

17. From the studies conducted by LcDoux we learn that _____.

    A. reactions of humans and animals to dangerous situations are often unpredictable

    B. memories of significant events enable people to control fear and distress

    C. people's unpleasant memories are derived from their feelings of fear

    D. the amygdale plays a vital part in human and animal responses to potential danger

18. From the passage we know that _____.

    A. a little worry will do us good if handled properly

B. a little worry will enable us to survive a recession

C. fear strengthens the human desire to survive danger

D. fear helps people to anticipate certain future events

19. Which of the following is the best way to deal with your worries according to Hallowell?

   A. Ask for help from the people around you.

   B. Use the belt-tightening strategies for survival.

   C. Seek professional advice and take action.

   D. Understand the situation and be fully prepared.

20. In Hallowell's view, people's reaction to the terrorist threat last fall was _____.

   A. ridiculous   B. understandable

   C. over-cautious   D. sensible

Passage Five

In the following article, some paragraphs have been removed. For Questions 21-25, choose the most suitable one from the list of A-F to fit into each of the numbered blank. Mark your answers on the ANSWER SHEET.

How Poison Ivy Works

According to the American Academy of Dermatology, an estimated 10 to 50 million people in this country have an allergic reaction to poison ivy each year. Poison ivy is often very difficult to spot. It closely resembles several other common garden plants, and can also blend in with other plants and weeds. But if you come into contact with it, you'll soon know by the itchy, blistery rash that forms on your skin. Poison ivy is a red, itchy rash caused by the plant that bears its name. Many people get it when they are hiking or working in their garden and accidentally come into direct contact with the plant's leaves, roots, or stems. The poison ivy rash often looks like red lines, and sometimes it forms blisters.

21. _____

About 85 percent of people are allergic to the urushiol in poison ivy, according to the American Academy of Dermatology. Only a tiny amount of this chemical — 1 billionth of a gram — is enough to cause a rash in many people. Some people may boast that they've been exposed to poison ivy many times and have never gotten the rash, but that doesn't necessarily mean they're not allergic. Sometimes the allergy doesn't emerge until you've been exposed several times, and some people develop a rash after their very first exposure. It may take up to ten days for the rash to emerge the first time.

22. _____

Here are some other ways to identify the poison ivy plant. It generally grows in a cluster of low, weed-like plants or a woody vine which can climb trees or fences. It is most often found in moist areas, such as riverbanks, woods, and pastures. The edges of the leaves are generally smooth or have tiny "teeth". Their color changes based on the season — reddish in the spring; green in the summer; and yellow, orange, or red in the fall. Its berries are typically white.

23. _____

The body's immune system is normally in the business of protecting us from bacteria, viruses, and other foreign invaders that can make us sick. But when urushiol from the poison ivy plant touches the skin, it instigates an immune response, called dermatitis, to what would otherwise be a harmless substance. Hay fever is another example of this type of response; in the case of hay fever, the immune system overreacts to pollen, or another plant-produced substance.

24. _____

The allergic reaction to poison ivy is known as delayed hypersensitivity. Unlike immediate hypersensitivity, which causes an allergic reaction within minutes of exposure to an antigen, delayed hypersensitivity reactions don't emerge for several hours or even days after the exposure.

25. _____

In the places where your skin has come into contact with poison ivy leaves or urushiol, within one to two days you'll develop a rash, which will usually itch, redden, burn, swell, and form blisters. The rash should go away within a week, but it can last longer. The severity of the reaction often has to do with how much urushiol you've touched. The rash may appear sooner in some parts of the body than in others, but it doesn't spread — the urushiol simply absorbs into the skin at different rates in different parts of the body. Thicker skin such as the skin on the soles of your feet, is harder to penetrate than thinner skin on your arms and legs.

A. Because urushiol is found in all parts of the poison ivy plant — the leaves, stems, and roots — it's best to avoid the plant entirely to prevent a rash. The trouble is, poison ivy grows almost everywhere in the United States (with the exception of the Southwest, Alaska, and Hawaii), so geography won't help you. The general rule to identify poison ivy, "leaflets three, let it be," doesn't always apply. Poison ivy usually does grow in groups of three leaves, with a longer middle leaf — but it can also grow with up to nine leaves in a group.

B.   Most people don't have a reaction the first time they touch poison ivy, but develop an allergic reaction after repeated exposure. Everyone has a different sensitivity, and therefore a slightly different reaction, to poison ivy. Sensitivity usually decreases with age and with repeated exposures to the plant.

C.   Here's how the poison ivy response occurs. Urushiol makes its way down through the skin, where it is metabolized, or broken down. Immune cells called T lymphocytes (or T-cells) recognize the urushiol derivatives as a foreign substance, or antigen. They send out inflammatory signals called cytokines, which bring in white blood cells. Under orders from the cytokines, these white blood cells turn into macrophages. The macrophages eat foreign substances, but in doing so they also damage normal tissue, resulting in the skin inflammation that occurs with poison ivy.

D.   Poison ivy's cousins, poison oak and poison sumac, each have their own unique appearance. Poison oak grows as a shrub (one to six feet tall). It is typically found along the West Coast and in the South, in dry areas such as fields, woodlands, and thickets. Like poison ivy, the leaves of poison oak are usually clustered in groups of three. They tend to be thick, green, and hairy on both sides. Poison sumac mainly grows in moist, swampy areas in the Northeast, Midwest, and along the Mississippi River. It is a woody shrub made up of stems with rows of seven to thirteen smooth-edged leaflets.

E.   The culprit behind the rash is a chemical in the sap of poison ivy plants called urushiol. Its name comes from the Japanese word "urushi", meaning lacquer. Urushiol is the same substance that triggers an allergic reaction when people touch poison oak and poison sumac plants. Poison ivy, Eastern poison oak, Western poison oak, and poison sumac are all members of the same family — Anacardiaceae.

F.   Call your doctor if you experience these more serious reactions:

Pus around the rash (which could indicate an infection).

A rash around your mouth, eyes, or genital area.

A fever above 100 degrees.

A rash that does not heal after a week.

山东大学2015年博士研究生入学考试英语试题（阅读部分）答案与解析

Passage One

1. A。词汇题。根据第一段最后两句：创造性思维和批判性思维对写作过程都起作用，但它们却不能work in parallel。本题的关键是对短语in parallel的理解。in parallel在文章中的意思是"同时"。因此，选项A符合题意。本题在不知道in parallel的意思的情况下，还可以采用排除法。选项B，C，D的意思都与第一段最后一句话的前半句的意思不符，因此排除。

2. C。细节题。本题问是什么阻止了连续写作。关键词prevents people from writing on 与第二段第一句中barrier意思相近，因此定位在第二段第一句。由此可知，试图边写作边修改写作内容可能是我们大多数人在写作时遇到的最大障碍。因此，选项C符合题意。

3. B。细节题。本题问写作第一阶段的主要目标是什么。根据关键词the chief objective of the first stage of writing，定位在第三段第二句：目标是不间断地写作。而不断地写的目标则是本段最后指出的：捕捉灵感。因此，选项B符合题意。

4. D。细节题。本题问关于free writing，作者们普遍关心的问题是什么。本题无法用关键词来定位，需要通过分析文章内容来定位。第三段主要说明了free writing的目的和方法。第四段说明了如何用the critical mind来修改free writing。第四段第二句提到很多人认为这样做会花费更多的时间。可见，作者们担心随后的修改很浪费时间。因此，选项D符合题意。

5. D。细节题。本题同样无法用关键词定位。但本题属于细节题，细节题出题的顺序与文章的顺序一致。上题已定位在第四段第二句，因此本题应定位在最后一段。最后一段说明了the critical mind的作用是修改完善写作。通过本段最后一句的后半句可知，通过批判性思维的修改，写作效果很可能比目前的练习好得多。也就是说，利用批判性思维能够精炼作者的作品使之更好。因此，选项D符合题意。

Passage Two

6. A。推断题。题干：根据作者的观点，大多数学生_____。文章第一段说，如果以"全球环境状况非常好"作为考试题，大多数学生会将试卷撕碎，并列出一大堆的抱怨，从烟雾到全球气候变暖，从砍伐森林到物种灭绝。由此可推断，大多数学生认为全球环境并不令人满意。因此，A项正确。

7. C。推断题。题干：全球产量和人口迅猛增长_____。文章第二段和第三段说，21世纪，全球人口是原来的三倍多，全球产量也有巨大的增长，因此你可能会认为地球会受到影响。的确，如果人们还像1900年或1950年甚至1980年那样居住、消费和生产，那么到现在，地球很可能是一个令人厌恶的地方。但人们没有这样做。注意此处的虚拟语气，由此可推断产量和人口的增长并没有对全球环境造成太大的影响，因此，应选C。

8. D。辨认事实题。题干：从长远来看，物价呈下降趋势原因之一是_____。文章第四段提到，每次当一种资源似乎要匮乏时，价格就会上升，相应地，人们会寻找新的资源，想方设法找到节省资源的方法或者寻找新的替代品。正因为如此，21世纪能源和矿产品的价格实质上已经下降了。故选D。

9. B。推断题。题干：鱼类资源不断减少的原因是_____。根据文章最后一段可知，市场并不能总是保持环境的健康发展。如果相关的资源不属于任何人，人们就没有兴趣保护它、培养它。鱼类资源就是一个最好的例子。因此，可推断B项正是鱼类减少的原因。

10. A。推断题。题干：解决环境问题的最主要的方法是_____。根据文章最后一段可知，在价格和市场手段不能正常运转的地方，这种良性的趋势就会动摇，就会出现环境能源等问题。让市场价格手段正常地发挥作用才是解决环境问题的方法，A项与文章的意思相符，故而正确。

Passage Three

11. B。推理题。文章第一段前半部分的大意是：低水平的刀耕火种方式并不会对雨林造成破坏。相反，它会给农民带来好处，并且提高森林土壤的质量。这是一位德国的土壤学家所提出的不同于正统观点的看法。既然"不会对雨林造成破坏"是不同于正统观点的看法，那么正统的观点就是"会对雨林造成破坏"。因此本题正确答案为B。

12. C。细节题。文章第二段第一句大意是：因为雨林土壤缺乏矿物质，因为当有机物质到达森林地面之后不到四年其中大部分就会遭到高温和强降水的破坏。所以大多数雨林土壤很贫瘠。因此，正确答案为C。

13. A。细节题。从文章中可知，Glazer的discovery是"刀耕火种有利于提高土壤肥力"。根据第二段"...has studied unexpected patches of fertile soils in the central Amazon"可知，他意外地在亚马孙雨林中部地区发现了大片肥沃的土壤，并进行了研究，所以他的发现途径对应选项A。

14. D。细节题。根据题干中的regrowth of rainforests定位到第五段第四句：And rainforests easily regrow after small-scale clearing. 很容易选出正确答案为D。

15. D。推理题。根据对主题的判断，可以排除A和C，因为这两个选项与主题相悖。

选项D "the richest in the world" 太绝对。文章最后三段表明，有很多证据都证明在亚马孙存在过城市文明，故本题答案为D。

Passage Four

16. B。细节题。从第一段第一句可知：从纯粹的生物学意义上来说，恐惧始于人类系统对可能伤害我们的东西做出的反应——即所谓的 "迎击或逃离反应"。故本题选B。

17. D。理解题。第二段陈述了LeDoux关于扁桃核功能的研究成果，以支撑第一段最后两句：在人与动物对潜在危险反应的过程中，起着核心作用的是一组位于大脑深处的神经元，这组神经元被称为 "扁桃核"。故本题答案为D。

18. A。主旨题。从倒数第三段可知：若应用得当，"担忧" 是一种不可思议的工具。毕竟，少量健康的 "担忧" 如能导致建设性的积极行动也并无大碍，比如让医生检查一下你背上那个奇怪的斑点。故本题答案为A。

19. D。细节题。从倒数第二段第一句可知：Howllowell坚持认为要以合理的方式对待 "担忧"，"永远不要独自忧愁，弄清问题真相，做出相应计划"。故选D，根据Hollowell的观点，对待worry的最佳方式是了解局势，做好充分准备。

20. B。主旨题。从最后一段可知：不幸的是，我们中很少有人对恐怖主义的威胁有应对经验，所以很难弄明白我们该如何反应。因此，Hallowell认为，去年秋天人们对医生索要抗炭坦病药物、购买防毒面具，那些沉溺于极端恐惧的行为并不离奇。故本题选B。

Passage Five

21. E。第一段末尾讲到毒藤往往引起类似红线的反应，有时还会起水泡。空格后的段落首句讲到85%的人都会对毒藤里面的urushiol过敏。因此空格处填入对urushiol的解释是顺理成章的。

22. A。由空格后的 "Here are some other ways to identify the poison ivy plant" 可知，空格处应该填入鉴别毒藤的一些方法。因此A选项是正确答案。

23. D。空格上文讲到如何鉴定判别毒藤，空格处应该顺承文意填入毒藤家族的其他成员。因此最佳答案为D。

24. B。上一段写到人们是在接触毒藤数小时甚至数天后才会出现过敏性症状，因此空格处填入不同的人对这种有毒物质出现的不同反应症状，故本题答案为B。

25. C。空格后的段落讲到身体的免疫系统是如何抵抗有毒物质的侵害的，可推测得知空格处应该是讲解毒藤的有毒物质是如何引起人类过敏的。因此C为正确答案。

云南大学2018年博士研究生入学考试英语试题
（阅读部分）

Passage One

When the government talks about infrastructure contributing to the economy the focus is usually on roads, railways, broadband and energy. Housing is seldom mentioned.

Why is that? To some extent the housing sector must shoulder the blame. We have not been good at communicating the real value that housing can contribute to economic growth. Then there is the scale of the typical housing project. It is hard to shove for attention among multibillion-pound infrastructure projects, so it is inevitable that the attention is focused elsewhere. But perhaps the most significant reason is that the issue has always been so politically charged.

Nevertheless, the affordable housing situation is desperate. Waiting lists increase all the time and we are simply not building enough new homes.

The comprehensive spending review offers an opportunity for the government to help rectify this. It needs to put historical prejudices to one side and take some steps to address our urgent housing need.

There are some indications that it is preparing to do just that. The Communities Minister, Don Foster, has hinted that George Osborne, Chancellor of the Exchequer, may introduce more flexibility to the current cap on the amount that local authorities can borrow against their housing stock debt. Evidence shows that 60,000 extra new homes could be built over the next five years if the cap were lifted, increasing GDP by 0.6%.

Ministers should also look at creating greater certainty in the rental environment, which would have a significant impact on the ability of registered providers to fund new developments from revenues.

But it is not just down to the government. While these measures would be welcome in the short term, we must face up to the fact that the existing £4.5bn programme of grants to fund new affordable housing, set to expire in 2015, is unlikely to be extended beyond then. The Labour party has recently announced that it will retain a large part of the coalition's spending plans if it returns to power. The housing sector needs to accept that we are very unlikely to ever return to era of large-scale public grants. We need to adjust to this changing climate.

1. The author believes that the housing sector _____.

    A. has attracted much attention

    B. involves certain political factors

    C. shoulders too much responsibility

    D. has lost its real value in economy

2. It can be learned that affordable housing has _____.

    A. increased its home supply

    B. offered spending opportunities

    C. suffered government biases

    D. disappointed the government

3. According to Paragraph 5, George Osborne may _____.

    A. allow greater government debt for housing

    B. stop local authorities from building homes

    C. prepare to reduce housing stock debt

    D. release a lifted GDP growth forecast

4. It can be inferred that a stable rental environment would _____.

    A. lower the costs of registered providers

    B. lessen the impact of government interference

    C. contribute to funding new developments

    D. relieve the ministers of responsibilities

5. The author believes that after 2015, the government may _____.

    A. implement more policies to support housing

    B. review the need for large-scale public grants

    C. renew the affordable housing grants programme

    D. stop generous funding to the housing sector

Passage Two

We tend to think of the decades immediately following World War II as a time of prosperity and growth, with soldiers returning home by the millions, going off to college on the G.I. Bill and lining up at the marriage bureaus.

But when it came to their houses, it was a time of common sense and a belief that less could truly be more. During the Depression and the war, Americans had learned to live with less, and that restraint, in combination with the postwar confidence in the future, made small, efficient housing positively stylish.

Economic condition was only a stimulus for the trend toward efficient living. The phrase "less is more" was actually first popularized by a German, the architect Ludwig Mies van der Rohe, who like other people associated with the Bauhaus, a school of design, emigrated to the United States before World War II and took up posts at American architecture schools. These designers came to exert enormous influence on the course of American architecture, but none more so that Mies.

Mies's signature phrase means that less decoration, properly organized, has more impact than a lot. Elegance, he believed, did not derive from abundance. Like other modern architects, he employed metal, glass and laminated wood—materials that we take for granted today but that in the 1940s symbolized the future. Mies's sophisticated presentation masked the fact that the spaces he designed were small and efficient, rather than big and often empty.

The apartments in the elegant towers Mies built on Chicago's Lake Shore Drive, for example, were, smaller—two-bedroom units under 1,000 square feet—than those in their older neighbors along the city's Gold Coast. But they were popular because of their airy glass walls, the views they afforded and the elegance of the buildings' details and proportions, the architectural equivalent of the abstract art so popular at the time.

The trend toward "less" was not entirely foreign. In the 1930s Frank Lloyd Wright started building more modest and efficient houses—usually around 1,200 square feet—than the spreading two-story ones he had designed in the 1890s and the early 20th century.

The "Case Study House" commissioned from talented modern architects by *California Arts & Architecture* magazine between 1945 and 1962 were yet another homegrown influence on the "less is more" trend. Aesthetic effect came from the landscape, new materials and forthright detailing. In his Case Study House, Ralph Rapson may have mispredicted just how the mechanical revolution would impact everyday life—few American families acquired helicopters, though most eventually got clothes dryers—but his belief that self-sufficiency was both desirable and inevitable was widely shared.

6. The postwar American housing style largely reflected the Americans' _____.

    A. prosperity and growth

    B. efficiency and practicality

    C. restraint and confidence

    D. pride and faithfulness

7. Which of the following can be inferred from Paragraph 3 about Bauhaus?

    A. It was founded by Ludwig Mies van der Rohe.

    B. Its designing concept was affected by World War II.

    C. Most American architects used to be associated with it.

    D. It had a great influence upon American architecture.

8. Mies held that elegance of architectural design _____.

    A. was related to large space

    B. was identified with emptiness

    C. was not reliant on abundant decoration

    D. was not associated with efficiency

9. What is true about the apartments Mies built on Chicago's Lake Shore Drive?

    A. They ignored details and proportions.

    B. They were built with materials popular at that time.

    C. They were more spacious than neighboring buildings.

    D. They shared some characteristics of abstract art.

10. What can we learn about the design of the "Case Study House"?

    A. Mechanical devices were widely used.

    B. Natural scenes were taken into consideration.

    C. Details were sacrificed for the overall effect.

    D. Eco-friendly materials were employed.

Passage Three

Will the European Union make it? The question would have sounded strange not long ago. Now even the project's greatest cheerleaders talk of a continent facing a "Bermuda triangle" of debt, population decline and lower growth.

As well as those chronic problems, the EU faces an acute crisis in its economic core, the 16 countries that use the single currency. Markets have lost faith that the euro zone's economies, weaker or stronger, will one day converge thanks to the discipline of sharing a single currency, which denies uncompetitive members the quick fix of devaluation.

Yet the debate about how to save Europe's single currency from disintegration is stuck. It is stuck because the euro zone's dominant powers, France and Germany, agree on the need for greater harmonization within the euro zone, but disagree about what to harmonize.

Germany thinks the euro must be saved by stricter rules on borrow spending and competitiveness, barked by quasi-automatic sanctions for governments that do not obey. These might include threats to freeze EU funds for poorer regions and EU mega-projects and even the suspension of a country's voting rights in EU ministerial councils. It insists that economic co-ordination should involve all 27 members of the EU club, among whom there is a small majority for free-market liberalism and economic rigour; in the inner core alone, Germany fears, a small majority favour French interference.

A "southern" camp headed by French wants something different: "European economic government" within an inner core of euro-zone members. Translated, that means politicians intervening in monetary policy and a system of redistribution from richer to poorer members, via cheaper borrowing for governments through common Eurobonds or complete fiscal transfers. Finally, figures close to the France government have murmured, euro-zone members should agree to some fiscal and social harmonization: e.g., curbing competition in corporate-tax rates or labor costs.

It is too soon to write off the EU. It remains the world's largest trading block. At its best, the European project is remarkably liberal: built around a single market of 27 rich and poor countries, its internal borders are far more open to goods, capital and labour than any comparable trading area. It is an ambitious attempt to blunt the sharpest edges of globalization, and make capitalism benign.

11. The EU is faced with so many problems that _____.

    A. it has more or less lost faith in markets

B. even its supporters begin to feel concerned

C. some of its member countries plan to abandon euro

D. it intends to deny the possibility of devaluation

12. The debate over the EU's single currency is stuck because the dominant powers _____.

A. are competing for the leading position

B. are busy handling their own crises

C. fail to reach an agreement on harmonization

D. disagree on the steps towards harmonization

13. To solve the euro problem, Germany proposed that _____.

A. EU funds for poor regions be increased

B. stricter regulations be imposed

C. only core members be involved in economic co-ordination

D. voting rights of the EU members be guaranteed

14. The French proposal of handling the crisis implies that _____.

A. poor countries are more likely to get funds

B. strict monetary policy will be applied to poor countries

C. loans will be readily available to rich countries

D. rich countries will basically control Eurobonds

15. Regarding the future of the EU, the author seems to feel _____.

A. pessimistic   B. desperate

C. conceited   D. hopeful

Passage Four

I was addressing a small gathering in a suburban Virginia living room—a women's group that had invited men to join them.

Throughout the evening one man had been particularly talkative, frequently offering ideas and anecdotes, while his wife sat silently beside him on the couch. Toward the end of the evening I commented that women frequently complain that their husbands don't talk to them. This man quickly nodded in agreement. He gestured toward his wife and said, "She's the talker in our family." The room burst into laughter; the man looked puzzled and hurt. "It's true," he explained. "When I come home from work I have nothing to say. If she didn't keep the conversation going, we'd spend the whole evening in silence."

This episode crystallizes the irony that although American men tend to talk more than women in public situations, they often talk less at home. And this pattern is wreaking havoc with marriage.

The pattern was observed by political scientist Andrew Hacker in the late 1970s. Sociologist Catherine Kohler Riessman reports in her new book *Divorce Talk* that most of the women she interviewed—but only a few of the men—gave lack of communication as the reason for their divorces. Given the current divorce rate of nearly 50 percent, that amounts to millions of cases in the United States every year — a virtual epidemic of failed conversation.

In my own research, complaints from women about their husbands most often focused not on tangible inequities, such as, having given up the chance for a career to accompany a husband to his or doing far more than their share of daily life-support work like cleaning, cooking, social arrangements and errands. Instead, they focused on communication: "He doesn't listen to me."

"He doesn't talk to me." I found, as Hacker observed years before, that most wives want their husbands to be, first and foremost, conversational partners but few husbands share this expectation of their wives.

In short, the image that best represents the current crisis is the stereotypical cartoon scene of a man sitting at the breakfast table with a newspaper held up in front of his face, while a woman glares at the back of it, wanting to talk.

16. What is most wives' main expectation of their husbands?

    A. Talking to them.
    B. Trusting them.
    C. Supporting their careers.
    D. Sharing housework.

17. Judging from the context, the phrase "wreaking havoc" (Paragraph 3) most probably means _____.

    A. generating motivation
    B. exerting influence
    C. causing damage
    D. creating pressure

18. All of the following are true EXCEPT _____.

    A. men tend to talk more in public than women

B. nearly 50 percent of recent divorces are caused by failed conversation

C. women attach much importance to communication between couples

D. a female tends to be more talkative at home than her spouse

19. Which of the following can best summarize the main idea of this text?

A. The moral decaying deserves more research by sociologists.

B. Marriage break-up stems from sex inequalities.

C. Husband and wife have different expectations from their marriage.

D. Conversational patterns between man and wife are different.

20. In the following part immediately after this text, the author will most probably focus on _____.

A. a vivid account of the new book *Divorce Talk*

B. a detailed description of the stereotypical cartoon

C. other possible reasons for a high divorce rate in the U.S.

D. a brief introduction to the political scientist Andrew Hacker

云南大学2018年博士研究生入学考试英语试题（阅读部分）答案与解析

Passage One

1. B。细节题。根据题干定位至第二段最后一句 "But perhaps the most significant reason is that the issue has always been so politically charged.（但或许最重要的原因是，这个问题一直以来都带有浓厚的政治色彩）"。由此可知 B 选项 involves certain political factors（涉及某些政治因素）符合题意。故答案为 B。

2. C。细节题。根据题干定位至第四段中的 "It needs to put historical prejudices to one side and take some steps to address our urgent housing need.（它需要把历史偏见放在一边，采取一些措施来解决我们迫切的住房需求）"。由此可知 C 选项 suffered government biases（遭受政府偏见）符合题意。故答案为 C。

3. A。细节题。根据题干定位至第五段第二句：The Communities Minister, Don Foster,

has hinted that George Osborne, Chancellor of the Exchequer, may introduce more flexibility to the current cap on the amount that local authorities can borrow against their housing stock debt.（社区部长唐·福斯特暗示，财政大臣乔治·奥斯本可能会对地方政府现有的住房债务上限引入更多的灵活性。）由此可知，A 选项 allow greater government debt for housing（允许政府增加住房债务）符合题意。故答案为 A。

4. C。推理题。根据题干定位至第六段：Ministers should also look at creating greater certainty in the rental environment, which would have a significant impact on the ability of registered providers to fund new developments from revenues.（部长们还应着眼于在租赁环境中创造更大的确定性，这将对已注册供应商从收入中为新开发项目提供资金的能力产生重大影响。）由此可知 C 选项正确。

5. D。细节题。根据题干定位至最后一段中的 "While these measures would be welcome in the short term, we must face up to the fact that the existing £4.5bn programme of grants to fund new affordable housing, set to expire in 2015, is unlikely to be extended beyond then.（尽管这些措施在短期内会受到欢迎，但我们必须正视这样一个事实：将于 2015 年到期的、为新保障性住房提供资金的现有 45 亿英镑资助计划不太可能在 2015 年之后延长。）" 以及文章最后提到的 "We need to adjust to this changing climate.（我们需要适应这个正在变化的形势。）"，this climate 指的也是政府将不会提供大规模拨款，由此可知 D 选项正确。

Passage Two

6. A。细节题。根据题干定位至第一段中的 We tend to think of the decades immediately following World War II as a time of prosperity and growth（我们倾向于认为二战后的几十年是繁荣和发展的时期）。由此可知 A 选项符合题意。

7. C。细节题。根据题干定位至第三段：The phrase "less is more" was actually first popularized by a German, the architect Ludwig Mies van der Rohe, who like other people associated with the Bauhaus, a school of design, emigrated to the United States before World War II and took up posts at American architecture schools.（"少即是多" 这个短语实际上是由一位德国人首次普及的，他就是建筑师路德维希·密斯·凡德罗。与其他和包豪斯设计学派有关的人物一样，他在二战前移居美国，并在美国的建筑学院担任职务。）由此可知 C 选项 Most American architects used to be associated with it（大多数美国建筑师曾与它有关）符合题意。故答案为 C。

8. C。细节题。根据题干定位至第四段：Mies's signature phrase means that less decoration, properly organized, has more impact than a lot. Elegance, he believed, did not

derive from abundance.（密斯的名言是，少装饰，合理组织，会产生更大的影响。他认为优雅并非来自丰富。）由此可知 C 选项 was not reliant on abundant decoration（不依赖丰富的装饰）正确。故答案为 C。

9. D。细节题。根据题干定位至第五段：But they were popular because of their airy glass walls, the views they afforded and the elegance of the buildings' details and proportions, the architectural equivalent of the abstract art so popular at the time.（但它们之所以受欢迎，是因为其通透的玻璃墙、所提供的视野以及建筑细节和比例的优雅，这是与当时流行的抽象艺术相当的建筑风格）。由此可知 D 选项正确。

10. A。细节题。根据题干定位至最后一段最后一句：In his Case Study House, Ralph Rapson may have mispredicted just how the mechanical revolution would impact everyday life—few American families acquired helicopters, though most eventually got clothes dryers—but his belief that self-sufficiency was both desirable and inevitable was widely shared.（在他研究的住宅案例中，拉尔夫·拉普森可能错误地预测了机械革命将如何影响日常生活——很少美国家庭拥有直升机，尽管大多数人最终都获得了干衣机——但他坚信自给自足既是可取的也是必然的，这一观点被广泛认同。）由此可知机械设备已经得到应用，因此选项 A 正确。

Passage Three

11. B。细节题。根据题干定位至第一段：Now even the project's greatest cheerleaders talk of a continent facing a "Bermuda triangle" of debt, population decline and lower growth.（现在，即便是该项目最坚定的支持者也在谈论一个面临"百慕大三角"困境的大陆——债务、人口减少和增长放缓。）由此可知欧盟的问题已经使得一些支持者都开始担心了，因此选项 B 正确。

12. C。细节题。根据题干定位至第三段：Yet the debate about how to save Europe's single currency from disintegration is stuck. It is stuck because the euro zone's dominant powers, France and Germany, agree on the need for greater harmonization within the euro zone, but disagree about what to harmonize.（然而，关于如何使欧洲单一货币免于解体的辩论却陷入了僵局。它之所以陷入困境，是因为欧元区的主导力量法国和德国一致认为有必要在欧元区内部加强协调，但对于协调哪些方面存在分歧。）由此可知 C 选项"未能就协调问题达成一致"正确，因此选 C。

13. B。细节题。根据题干定位至第四段：Germany thinks the euro must be saved by stricter rules on borrow spending and competitiveness, barked by quasi-automatic sanctions for governments that do not obey.（德国认为必须通过对借贷支出和竞争力的严格规定来拯

救欧元，对不遵守规定的政府实行准自动制裁。）由此可知，选项 B "实行更严格的规定"正确。故答案为 B。

14. D。细节题。根据题干定位至第五段中的：Translated, that means politicians intervening in monetary policy and a system of redistribution from richer to poorer members, via cheaper borrowing for governments through common Eurobonds or complete fiscal transfers.（换句话说，这意味着政客们干预货币政策，以及一个从较富裕成员国向较贫穷成员国进行再分配的体系，途径是政府通过发行共同欧元债券或完全的财政转移，以较低成本借入资金）。因此选项 D 正确。

15. D。细节题。根据题干定位至最后一段：It is too soon to write off the EU. It remains the world's largest trading block. At its best, the European project is remarkably liberal: built around a single market of 27 rich and poor countries, its internal borders are far more open to goods, capital and labour than any comparable trading area.（现在把欧盟一笔勾销还为时过早。它仍然是世界上最大的贸易集团。在最好的情况下，欧洲计划是非常自由的：建立在一个由 27 个富国和穷国组成的单一市场上，其内部边界对商品、资本和劳动力的开放程度远远超过任何类似的贸易区。）由此可知作者对于欧盟的态度还是积极的，因此选项 D 正确。

Passage Four

16. A。推理题。根据题干定位至第二段：Toward the end of the evening I commented that women frequently complain that their husbands don't talk to them. This man quickly nodded in agreement.（晚上快结束的时候，我评论说，女人经常抱怨她们的丈夫不跟她们说话。这位男士立刻点头表示同意。）由此可知，大多数妻子都希望丈夫能和她们多多沟通，因此选项 A 正确。

17. C。语义题。根据句意：这种模式正在对婚姻造成严重破坏。由此可知 wreaking havoc 和 causing damage（造成损害）意义最接近，因此选项 C 正确。

18. B。细节题。根据题干定位至第四段：Given the current divorce rate of nearly 50 percent, that amounts to millions of cases in the United States every year — a virtual epidemic of failed conversation.（考虑到目前美国近 50% 的离婚率，每年在美国就会有数百万起这样的案例——这简直是一种谈话失败的流行病。）美国有近 50% 的离婚率，但并不都是缺少交流引起的，因此选项 B 正确。

19. D。主旨题。整篇文章由一个真实场景引出婚姻中的谈话沟通，提及了美国部分家庭的婚姻现状，主要探讨妻子和丈夫对于沟通的不同看法以及做法，丈夫在外健谈、在家很少说话的交谈模式以及妻子想和丈夫谈话的迫切需求使得婚姻出现裂痕。选项 D 符合文意。

20．B。推理题。文章最后一段提到能代表当前危机的形象是一个典型的卡通场景，可以推断作者接下来可能会对这个卡通场景的一些细节展开论述，因此选项 B 符合题意。

中南大学2019年博士研究生入学考试英语试题
（阅读部分）

Passage One

The motivation for deep-space travel is shifting from discovery to economics. The past year has seen a flurry of proposals aimed at bringing celestial riches down to Earth. No doubt this will make a few billionaires even wealthier, but we all stand to gain: the mineral bounty and spin-foo technologies could enrich us all.

But before the miners start firing up their rockets, we should pause for thought. At first glance, space mining seems to sidestep most environmental concerns: there is (probably!) no life on asteroids, and thus no habitats to trash. But its consequences—both there on Earth and in space—merit careful consideration.

Part of this is about principles. Some will argue that space's "magnificent desolation" is not ours to despoil, just as they argue that our own planet's pole should remain pristine. Others will suggest that glutting ourselves on space's riches is not an acceptable alternative to developing more sustainable ways of earthly life.

History suggests that those will be hard lines to hold, and it may be difficult to persuade the public that such barren environments are worth preserving. After all, they exist in vast abundance, and even fewer people will experience them than have walked through Antarctica's icy landscapes.

There's also the emerging off-world economy to consider. The resources that are valuable in orbit and beyond may be very different to those we prize on Earth. Questions of their stewardship have barely been broached—and the relevant legal and regulatory framework is fragmentary, to put it mildly.

Space miners, like their earthly counterparts, are often reluctant to engage with such questions. One speaker at last week's space-mining forum in Sydney, Australia, concluded with a plea that regulation should be avoided. But miners have much to gain from a broad agreement on the for-profit exploitation of space. Without consensus, claims will be disputed, investment risky, and the gains made insecure. It is in all of our long-term interests to seek one out.

41. The central claim of the passage is that space mining has positive potential but _____.

    A. it will end up encouraging humanity's reckless treatment of the environment

    B. its effects should be thoughtfully considered before it becomes a reality

    C. such potential may not include replenishing key resources that are disappearing of Earth

    D. experts disagree about the commercial viability of the discoveries it could yield

42. As used in the sentence underlined (Paragraph 4), "hold" most nearly means _____.

    A. maintain   B. grip

    C. restrain   D. withstand

43. According to the passage the off-planet economy such as the future of space mining in future _____.

    A. is inconsistent with the sustainable use of space resources

    B. will be difficult to bring about in the absence of regulations

    C. cannot be attained without technologies that do not yet exist

    D. seems certain to affect Earth's economy in a negative way

44. Which of the following statements provides the best evidence for the answer to the previous question?

    A. Some will argue that space's "magnificent desolation" is not ours to despoil, just as they argue that our own planet's pole should remain pristine.

    B. The resources that are valuable in orbit and beyond may be very different to those we prize on Earth.

    C. One speaker at last week's space-mining forum in Sydney, Australia, concluded with a plea that regulation should be avoided.

    D. Without consensus, claims will be disputed, investments risky, and the gains made insecure.

Passage Two

No one can be a great thinker who does not realize that as a thinker it is his first duty to follow this intellect to whatever conclusions it may lead. Truth gains more even by the errors of one who, with due study and preparation, thinks for himself, than by the true opinions of those who only hold them because they do not suffer themselves to think. Nor that it is solely, or chiefly to form great thinkers that freedom of thinking is required. On the contrary, it is as much or even more indispensable to enable average human beings to attain the mental stature which they are capable of. There have been, and may again be, great individual thinkers in a general atmosphere of mental slavery. But there never has been, nor ever will be, in that atmosphere an intellectually active people. Where any people has made a temporary approach to such a character, it has been because the dread of heterodox speculation was for a time suspended. Where there is a tacit convention that principles are not to be disputed, where the discussion of the greatest questions which can occupy humanity is considered to be closed, we cannot hope to find that generally high scale of mental activity which has made some periods of history so remarkable. Never when controversy avoided the subjects which are large and important enough to kindle enthusiasm as the mind of a people stirred up from its foundations and the impulse given which raised even persons of the most ordinary intellect to something of the dignity of thinking beings.

He who knows only his own side of the case knows little of that. His reasons may be good, and no one may have been able to refute them. But if he is equally unable to refute the reasons on the opposite side; if he does not so much as know what they are, he has no ground of preferring either opinion. The rational position for him would be suspension of judgment and unless he contents himself with that, he is either led by authority, or adopts, like the generality of the world, the side to which he feels the most inclination. Nor is it enough that he should hear the arguments of adversaries from his own teachers, presented as they state them, and accompanied by what they offer as refutations. That is not the way to do justice to the arguments, or bring them into real contact with his own mind. He must be able to hear them from persons who actually believe them, who defend them in earnest, and do their very utmost for them. He must know them in their most plausible and persuasive form, he must feel the whole force of the difficulty which the true view of the subject has to encounter and dispose of, else he will never really possess himself of the portion of truth which meets and removes that difficulty. Ninety-nine in a hundred of what are called educated men are in this condition, even of those who can argue fluently for their opinions. Their conclusion may be true, but it might be false for anything they know: they have never thrown themselves into the mental position of those who think differently from them and considered what such persons may have to say, and consequently they do not, in any proper sense of the word, know the doctrines which they themselves profess. They do not know those parts of it which explain and justify the remainder; the considerations which show that a fact which seemingly conflicts with another is reconcilable with it, or that, of two apparently strong reasons, one and not the other ought to be preferred.

45. The best title for this passage is _____.

    A. The Age of Reason

    B. The Need for Independent Thinking

    C. The Value of Refutation

    D. How People Think

46. According to the author, it is always advisable to _____.

    A. have opinion which cannot be refuted

    B. adopt the point of view to which he feels the most inclination

    C. be acquainted with the arguments favoring the point of view with which he disagrees

    D. ignore the accepted opinions of the vast majority

47. According to the author, which of the following statements is true?

    A. Most educated people study both sides of a question.

    B. Heterodox speculation will lead to many errors in thinking.

    C. The vast majority of people who argue fluently are acquainted with only one side of an issue.

    D. It is wise to get both sides of a debatable issue from one's teachers.

48. It can be inferred from the passage that the author would be most likely agree with which of the following statements?

    A. Excessive controversy prevents clear thinking.

    B. Periods of intellectual achievement are periods of heterodox speculation.

    C. The refutation of accepted ideas can best be provided by one's own teachers.

    D. In a period mental slavery, no true intellectual thought is possible.

Passage Three

Contending for the rights of woman, my main argument is built on this simple principle, that if she be not prepared by education to become the companion of man, she will stop the progress of knowledge and virtue; for truth must be common to all, or it will be inefficacious with respect to its influence on general practice. And how can woman be expected to co-operate unless she knows why she ought to be virtuous?

Unless freedom strengthens her reason till she comprehends her duty, and sees in what manner it is connected with her real good? If children are to be educated to understand the true principle of patriotism, their mother must be a patriot; and the love of mankind, from which an orderly train of virtues spring, can only be produced by considering the moral and civil interest of mankind; but the education and situation of woman, at present, shuts her out from such investigations.

Consider, sir, dispassionately, these observations — for a glimpse of this truth seemed to open before you when you observed, "that to see one half of the human race excluded by the other from all participation of government, was a political phenomenon that, according to abstract principles, it was impossible to explain." If so, on what does your constitution rest? If the abstract rights of man will bear discussion and explanation, those of woman, by a parity of reasoning, will not shrink from the same test: though a different opinion prevails in this country, built on the very arguments which you use to justify the oppression of woman — prescription.

Consider — I address you as a legislator — whether, when men contend for their freedom, and to be allowed to judge for themselves respecting their own happiness, it be not inconsistent and unjust to subjugate women, even though you firmly believe that you are acting in the manner best calculated to promote their happiness? Who made man the exclusive judge, if woman partake with him the gift of reason?

In this style, argue tyrants of every denomination, from the weak king to the weak father of a family; they are all eager to crush reason; yet always assert that they usurp its throne only to be useful. Do you not act a similar part, when you force all women, by denying them civil and political rights, to remain immured in their families groping in the dark?

49. According to the passage, in order for society to progress, women must _____.

    A. enjoy personal happiness and financial security

B. follow all currently prescribed social rules

C. replace men as figures of power and authority

D. receive an education comparable to that of men

50. In the passage, the author claims that freedoms granted by society's leaders have _____.

A. privileged one gender over the other

B. resulted in a general reduction in individual virtue

C. caused arguments about the nature of happiness

D. ensured equality for all people

51. The author would most likely agree with which of the following statements about women in the eighteenth century?

A. Their natural preferences were the same as those of men.

B. They needed a good education to be successful in society.

C. They were just as happy in life as men were.

D. They generally enjoyed fewer rights than men did.

52. The intention for the passage is to dispute the idea that _____.

A. women seem to be not naturally suited for the exercise of civil political rights

B. men and women possess similar degrees of reasoning ability

C. women do not need to remain confined to their traditional family duties

D. the principles of natural law should not be invoked when considering gender roles

Passage Four

The history of mammals dates back at least to Triassic time. Development was retarded, however, until the sudden acceleration of evolional change that occurred in the oldest Paleogene. This led in Eocene time to increase in average size, larger mental capacity, and special adaptations for different modes of life. In the Oligocene Epoch, there was further improvement, with some appearance of some new lines and extinction of others. Miocene and Pliocene time was marked by culmination of several groups and continued approach toward modern characters. The peak of the career of mammals in variety and average large size was attained in the Miocene.

The adaption of mammals to almost all possible modes of life parallels that of the reptiles in Mesozoic time, and except for greater intelligence, the mammals do not seems to have done much better than corresponding reptilian forms. The bat is doubtless a better flying animal than the pterosaur, but the dolphin and whale are hardly more fishlike than the ichthyosaur. Many swift-running mammals of the plains, like the horse and the antelope, must excel any of the dinosaurs. The tyrannosaurs was a more ponderous and powerful carnivore than any flesh-eating mammals, but the lion or tiger is probably a more efficient and dangerous beast of prey because of a superior brain. The significant point to observe is that different branches of the mammals gradually filled themselves for all sorts of life, grazing on the plains and able to run swiftly (horse, deer, bison), living in rivers and swamps (hippopotamus, beaver), dwelling in trees (sloth, monkey), digging underground (mole, rodent), feeding on flesh in the forest (tiger) and on the plain (wolf), swimming in the sea (dolphin, whale, seal) and flying in the air (bat). Man is able by mechanical means to conquer the physical world and to adapt himself to almost any set of conditions.

This adaptation produces gradual changes of form and structure. It is biologically characteristic of the youthful, plastic stage of group. Early in its career, an animal assemblage seems to possess capacity for change, which, as the unit becomes old and fixed, disappears. The generalized types of organisms retain longest the ability to make adjustments when required, and it is from them that new, fecund stocks take origin — certainly not from any specialized end products. So, in the mammals, we witness the birth, plastic spread in many directions, increasing specialization, and in some branches, the extinction, which we have learned from observation of the geologic record of life is a characteristic of the evolution of life.

53. In chronological order, the geologic periods are _____.

    A. Paleogene, Miocene, Triassic, Mesozoic

    B. Mesozoic, Triassic, Paleogene, Miocene

    C. Miocene, Paleogene, Triassic, Mesozoic

    D. Triassic, Mesozoic, Paleogene, Miocene

54. From this passage, we may conclude that the pterosaur _____.

    A. resembled the bat

    B. was a mammal that lived in the Mesozoic period

    C. was a flying reptile

D. evolved during the Miocene period

55. That the mammals succeeding the reptile in geologic time were superior is illustrated by the statement that _____.

      A. the tiger has a brain that surpasses that of the tyrannosaur

      B. the deer runs more swiftly than the lion

      C. the whale is more fishlike than the ichthyosaur

      D. the tiger is more powerful than the carnivorous reptile

56. The statements made by the writer are based on evidence _____.

      A. found by studying fossil remains

      B. found by comparing animals and reptiles

      C. found by going to different time periods

      D. that cannot be definitely established

Passage Five

Socrates gives us a basic insight into the nature of teaching when he compares the art of teaching to the ancient craft of the midwife. Just as the midwife assists the body to give birth to new life, so the teacher assists the mind to deliver itself of ideas, knowledge, and understanding. The essential notion here is that teaching is a humble, helping art. The teacher does not produce knowledge or stuff ideas into an empty, passive mind. It is the learner, not the teacher, who is the active producer of knowledge and ideas.

The ancients distinguish the skills of the physician and the farmer from those of the shoemaker and the house builder. Aristotle calls medicine and agriculture cooperative arts, because they work with nature to achieve results that nature is able to produce by itself. Shoes and houses would not exist unless men produced them, but the living body attains health without the intervention of doctors, and plants and animals grow without the aid of farmers. The skilled physician or farmer simply makes health or growth more certain and regular.

Teaching, like farming and healing, is a cooperative art which helps nature do what it can do itself—though not as well without it. We have all learned many things without the aid of a teacher. Some exceptional individuals have acquired wide learning and deep insight with very little formal schooling. But for most of us the process of learning is made more certain and less painful when we have a teacher's help.

One basic aspect of teaching is not found in the other two cooperative arts that work with organic nature. Teaching always involves a relation between the mind of one person and mind of another. The teacher is not merely a talking book, a living phonograph record, broadcast to an unknown audience. He enters into a dialogue with his student. This dialogue goes far beyond mere "talk", for a good deal of what is taught is transmitted almost unconsciously in the personal interchange between teacher and student. We might get by with encyclopedias, phonograph records, and TV broadcasts if it were not for this intangible element, which is present in every good teacher-students relation.

Speaking simply and in the broadest sense, the teacher shows the student how to find out, evaluate, judge, and recognize the truth. He does not impose a fixed content of ideas and doctrines that the student must learn by rote. He teaches the student how to learn and think for himself. He encourages rather than suppresses a critical and intelligent response.

The student's response and growth is the only reward suitable for such a labor of love. Teaching, the highest of the cooperative arts, is devoted to the good of others. It is an act of supreme generosity. St. Augustine calls it the greatest act of charity.

57. Socrates compares the art of teaching to the ancient craft of the midwife because _____.

 A. both teaching and midwifery are lowly professions

 B. the teacher delivers knowledge while the midwife delivers the baby

 C. both the body and the mind are of equal importance

 D. both the teacher and the midwife play helping role

58. The skills of the physician and the farmer differ from those of the shoemaker and the house builder in that _____.

 A. healing and farming demand greater skills

 B. healing and farming play more important role in society

 C. healing and farming need the cooperation of nature

 D. healing and farming command more respect

59. The chief difference between a teacher and a farmer is that _____.

 A. teaching involves interaction between two minds

 B. farming involves working with organic nature

 C. teaching transmits knowledge which is intangible

D. farming produces crops which are tangible

60. According to the passage the role of a teacher is _____.

A. to evaluate, judge, and recognize the truth

B. to make the student memorize what he teaches

C. to impose his ideas and doctrines on the student

D. to encourage critical thinking in the student

中南大学2019年博士研究生入学考试英语试题（阅读部分）答案与解析

Passage One

41．B。主旨题。第一段大意为"太空深度开发的经济意义"，第二段首句"But before the miners start firing up their rockets, we should pause for thought"则认为太空开发需要三思而后行，后面的内容是在阐述为什么要这样做。因此本文的主旨大意为B选项（在变成现实之前要仔细思考）。

42．A。词汇题。作者在第三段先提到反对太空开发的环境顾虑，接着讲在面对太空开发的经济回报时，那些环境顾虑就很难再坚持下去。maintain维持，grip握住，restrain克制，withstand忍受，由此可知A选项是正确答案。

43．B。细节题。从文中最后一段可知"Without consensus, claims will be disputed, investment risky, and the gains made insecure"，即如果没有达成一致，所有权将有争议，投资风险重重，收益也会毫无保障。这个结果是上一句话中a regulation should be avoided会带来的，由此可推理，规则是必须有的。

44．D。推理题。从上题的解析可知"Without consensus, claims will be disputed, investment risky, and the gains made insecure"，没有提到regulation的后果，因此本题正确答案为D。

Passage Two

45．B。主旨题。从第一段可知，进行独立思考的人即使犯错误，真理也能因此得到发展，而那些懒于思考的人，即使持有正确的观点，真理也难以得到发展。第一段还点明思想禁锢时期，即不能进行独立思考时期，难以讨论重大议题，产生不了活跃的人民，绝不会出现类似辉煌的文艺复兴那种时期。第二段也是围绕独立思考而写，只是从具体点着眼：人只知自己，不知对方，无法获得真理，只有独立思考，才能不为权威所左右，不会跟着自己的感觉走，最终知道自己的真正主张。

46．C。态度题。这是作者在第二段讲述的重要论点。他认为一个人只知自己一方，推理极好，无人能反驳，却不知对方的推理，也不能够予以反驳的话，他就无权选择对方的任一论点，应理性停止判断。否则他就会（像世界上芸芸众生那样）听命于权威，或者跟着感觉（的倾向）走。其二，作者提出，光听自己的老师讲述对立面的论点，以及他们所提出的反驳论点，是不够的，必须倾听那些人（他们真正相信对立的观点）的论点，并为此积极热情、竭尽全力地辩护，才能使自己的思想和对立论点接触，并做出公正的判断。

47．C。推理题。从第一段中可知，作者想表明独立思考的人所提出的即使是错误的见解，也比那些未经过自己思索的人所持有的正确意见对发展真理有更大的作用，作者并未说heterodox（异端）就一定会让思想犯错，因此B选项不对。从最后一段可知，他也不应该单听自己的老师陈述对手的论点并由老师加以批驳，单凭这种方式不能够对对方的论点做出公正的评判，他必须直接听到过那些真正持有这些论点，并且竭尽全力真诚维护这些论点的人陈述这些论点。因此D选项不正确。仍然在最后一段：大多数有教养的人（educated people），包括那些能够口若悬河地为自己的见解辩护的人……结论可能是真实的，但是说不定也是虚假的，因此A选项不对。故只有C选项符合最后一段的观点。

48．B。态度题。A选项"过度的辩论会制止清晰的思考"，B选项"思想有长足进步的时期就是进行反正统思考的时期"，C选项"一个人的老师最能提供所接受观点的反驳"，D选项"思想禁锢时期，不可能出现真正的思想家"。全文都在提倡真正的辩论和思考，因此A选项不对。文中最后一段很明确地表示，一个人不能从老师那里获得一个问题的多面看法，C选项不对。从第一段可知，在思想禁锢的气氛中，曾经产生过真正的思想家，因此D选项也不对。故本题正确答案为B，符合全文大意。

Passage Three

49．D。细节题。从第一段可知作者观点：为了争取女性的权利，我的主要论点是建立在这个简单的原则上的。即：如果女性不接受教育就成为男性的伴侣，她将会阻碍知识和美德的进步。由此可知，为了社会的进步，女性必须接受与男性同等的教育。

50．A。推理题。从倒数第二段可知，法律允许男性主张追求幸福的自主权，却压制女性（subjugate women），从而可推知A选项（性别不平等）为正确答案。

51．D。态度题。A选项"与男性的自然偏好一样"，B选项"她们需要良好的教育才能在社会获得成功"，C选项"她们和男性一样幸福"，D选项"她们的权利少于男性"。题干中问到most likely agree（最有可能）同意的说法，可知D选项与全文最后一句是吻合的——作者质问男性"当你通过剥夺所有女性的公民权利和政治权利，将她们禁锢于家庭，在黑暗中摸索时，你难道没有扮演类似的角色吗？"

52．A。主旨题。A选项"女性天生不适合享有民权"，B选项"男女拥有类似的推理能力"，C选项"女性无须局限在传统的家庭里"，D选项"当考虑性别角色时不应该援引自然法的基本原则"。全文的中心思想是作者（演讲者）对女性权利及地位的支持，B和C应该是作者同意而不是dispute（反对）的内容。文章并未讨论自然法的基本原则与性别角色的关系。因此A选项为正确答案。

Passage Four

53．D。细节题。从第一段可知：哺乳动物的历史至少可以追溯到三叠纪（Triassic）。然而，在最古老的古近纪（Paleogene）发生的进化变化突然加速之前，发展是缓慢的。这导致始新世（Eocene）时期的平均体型增大，脑容量增大，对不同生活方式的特殊适应。在渐新世（Oligocene），哺乳动物的进化很有趣，有些新的进化路线出现了，有些则消失了。中新世（Miocene）和上新世（Pilonce）时期的特点是多个群体的鼎盛时期和不断接近现代特征。中新世（Miocene）是哺乳动物多样性和平均大型化发展的高峰期。不难看出，中新世（Miocene）为最接近近现代的，为最后一个，可排除A选项和C选项。从首句可以看出，哺乳动物最早可以追溯到Triassic，这是最早出现的地质层。综合来看，D为正确选项。

54．D。推理题。通过pterosaur定位到第二段第二句。该段前两句的大意为：哺乳动物对几乎所有可能的生活方式的适应与中生代的爬行动物相似，除了更高的智力，哺乳动物似乎没有比相应的爬行动物做得更好。蝙蝠无疑是一种比翼龙更好的飞行动物，但海豚和鲸鱼几乎不比鱼龙更像鱼。由此可知，pterosaur是中生代的爬行动物。故D为正确答案。

55．A。细节题。用选项中的各种动物的名字可定位到第三段。A选项"老虎的大脑比霸王龙的发达"对应文中"霸王龙是一种比任何食肉哺乳动物都更笨重和强大的食肉动物，但狮子或老虎可能是一种更高效、更危险的猛兽，因为它有着更优越的大脑"，因此A选项是正确答案。

56．A。推理题。A选项"通过研究化石遗骸"找到的证据，B选项"通过对比动物和爬行动物"找到的证据，C选项"通过去不同的年代"找到的证据，D选项"不能被确证"的证据。通过最后一句话"这是我们从观察生命的地质记录中学到的生命进化的一个特征"可知，地质记录即为化石。其他几个选项与第二段内容均不一致，故A选项为正确答案。

Passage Five

57．D。理解题。第一段讲到苏格拉底将教学艺术和助产士的技艺相提并论，essential notion（核心思想）是"教学是一种虚心助人的艺术"。教师不会凭空产生思想和知识，而学习者才是积极的思想和知识制造者。这与助产士的工作是相通的。故正确答案为D。B选项（教师传递知识，助产士接生婴儿）有混淆性，错在教师帮助大脑获取知识，助产士帮助产妇自己生下孩子，主被动的角色出现问题。

58．C。通过第二段中的"Aristotle calls medicine and agriculture cooperative arts, because they work with nature to achieve results that nature is able to produce by itself"可知，亚里士多德把医学和农业称为合作艺术，因为它们与自然一起工作，以达到自然自身能够产生的结果。本题正确答案为C。

59．A。细节题。通过第四段中的"Teaching always involves a relation between the mind of one person and mind of another"可知，教学有一个基本特质在其他两种与自然协同工作的合作艺术中找不到，即教学总是涉及一个人和另一个人思想之间的关系。故A选项可与之对应。C选项"教学传递的知识是无形的"，其问题在于，文中谈到的intangible指向的是这个互动过程是看不见的。

60．D。细节题。从倒数第二段可知，教师展示给学生如何发现、评价、判断、辨认真理，而非教师本人去做上述事情，可知A选项偷换了主体。教师没有把死记硬背的思想等固化内容强加于人。他教学生如何自学和思考。他鼓励而不是压制批判性和智性反馈。B选项和C选项与其背道而驰。D选项（鼓励学生的批判性思维）是对原文的正确总结。

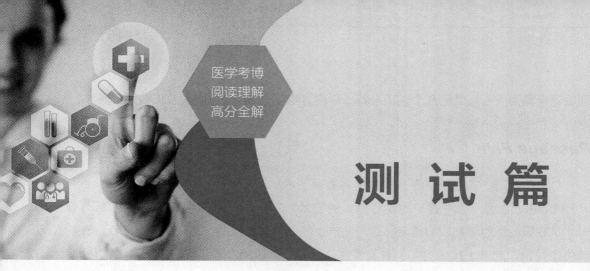

测 试 篇

Model Test 1

Passage One

This year marks exactly two countries since the publication of *Frankenstein; or, The Modern Prometheus*, by Mary Shelley. Even before the invention of the electric light bulb, the author produced a remarkable work of speculative fiction that would foreshadow many ethical questions to be raised by technologies yet to come.

Today the rapid growth of artificial intelligence (AI) raises fundamental questions: "What is intelligence, identify, or consciousness? What makes humans humans?"

What is being called artificial general intelligence, machines that would imitate the way humans think, continues to evade scientists. Yet humans remain fascinated by the idea of robots that would look, move, and respond like humans, similar to those recently depicted on popular sci-fi TV series such as "Westworld" and "Humans".

Just how people think is still far too complex to be understood, let alone reproduced, says David Eagleman, a Stanford University neuroscientist. "We are just in a situation where there are no good theories explaining what consciousness actually is and how you could ever build a machine to get there."

But that doesn't mean crucial ethical issues involving AI aren't at hand. The coming use of autonomous vehicles, for example, poses thorny ethical questions. Human drivers sometimes must make split-second decisions. Their reactions may be a complex combination of instant reflexes, input from past driving experiences, and what their eyes and ears tell them in that moment. AI "vision" today is not nearly as sophisticated as that of humans. And to anticipate every imaginable driving situation is a difficult programming problem.

Whenever decisions are based on masses of data, "you quickly get into a lot of ethical questions," notes Tan Kiat How, chief executive of a Singapore-based agency that is helping the government develop a voluntary code for the ethical use of AI. Along with Singapore, other governments and mega-corporations are beginning to establish their own guidelines. Britain is setting up a data ethics center. India released its AI ethics strategy this spring.

On June 7 Google pledged not to "design or deploy AI" that would cause "overall harm," or to develop AI-directed weapons or use AI for surveillance that would violate international norms. It also pledged not to deploy AI whose use would violate international laws or human rights.

While the statement is vague, it represents one starting point. So does the idea that decisions made by AI systems should be explainable, transparent, and fair.

To put it another way: How can we make sure that the thinking of intelligent machines reflects humanity's highest values? Only then will they be useful servants and not Frankenstein's out-of-control monster.

1. Mary Shelley's novel *Frankenstein* is mentioned because it _____.

    A. fascinates AI scientists all over the world

    B. has remained popular for as long as 200 years

    C. involves some concerns raised by AI today

    D. has sparked serious ethical controversies

2. In David Eagleman's opinion, our current knowledge of consciousness _____.

    A. helps explain artificial intelligence

    B. can be misleading to robot making

    C. inspires popular sci-fi TV series

    D. is too limited for us to reproduce it

3. The solution to the ethical issues brought by autonomous vehicles _____.

    A. can hardly ever be found   B. is still beyond our capacity

    C. causes little public concern   D. has aroused much curiosity

4. The author's attitude toward Google's pledge is one of _____.

    A. affirmation   B. skepticism

    C. contempt   D. respect

5. Which of the following would be the best title for the text?

    A. AI's Future: In the Hands of Tech Giants

B. Frankenstein, the Novel Predicting the Age of AI

C. The Conscience of AI: Complex But Inevitable

D. AI Shall Be Killers Once out of Control

Passage Two

It was the worst tragedy in maritime history, six times more deadly than the Titanic. When the German cruise ship Wilhelm Gustloff was hit by torpedoes fired from a Russian submarine in the final winter of World War II, more than 10,000 people — mostly women, children and old people fleeing the final Red Army push into Nazi Germany — were packed aboard. An ice storm had turned the decks into frozen sheets that sent hundreds of families sliding into the sea as the ship tilted and began to go down. Others desperately tried to put lifeboats down. Some who succeeded fought off those in the water who had the strength to try to claw their way aboard. Most people froze immediately. "I'll never forget the screams," says Christa Ntitzmann, 87, one of the 1,200 survivors. She recalls watching the ship, brightly lit, slipping into its dark grave — and into seeming nothingness, rarely mentioned for more than half a century.

Now Germany's Noble Prize — winning author Gtiner Grass has revived the memory of the 9,000 dead, including more than 4,000 children — with his latest novel *Crab Walk*, published last month. The book, which will be out in English next year, doesn't dwell on the sinking; its heroine is a pregnant young woman who survives the catastrophe only to say later, "Nobody wanted to hear about it, not here in the West of Germany and not at all in the East." The reason was obvious. As Grass put it in a recent interview with the weekly *Die Woche*, "Because the crimes we Germans are responsible for were and are so dominant, we didn't have the energy left to tell of our own sufferings."

The long silence about the sinking of the Wilhelm Gustloff was probably unavoidable — and necessary. By unreservedly owing up to their country's monstrous crimes in the Second World War, Germans have managed to win acceptance abroad, marginalize the neo-Nazis at home and make peace with their neighbors. Today's unified Germany is more prosperous and stable than at any time in its long, troubled history. For that, a half century of willful forgetting about painful memories like the German Titanic was perhaps a reasonable price to pay. But even the most politically correct Germans believe that they've now earned the right to discuss the full historical record. Not to equate German suffering with that of its victims, but simply to acknowledge a terrible tragedy.

6. Why does the author say the sinking of the Wilhelm Gustloff was the worst tragedy in maritime history?

    A. It was attacked by Russian torpedoes.

    B. It caused the largest number of casualties.

    C. Most of its passengers were frozen to death.

    D. Its victims were mostly women and children.

7. Hundreds of families dropped into the sea when _____.

    A. the badly damaged ship leaned toward one side

    B. a strong ice storm tilted the ship

    C. the cruise ship sank all of a sudden

    D. the frightened passengers fought desperately for lifeboats

8. The Wilhelm Gustloff tragedy was little talked about for more than half a century because Germans _____.

    A. were eager to win international acceptance

    B. had been pressured to keep silent about it

    C. were afraid of offending their neighbors

    D. felt guilty for their crimes in World War II

9. How does Gunter Grass revive the memory of the Wilhelm Gustloff tragedy?

    A. By describing the ship's sinking in great detail.

    B. By giving an interview to the weekly *Die Woche*.

    C. By presenting the horrible scene of the torpedo attack.

    D. By depicting the survival of a young pregnant woman.

10. It can be learned from the passage that Germans no longer think that _____.

    A. the Wilhelm Gustloff tragedy is a reasonable price to pay for the nation's past misdeeds

    B. Germany is responsible for the horrible crimes it committed in World War II

    C. they will be misunderstood if they talk about the Wilhelm Gustloff tragedy

    D. it is wrong to equate their sufferings with those of other countries

Passage Three

A new survey by Harvard University finds more than two-thirds of young Americans disapprove of President Trump's use of Twitter. The implication is that Millennials prefer news from the White House to be filtered through other source, Not a president's social media platform.

Most Americans rely on social media to check daily headlines. Yet as distrust has risen toward all media, people may be starting to **beef up** their media literacy skills. Such a trend is badly needed. During the 2016 presidential campaign, nearly a quarter of web content shared by Twitter users in the politically critical state of Michigan was fake news, according to the University of Oxford. And a survey conducted for BuzzFeed News found 44 percent of Facebook users rarely or never trust news from the media giant.

Young people who are digital natives are indeed becoming more skillful at separating fact from fiction in cyberspace. A Knight Foundation focus-group survey of young people between ages 14 and 24 found they use "distributed trust" to verify stories. They cross-check sources and prefer news from different perspectives — especially those that are open about any bias. "Many young people assume a great deal of personal responsibility for educating themselves and actively seeking out opposing viewpoints," the survey concluded.

Such active research can have another effect. A 2014 survey conducted in Australia, Britain, and the United States by the University of Wisconsin-Madison found that young people's reliance on social media led to greater political engagement.

Social media allows users to experience news events more intimately and immediately while also permitting them to re-share news as a projection of their values and interests. This forces users to be more conscious of their role in passing along information. A survey by Barna research group found the top reason given by Americans for the fake news phenomenon is "reader error", more so than made-up stories or factual mistakes in reporting. About a third say the problem of fake news lies in "misinterpretation or exaggeration of actual news" via social media. In other words, the choice to share news on social media may be the heart of the issue. "This indicates there is a real personal responsibility in countering this problem," says Roxanne Stone, editor in chief at Barna Group.

So when young people are critical of an over-tweeting president, they reveal a mental discipline in thinking skills — and in their choices on when to share on social media.

11. According to the Paragraphs 1 and 2, many young Americans cast doubts on _____.

    A. the justification of the news-filtering practice

    B. people's preference for social media platforms

    C. the administrations ability to handle information

    D. social media was a reliable source of news

12. The phrase "beef up" (Line 2, Para. 2) is closest in meaning to _____.

    A. sharpen   B. define   C. boast   D. share

13. According to the Knight Foundation survey, young people _____.

    A. tend to voice their opinions in cyberspace

    B. verify news by referring to diverse resources

    C. have s strong sense of responsibility

    D. like to exchange views on "distributed trust"

14. The Barna survey found that a main cause for the fake news problem is _____.

    A. readers' outdated values   B. journalists' biased reporting

    C. readers' misinterpretation   D. journalists' made-up stories

15. Which of the following would be the best title for the text?

    A. A Rise in Critical Skills for Sharing News Online

    B. A Counteraction Against the Over-tweeting Trend

    C. The Accumulation of Mutual Trust on Social Media

    D. The Platforms for Projection of Personal Interests

Passage Four

Kids heading back to enlightened schools this fall may find nutrition and exercise on the agenda even in math class. In an effort to reverse the alarming increase of obesity in children, some schools have found ways to encourage healthful lifestyle changes without emphasizing the negative — too much body weight. Planet Health, developed by Harvard University researchers and now used in hundreds of schools throughout the country, integrates obesity prevention lessons into the science, math, and social studies curricula, for example. Students come to appreciate the importance of reducing TV time by calculating during math class the amount of their lifetime they've spent in front of the set. In gym, they

医学考博阅读理解高分全解

decide on goals for subbing in physical activity instead.

The program costs only about $15 per student annually, a bargain, considering the payoffs: A 2005 study published in the *Archives of Pediatric and Adolescent Medicine* found that middle-school girls who had Planet Health in their schools were half as likely to purge or use diet pills as those in schools without it. "It really focuses on the positive, and that's why we think it's protective against these dangerous behaviors," says study author Bryn Austin, an assistant professor of pediatrics at Harvard Medical School.

A second program adopted by 7,000 elementary schools nationwide, the Coordinated Approach to Child Health (CATCH), similarly puts the focus on good health habits instead of weight. In class, students use a traffic-light system to identify "go" "slow", and "whoa" foods and take breaks to do jumping jacks. In the cafeteria, fruits, vegetables, low-fat milk, and whole-grain starches are labeled with green-light tags, and pizza gets a yellow light. Gym activities are designed to keep students constantly moving. "Every kid gets a ball to dribble or a hula hoop; there's no lining up and waiting to take a turn," says Phil Nader, professor of pediatrics emeritus at the University of California — San Diego, who helped develop CATCH.

A three-year study comparing CATCH schools with others without the program found that CATCH increased the proportion of gym class spent in motion, from 40 percent to 50 percent, and reduced the consumption of fat in schools from 39 percent of total calories to 32 percent. A second study found that the program prevented the growth in the number of overweight students that normally occurs from Grade 3 to Grade 5. CATCH students in El Paso, Texas (with one of the highest obesity rates in the nation), held the line between those grades, but in schools without the program, the share of overweight girls increased from 26 percent to 40 percent and of overweight boys from 29 percent to 39 percent.

Glen Cove Elementary School, near El Paso in Ysleta, was one of the first schools to adopt CATCH, and parents there have learned to eat better and exercise more along with their kids. "We have a day when everyone comes to fly kites and Wellness Wednesdays when family members run around for 20 minutes with their kids," says physical education teacher Ben Avalos, who brought the program to Glen Cove in 1998. "Parents also tell me their kids have gotten them to throw out the 'whoa' foods in the house." Avalos uses walking sticks, pogo sticks, and Chinese yo-yos in gym class — and nobody relaxes on the sidelines.

16. The study published in the *Archives of Pediatric and Adolescent Medicine* shows
_____.

    A. that girls who had Planet Health were less obese than those who didn't have

B. that girls who had Planet Health led a healthier lifestyle than those who didn't have

C. that girls who had Planet Health were more confident than those who didn't have

D. that girls who had Planet Health were more used to controlling weight in positive means than those who didn't have

17. The word "whoa" (Paragraph 3) most probably means _____.

   A. fast   B. stop   C. pause   D. no

18. In the CATCH, pizza is a kind of _____ food.

   A. dangerous   B. yellow-light

   C. highly-nutritious   D. less healthy

19. According to the second study of comparing CATCH schools with others without the program, CATCH students in EL Pasco _____.

   A. were not growing weight from Grade 3 to Grade 5

   B. were prevented from normal weight growth from Grade 3 to Grade 5

   C. were not growing overweight from Grade 3 to Grade 5

   D. were growing overweight from Grade 3 to Grade 5

20. Which of the following statements is TRUE of Glen Cove Elementary School?

   A. The school adopts CATCH in order to change the lifestyle of the school children's family.

   B. The school applied CATCH to the school children's parents.

   C. The school wanted to help children to form good health habits with the help of their parents.

   D. The CATCH school children also teach their family how to live healthily.

Passage Five

Two real-world studies from Europe demonstrate the health damage done by automotive air pollution, especially the kind emitted by diesel engines. An 11-year period of improving air quality in Switzerland, which started with some of the cleanest air in Europe, produced measurable benefits in lung function for adults as they aged, according to a report in the Dec. 6 issue of the *New England Journal of Medicine*. "Even with small improvements in air quality, you get measurable health benefits," said Dr. Ursula Ackermann-Liebrich, a professor of public health at the University of Basel. "That is true at levels even which are quite low."

And an unusual collaborative study by American and British researchers, reported in the same issue of the journal, showed that people with asthma who walked along a street used by diesel-powered traffic experienced loss of breathing much greater than those who strolled through a traffic-free park. "The unique feature of this study in real-world conditions was that we have demonstrated that typical urban levels of air pollution with diesel-rich powered vehicles have measurable effects," said Dr. Junfeng Zhang, chairman of environmental and occupational health at the New Jersey School of Public Health and an American member of the research team. "There have been theories or hypotheses of diesel exhaust or particle matter and also laboratory studies with animals, but this was a study in the real world with real people."

The study had 60 adults with mild or moderate asthma walk for two hours along two London locales — busy, exhaust-filled Oxford Street or the more bucolic Hyde Park. The Oxford Street walk produced a 5 percent to 6 percent reduction in lung function, "and asthmatics already have compromised lung function," Zhang said. The reduction in lung function was "significantly larger" than what was measured after the Hyde Park walk and was accompanied by an increase in biomarkers of lung inflammation. The negative effect on the lung was greater than has been seen in animal studies using breathing chambers, Zhang said.

The Swiss study found a decrease in the amount of airborne fine particulate pollutants, a major feature of diesel emissions. That improvement in Swiss air quality was accompanied by a slowing in the rate of the loss of breathing function that occurs as people age, Ackerman-Liebrich said. The journal report attributed the healthful effect to "decreasing exposure to airborne particulates." "There seems to be something more potent than other forms of air pollution in diesel exhausts," said Dr. Morton Lippman, a professor of environmental medicine at New York University. "It is something many other studies have pointed to."

The issue of diesel pollution is of growing interest because "new diesel technologies are increasingly coming on the market," Lippmann said. Diesel automobiles are much more common in Europe than in the United States but are gaining attention because of their greater fuel efficiency, he noted.

The two studies are welcome because they assess the effect of diesel emissions at relatively low levels, Lippmann said. "That remains a complex issue," he said. "Getting statistically significant information on a small average effect on a large population is not easy.

There are a lot of unknowns. Most effects are associated with particles rather than gases in the mixture, but there is no data on which part of the components is particularly nasty."

21. By saying "That is true at levels even which are quite low.", Dr. Ursula Ackermann-Liebrich meant _____.

    A. people could really get health benefits even though the benefits were at low levels

    B. people could get measurable health benefits with air quality improved slightly even at the region in low latitude

    C. people could get measurable health benefits even in the region with low levels of air pollution

    D. people could get health benefits with air quality improved slightly even in the region with low levels of air pollution

22. The collaborative study by American and British researchers was unusual in that _____.

    A. it was a study in the real world with real people living in urban levels of air pollution

    B. it proved that air pollution by diesel-rich powered vehicles have measurable effects

    C. it verified that people in the city are generally affected by air pollution with diesel-engined automobiles

    D. it demonstrated the real negative effect was greater than that of laboratory studies

23. According to the collaborative study by American and British researchers, people strolling in Hyde Park _____.

    A. had an increase in biomarkers of lung inflammation

    B. had a greater reduction in lung function than animals under the same condition

    C. had a larger reduction in lung function than walking in a busy street

    D. were, as a matter of fact, affected by the air pollution

24. According to Dr. Morton Lippman, the more potent form of air pollution many other studies have pointed to was _____.

    A. airborne particulates in diesel exhausts

    B. airborne fine particulate pollutants

C. particular mixture from diesel emissions

D. some other forms of air pollution

25. Which of the following statements is TRUE of the Swiss study?

A. The study is aimed to produce a pleasant air quality for people as they age.

B. The study proves that people could enjoy healthful effect as they seldom expose themselves to the airborne particulates.

C. The study is conducted in the least polluted region in Europe.

D. The study is aimed to make people own the clearest air in Europe.

Passage Six

Scientists have developed a slimming drug that successfully suppresses appetite and results in a dramatic loss of weight without any apparent ill effects. The drug interferes with appetite control and prevents the build-up of fatty tissue. More importantly, the drug appears to prevent a serious decline metabolic rate — causing tiredness and lethargy — which is typically associated with living on a starvation diet. As a result, mice taking the drug lost 45 percent more weight than mice fed the same amount of food, which compensate for the lack of food by becoming more sluggish.

The scientists, from the Johns Hopkins University in Baltimore, said that C75 is likely to produce a similar effect on humans because appetite control in the brain is thought to be based largely on the same chemical pathways as those in mice. "We are not claiming to have found the fabled weight-loss drug. What we have found, using C75, is a major pathway in the brain that the body uses naturally in regulating appetite at least in mice," said Francis Kuhajda, a pathologist and senior team member. "We badly need effective drugs for weight loss. Obesity is a huge problem. We're hoping to explore the possibilities of this new pathway," he said.

Discovering a biochemical pathway in the brain that controls appetite raises new prospects for eloping slimming aids. Research on leptin, a hormone produced in fatty tissue for controlling fat deposits, has so far failed to produce the expected slimming drug break-through. The latest study, published in the journal *Science*, showed that even moderate doses of C75 produced a significant loss of appetite, which returned to normal after a few months.

The scientists believe that C75, which they produced synthetically in the laboratory, binds to an enzyme called fatty acid synthase, which is involved in storing excess food intake as fat. Inhibiting enzyme causes a build-up of a chemical in the liver which acts as a precursor to fat deposition. This precursor is thought to have an indirect effect on the brain, causing appetite suppression.

Normally, when animals fast, a hormone called neuropeptide Y increases sharply in the appetite control centers of the brain, stimulating the desire for food. However, when animals are given C75, levels of this hormone fall, leading to a loss of interest in food. Dr. Kuhajda said discovering that C75 has no effect on metabolic rate is one of the most significant findings of the study. "If you try to lose weight by starving, your metabolism slows down after a few days," he said. "It's a survival mechanism that sabotages many diets. We see this in fasting mice. Yet metabolic rate in the C75-treated mice doesn't slow down at all." Further animals studies will be needed before C75 could be tested on humans.

26. Living on a starvation diet may result in _____.

    A. a dramatic loss of weight without any ill effects

    B. a long-term loss of interest in eating

    C. a slowdown of fat deposition

    D. fatigue and inactivity

27. The scientists from the Johns Hopkins University said that C75, the slimming drug proved effective in mice, is likely to work on humans because _____.

    A. the chemical pathway responsible for appetite control in humans is believed to be the same as that in mice

    B. it is a major pathway in the brain which is activated to regulate appetite

    C. it is especially effective in the battle against obesity

    D. its effect has also been proved by human studies

28. Leptin _____.

    A. refers to a new biochemical pathway in the brain that controls appetite

    B. raises new prospects for developing slimming drugs

    C. is a hormone produced in fatty tissue for controlling fat build-up

    D. has turned to a breakthrough in the search for effective slimming drugs

29. The newly-found slimming drug can successfully suppress appetite because _____.

    A. C75 made synthetically in the laboratory works effectively on human body

    B. fatty acid sythase is involved in storing excess food intake as fat

C. C75 inhibits the activity of an enzyme called fatty acid synthase

D. it increases a hormone called neuropeptide Y in the appetite-control centers of the brain

30. What is the most remarkable about the new slimming drug C75?

A. It successfully suppresses appetite.

B. It encourages the scientists to study slimming drugs from new perspectives.

C. It generates a new hormone that may prove to be the key to overweight.

D. It doesn't affect the metabolic rate, a survival mechanism in living beings.

Model Test 2

Passage One

Playing violent video games can have immediate and lasting effects on a person's thoughts and behavior, new research show. In fact, researchers report that the interactive and increasingly graphic nature of some video games makes them "potentially more dangerous" than violence-charged television and movies.

Psychologists Anderson and Dill conducted two studies. In one study of 227 college students, the investigators found that students who more frequently played violent video games during junior high and high school were more likely to have engaged in "aggressive behavior". A second study in which 210 college students played either a violent or non-violent video game revealed that the violence-packed game increased subjects' aggression immediately afterwards.

In the first study, the investigators questioned students on their natural levels of aggression and irritability, and their delinquent(犯法的）behavior — for instance whether they had bit other students in the past year. The investigators found that students with aggressive personalities and those who more often played violent video games were more prone to real-life aggression. Students who considered themselves aggressive were also more likely to play violent video games. Since aggressive people may seek out violet games, coming to the conclusion that the video games caused real-life delinquency is too risky.

However, the second study lined video-game violence with immediate increases in aggression. Anderson and Dill had students play either a violent game or a nonviolent game and let the students believe they were playing against an opponent in another room. After completing the video game, participants played a competitive-reaction game with their imaginary opponents. In this game the winner was allowed to publish the loser with a noise blast（响亮的噪音）. The researchers found that students who were fresh from the violent video game blasted their opponents longer than those who played the nonviolent game.

Because video games show short-term and long-term effects, Anderson and Dill suppose that video-game violence influences behavior not by arousing aggressive feelings, but by teaching players to find "aggressive solutions" to problems. Unlike TV, many video games demand that player identify with the aggressor and actively participate in violence.

1. According to the passage, violent video games may be more dangerous than violent movies or TV programs because video games _____.

    A. tend to be more violent

    B. lay more emphasis on violent acts

    C. require active involvement of players

    D. arouse aggressive feelings more quickly

2. The purpose of the first study was to try to establish a cause-effect relationship between _____.

    A. aggressive personality and real-life violence

    B. violent behavior in the past and violent behavior at present

    C. aggressive personality and more involvement in playing violent video games

    D. more involvement in playing violet video games and aggressive behavior

3. In order to find out the short-term effect of violent video game, researchers _____.

    A. asked game players to blast the loser in the violent video games

    B. observed the behavior of game players when playing violent video games

    C. put game players into a real fight in a small room with aggressive opponents

    D. observed game players' reaction to their imaginary opponents in competitive games

4. Which of the following statements is NOT true, according to the passage?

    A. Violent video games arouse aggressive feelings in game players.

    B. Violent video games inevitably result in delinquent behavior of game players.

    C. Violent video games teach players to solve problems in an aggressive ways.

    D. Violent video games have short-term and long-term effects on game players.

5. The best title of this passage can be _____.

   A. Effects of Violent Video Games

   B. Video Games Increase Crimes

   C. Video Games and Psychology

   D. New Research Findings of Video Games

Passage Two

The belief that the mind plays an important role in physical illness goes back to the earliest days of medicine. From the time of the ancient Greeks to the beginning of the 20th century, it was generally accepted by both physician and patient that the mind can affect the course of illness, and it seemed natural to apply this concept in medical treatments of disease. After the discovery of antibiotics, a new assumption arose that treatment of infectious or inflammatory disease requires only the elimination of the foreign organism or agent that triggers the illness. In the rush to discover antibiotics and drugs that cure specific infections and diseases, the fact that the body's own responses can influence susceptibility to disease and its course was largely ignored by medical researchers.

It is ironic that research into infectious and inflammatory disease first led 20th-century medicine to reject the idea that the mind influences physical illness, and now research in the same field — including the work of our laboratories and of our collaborators at the National Institutes of Health — is proving the contrary. New molecular and pharmacological tools have made it possible for us to identify the intricate network that exists between the immune system and the brain, a network that allows the two systems to signal each other continuously and rapidly. Chemicals produced by immune cells signal the brain, and the brain in turn sends chemical signals to restrain the immune system. These same chemical signals also affect behavior and the response to stress. Disruption of this communication network in any way, whether inherited or through drugs, toxic substances or surgery, exacerbates the diseases that these systems guard against: infectious, inflammatory, autoimmune, and associated mood disorders.

The clinical significance of these findings is likely to prove profound. They hold the promise of extending the range of therapeutic treatments available for various disorders, as drugs previously known to work primarily for nervous system problems are shown to be effective against immune maladies, and vice versa. They also help to substantiate the popularly held impression (still discounted in some medical circles) that our state of mind can influence how well we resist or recover from infectious or inflammatory diseases.

The brain's stress response system is activated in threatening situations. The immune system responds automatically to pathogens and foreign molecules. These two response systems are the body's principal means for maintaining an internal steady state called homeostasis. A substantial proportion of human cellular machinery is dedicated to maintaining it.

When homeostasis is disturbed or threatened, a repertoire of molecular, cellular and behavioral responses comes into play. These responses attempt to counteract the disturbing forces in order to reestablish a steady state. They can be specific to the foreign invader or a particular stress, or they can be generalized and nonspecific when the threat to homeostasis exceeds a certain threshold. The adaptive response may themselves turn into stressors capable of producing disease. We are just beginning to understand the interdependence of the brain and the immune system, how they help to regulate and counterregulate each other and how they themselves can malfunction and produce disease.

6. The passage supplies information to suggest that _____.

    A. it has always been the belief of both physician and patient that one's state of mind can affect physical disease

    B. the popular belief that stress exacerbates inflammatory illness has always been discredited by the doctors

    C. the discovery of antibiotics sheds light on people's understanding of the mind-body interaction in disease

    D. there is a new understanding of the communication between the brain and immune system

7. Which of the following best states the mind-body interaction in disease?

    A. The brain and immune systems send signals to each other.

    B. The immune and central nervous systems are organized in very different ways to affect the course of illness.

    C. Disruption of the communication of the brain and immune system can cure certain disease.

    D. The immune system and the brain share a lot of hormones to facilitate their communication.

8. Which of the following statements about clinical significance of the new findings can be best supported by the passage?

    A. The responsive stress is genetically determined.

    B. The treatment of immune maladies can be consciously controlled.

    C. Psychoactive drugs may in some cases be used to treat inflammatory diseases.

    D. Social interactions can lessen psychological stress and alter immune responses.

9. Which of the following statements can be inferred from the passage?

    A. Taking the cure at a mountain sanatorium doesn't work for the treatment for many chronic diseases.

    B. The relaxing effects of hot-springs spa can help restore the communication between the brain and immune system.

    C. The disruption of the brain's stress response reduces the body's response.

    D. Depression is also associated with inflammatory disease.

10. According to the passage, in order to maintain an internal steady state called homeostasis, _____.

    A. sometimes the stress response needs to go to the extreme

    B. the stress response has to bar the foreign pathogens from the body

    C. both the stress and immune responses need to be regulated

    D. the immune system promotes physiological and behavioral changes

Passage Three

Genetically modified crops and foods having been launched by big companies bent on taking over agriculture, this new breakthrough in science poses a new problem — whether it's safe for people to eat them. Experts say that much of the current angst over genetically modified foods is unnecessary. If research and development are allowed to continue, the products will be there for all to appreciate.

New varieties of rice and other crops, resistant to insects and diseases, will have replaced those cultivated today. Farmers will no longer lose substantial proportions of their harvests. The impact of these advances will be felt in the less developed countries. Health benefits will also come from plants genetically engineered to be more balanced nutritionally than those that have evolved through natural selection or been bred by traditional methods.

The potential medical spin-offs from plant biotechnology are considerable. A new generation of more potent vaccines, many against illness for which no vaccines have been available, will be grown in plants such as maize and bananas.

Malnutrition could be banished. Biotechnology can improve efficiency of food production and generate more nourishing crops.

Throughout the world, gardeners, vegetarians, and consumers will benefit from plant varieties resistant to spoilage, foods which reduce our dependence on animals, and cheaper and/or tastier products.

We should not, however, overlook potential hazards in altering our diets by genetic engineering. As with all other applications of science to human welfare, biotechnology is likely to have risks. Mistakes will probably be made.

Nevertheless, any analysis of the new techniques for ferrying genes between plants must surely conclude that they are being applied and controlled more stringently than any technology ever before.

Nearly 25 years ago, when scientists first learned to combine DNA from different sources, commentators warned of the iniquity of "opening Pandora's box". Among their horrific forecast were unstoppable epidemics and worldwide pestilence. None of these has come to pass, partly because genetic manipulation has not proved inherently dangerous.

In addition, regulatory committees have been set up to ensure that experiments are conducted in appropriately safe conditions.

The regulators' task is not simply to allow research to go ahead unless potential hazards are obvious. It is to consider risks that could come to light later. Will a gene, introduced into rape to protect it against virus attack, also make the pollen grains more likely to cause hay fever? All proposals have to survive positive vetting of this sort before they are sanctioned.

Genetic engineering is far more precise — and thus predictable — than the gene movements which occur in nature. When plants fertilize and cross-fertilize in the wild, large numbers of genes are transferred in a haphazard fashion.

Biotechnology allows individual genes to be moved with precision from one plant to another. It is much easier to know how one gene will work in its new setting. The likelihood of unexpected consequences and the margin of error are correspondingly reduced.

There is a chance, however remote, that a gene introduced into a particular plant at one time and location might have adverse.

Consequences if it eventually gets into another plant distant in space and time.

Given the astronomical amount of random gene transfer which occurs through the biosphere such extreme caution is unwarranted. I believe most food producers — and eaters — would agree.

11. The expression "spin-offs" in Para. 3 refers to _____.

    A. byproducts

    B. by-work

    C. side effects

    D. consequences

12. In his defense of genetic technology, the author shows us the benefits produced by genetic technology EXCEPT in _____.

    A. high-tech

    B. health

    C. medicine

    D. agrarian production

13. Despite the possibility of introduction of a gene into a particular plant at one time and location, the author contends that such extreme caution about genetic technology is unwarranted because _____.

    A. there are regulatory committees

    B. in labs gene ferrying is being applied and controlled stringently

    C. genetic engineering is far more precise than the natural gene movements

    D. the possibility of such an event is too small

14. According to your common sense, which of the following techniques does not belong to the field of genetic engineering?

    A. Cloning.

    B. Artificial insemination.

    C. Invitro fertilization.

    D. Heart bypasses.

15. What is your understanding of the quotation of the Creek myth "opening Pandora's box"?

    A. Something appears valuable, but is actually a curse.

    B. A box contains all the evils and miseries.

    C. Some media argue that the combination DNA from different sources would cause a lot of problems and plagues that did not exist or were not known before.

    D. Pandora possessed a gift that was never to be opened. When it was, all the evils of the world were released.

Passage Four

People from around the world flock to the United States expecting to find a better life. But to scientists' surprise, a growing body of evidence indicates that increasing familiarity with U.S. culture and society renders immigrants and their children far more susceptible to many mental and physical ailments, even if they attain financial success.

The latest study of this phenomenon, directed by epidemiologist William A. Vega of the University of Texas, San Antonio, finds much higher rates of major depression, substance abuse, and other mental disorders in U.S.-born Mexican-Americans compared with both recent and long-standing Mexican-American immigrants. This pattern held regardless of education or income levels.

Vega's results appear at the same time as the release of a national report on declining physical and mental health in children of immigrant families. A panel convened by the National Research Council and the Institute of Medicine, both in Washington, D. C., reviewed previous studies and concluded that assimilation into a U.S. lifestyle may undermine the overall health of immigrant children much more than being poor does.

In contrast, studies of nonimmigrant U.S. residents usually link poverty to poor physical and mental health.

"The material on immigrant health shocked me when we first reviewed it," says panel member Arthus M. Kleinman, a psychiatrist and anthropologist at Harvard Medical School in Boston. "Vega's study is consistent with the panel's conclusion that immigrants' health deteriorates with assimilation to U.S. society, declining toward general U.S. norms," says Kleinman. Other studies have indicated that citizens of many countries, including Mexico, are healthier overall than U.S. citizens.

Vega's team interviewed 3,012 adults of Mexican origin, ages 18-59, living Fresno County, Calif. Of that number, 1,810 people identified themselves as immigrants. Interviews were in English or Spanish. Interviewers expressed an interest in health issues only and tried to minimize any tendency of participants to lie — due to U.S. residency concerns — about having immigrated.

Nearly one-half of U.S.-born Mexican-Americans had suffered from at least one of 12 psychiatric disorders at some time in their lives, compared with only one-quarter of the immigrants. Common mental conditions in U.S.-born individuals included major depression, phobias and other anxiety disorders, and substance abuse and dependence.

Prevalence rates for mental disorders were lowest for those who had immigrated within the past 13 years. The higher rates found among immigrants of 13 or more years still fell considerably below those for the native-born group.

16. Vega's group was surprised to find worse physical and mental health in _____.

    A. both recent and long-standing Mexican-American immigrants

    B. the immigrants who received fewer years of education

    C. the financially disadvantaged immigrants

    D. U.S.-born Mexican-Americans

17. The scientists found that the immigrants' declining physical and mental health is linked to _____.

    A. being reluctant to be assimilated into the U.S. lifestyle

    B. blending with U.S. culture and society

    C. working hard for a better life

    D. being poor

18. Vega and Kleinman _____.

    A. are divided over the phenomenon

    B. ascribe the phenomenon to racial discrimination

    C. puzzle over the phenomenon

    D. seem to see eye to eye on the phenomenon

19. Vega's team interviewed the immigrants _____.

    A. for their U.S. residency concerns

    B. for their identifications

    C. for their health issues

    D. all of the above

20. Which of the following groups is least susceptible to mental disorders?

    A. The U.S.-born Mexican-Americans.

    B. The immigrants of 13 or more years.

    C. The immigrants of financial success.

    D. The immigrants of less than 13 years.

Passage Five

Although speech and writing are the special means of communicating of humans, the interchange also takes place in many other ways. A person may relay his or her feelings, thoughts, and reactions through body positioning, body contact, body odors, eye contact, responsive actions, habits, attitudes, interests, state of health, dress and grooming, choice of life-style, and use of talents—in fact, through everything the individual says or does.

In turn, every person is constantly receiving multitudes of external and internal messages through his or her five senses and personal biorhythm system. An individual screens, selects, regulates, and controls specific aspects of this information through a process of mental choices. Some of these choices are automatic; some are subconscious because of habit, block, or lack of development; and some are made by a conscious process. The degree to which a person is able to communicate depends upon the extent of his or her conscious awareness, priority of need, and control of this process.

The person with a behavior disorder is shut off from the communicative flow that normally exists among humans. His or her mind is confused, and he or she may feel unable to express personal thoughts, needs, and emotions, and unable to make himself or herself understood. Sometimes the person may feel that he or she is communicating clearly but that others cannot or will not understand. Because the person is thus isolated in internal problems, he or she is interested only in these problems and cannot focus attention on the messages of others. The person often projects fears and fantasies onto others, so that no matter what the real content is of the messages that others relay, the messages received are threatening ones.

The causes of such communicative shutoffs are blocks in the neural pathways of the person's processing of information. Sometimes a block is physical, as in deafness, mental retardation, brain tumor, or hardening of the cerebral arteries. However, the most common causes of blocks are injuries to a person's emotional system.

Emotional blocks occur to some degree in all human beings. They usually occur in childhood before good communicative skills are learned, and they are connected to individual symbolism. Unless such a block is removed shortly after happening, it can have profound and complicating effects that will distort emotional and mental growth and arrest the development potential of the individual. Even though a child with blocks will appear to grow and to seem mature in some ways, he or she will show the evidence of emotional blocking in efforts to communicate.

21. The concluding phrase of the first paragraph implies that human communication _____.

    A. is characterized by two features, form and meaning

    B. is mainly conducted through speech and writing

    C. is of two functions, stimulation and response

    D. takes two forms, verbal and nonverbal

22. In the second paragraph the author is mainly concerned with _____.

    A. communicative ability

    B. external and internal messages

    C. information and mental processing

    D. conscious and subconscious awareness

23. Shut off from the communicative flow, the person with a behavior disorder _____.

    A. is unable to focus attention on internal problems

    B. is isolated in internal problems

    C. relays threatening messages

    D. all of the above

24. Which of the following is universal according to the passage?

    A. Neural blocks.   B. Physical blocks.

    C. Cerebral blocks.   D. Emotional blocks.

25. The passage ends with _____.

    A. the contributing factors to emotional and mental disorders

    B. the importance of acquiring good communicative skills

    C. the significance of eliminating early emotional blocks

    D. the warning of emotional blocks common in childhood

Passage Six

Depression is a state of low vitality and discontent with life in which the individual withdraws from normal life activities even to the point of considering death as an attractive alternative.

Although everyone experiences "the blues" or periods of low spirits when nothing in life seems to go well, when everything seems to be an effort, and when efforts lead to frustration, these periods are usually brief and are likely to occur when the person is tired, hungry, lonely, or sick. Rest, good food, talking with friends, some fun, or an end to the sickness are usually enough to cure the blues. But when the low spirits persist, or when there are large swings in mood from elation to desolation, when nothing seems to catch the interest of the person, when relatives or friends cannot cheer the person and he or she continues to withdraw, then the person is depressed.

Even such depression is normal under certain circumstances. Anyone who is faced with a serious and painful illness or the loss of a limb, is exhausted by repeated narrow escapes from death (such as occurs in wartime), has been exposed to a dehumanizing environment (such as occurred with the Jews in Nazi Germany), has had an overwhelming series of stressful setbacks, or has experienced the death of several family members within a short time is expected to be depressed.

However, there are many depressed people who seem to the casual observer to have no reason to be depressed. Depression under these circumstances stems from severe behavior disturbance in which the person sees himself or herself as worthless. Such an image is usually the result of the psychosocial conditioning of a childhood deprived of a parental role model of security, love, care, and attention essential for the development of trusting relationships. The depressed person needs to build a new image of himself or herself as a useful and needed person. Psychotherapy is often helpful in restoring natural inner confidence and capacity for meaningful and trusting relationships.

Although it often takes years of psychotherapy for the individual to work through the underlying suspicion and anger of his or her problems, acceptance by another will get through to even the most deeply depressed person if the other is sincere. An attitude of matter-of-fact hopefulness on the part of those around the depressed person can reassure him or her of eventual recovery.

The disturbed thoughts of the depressed person cannot be forgotten until they are replaced by other thoughts. Yet, in depression, the person does not see that he or she has choices about what thoughts occupy his or her mind. The person needs to explore alternatives for thoughts and actions and learn to care for himself or herself enough to modify his or her own behavior.

26. Unlike others, according to the passage, a depressed person _____.

   A. is likely to recover in a short period of time

B. does not reveal any underlying cause

C. is characteristic of self-hatred

D. tends to stay with "the blues"

27. From a serious and painful illness to the death of several family members, the author is trying to tell us that _____.

    A. depression can potentially be detrimental to mental health

    B. the severity of depression varies with individuals

    C. depression is overwhelmingly prevailing

    D. depression is sometimes inescapable

28. Those who present no reason to be depressed, according to the passage, _____.

    A. need to protect their self-images

    B. need a parental role model at home

    C. can be helped psychologically to be useful and needed persons

    D. can be helped to restore their trusting relationships with their parents

29. The author implies that what the depressed person needs most is _____.

    A. sincerity   B. acceptance

    C. reassurance   D. all of the above

30. Under psychotherapy, the depressed person is encouraged _____.

    A. to free his or her mind of any thought

    B. to find substitutes for the disturbed thoughts

    C. to reassure himself or herself of early recovery

    D. to explore as many therapeutic approaches as possible

Model Test 3

Passage One

Behaviors that we do not understand often become nearly invisible — even when, in retrospect, we see how truly strange they are.

When I was a psychiatric resident, we had a faculty member who was famous for his messy office: stacks of papers and old journals covered every chair and table as well as much of the floor. One day, as I walked past the open office door with one of my supervisors, he murmured mildly, "Odd duck." And that was as far as anyone seemed to reflect on this peculiar state of affairs within an institution staffed by psychiatrists. Eventually, the faculty member had to be given another office in which to see patients.

Not surprisingly, the psychiatric diagnostic manual does not list "messy room" in the index. But it does mention a tantalizing symptom: inability "to discard worn-out or worthless objects even when they have no sentimental value". It comes under the diagnosis obsessive-compulsive personality disorder, an obscure cousin of the more famous obsessive-compulsive disorder.

I was barely aware of the diagnosis. Every era has mental disorders that for cultural or scientific reasons become popular. In Freud's day it was hysteria. Currently, depression has moved to center stage. But other ailments go relatively ignored, and this disorder was one.

It came with a list of additional symptoms that appeared to be peculiar: anxiety about spending money, excessive devotion to work to the exclusion of leisure activities, rigidity about following rules, perfectionism in doing tasks — at times to the point of interfering with finishing them.

In moderation, the symptoms seemed to fit right in with our workaholic culture — perhaps explaining the low profile of the diagnosis. Relentless work orientation and perfectionism may even be assets in rule- and detail-oriented professions like accounting or law.

But when the symptoms are too intense or pervasive, they become crippling. Beneath the seemingly adaptive behaviors lies a central disability. People with this diagnosis have enormous difficulty making decisions. They lack the internal sense of completion that most of us experience at the end of a choice or a task, even one as simple as throwing something out or making a purchase. In obsessive-compulsive personality disorder, this feeling occurs only after endless deliberation and revision, if at all.

The need to come up with the "correct" answer, the best purchase or the perfect proposal leads to excess rumination over each decision. It can even lead to complete paralysis. For such people, rules of all kinds are a godsend — they represent premade decisions. Open-ended assignments, like writing papers, are nightmares.

For such a patient or for a psychiatrist, understanding a cluster of diagnostic symptoms can be a revelation. The picture leaps out from the previously disorganized background. But undoubtedly, at times we can become too reductionistic, seeing patterns where none exist: sometimes a messy room is just a messy room.

1. Which of the following best describes people's attitude towards the faculty member?

   A. They disliked him, and that's why he got his separate room to see patients.

   B. They thought he was a little strange, but didn't pay much attention to his behavior.

   C. They were interested in his behavior, as they were all psychiatrists.

   D. They thought he had some mental retardedness.

2. The popular mental disorder of current time, according to the author, is _____.

   A. hysteria   B. depression

   C. messiness   D. obsessive compulsive disorder

3. The reason why symptoms of the "obsessive-compulsive disorder" go unnoticed is that _____.

   A. they are highly thought of according to law

   B. some of the mild symptoms fit in with a workaholic culture

   C. they have a low profile

   D. they take a long time to become intense or pervasive

4. Rules are a godsend to persons with the obsessive-compulsive personality disorder because _____.

   A. they do not involve decision-making

   B. they are open-ended assignments

   C. they lead to complete paralysis

   D. they are made by others

5. From the last paragraph we can see that the author's view is that _____.

   A. a messy room is just a messy room

   B. a messy room is an indication of the obsessive-compulsive personality disorder

   C. psychiatrists should pay attention to a messy room

   D. psychiatrists should see patterns of seemingly disorganized behaviors, but shouldn't be too reductionistic

Passage Two

Cancer has always been with us, but not always in the same way. Its care and management have differed over time, of course, but so, too, have its identity, visibility, and meanings. Pick up the thread of history at its most distant end and you have cancer the crab — so named either because of the ramifying venous processes spreading out from a tumor or because its pain is like the pinch of a crab's claw. Premodern cancer is a lump, a swelling that sometimes breaks through the skin in ulcerations producing foul-smelling discharges. The ancient Egyptians knew about many tumors that had a bad outcome, and the Greeks made a distinction between benign tumors (oncos) and malignant ones (carcinos). In the second century A. D., Galen reckoned that the cause was systemic, an excess of melancholy or black bile, one of the body's four "humors", brought on by bad diet and environmental circumstances. Ancient medical practitioners sometimes cut tumors out, but the prognosis was known to be grim. Describing tumors of the breast, an Egyptian papyrus from about 1600 B. C. concluded: "There is no treatment."

The experience of cancer has always been terrible, but, until modern times, its mark on the culture has been light. In the past, fear coagulated around other ways of dying: infectious and epidemic diseases (plague, smallpox, cholera, typhus, typhoid fever); "apoplexies" (what we now call strokes and heart attacks); and, most notably in the nineteenth century, "consumption" (tuberculosis). The agonizing manner of cancer death was dreaded, but that fear was not centrally situated in the public mind — as it now is. This is one reason that the medical historian Roy Porter wrote that cancer is "the modern disease par excellence", and that Mukherjee calls it "the quintessential product of modernity".

At one time, it was thought that cancer was a "disease of civilization", belonging to much the same causal domain as "neurasthenia" and diabetes, the former a nervous weakness believed to be brought about by the stress of modern life and the latter a condition produced by bad diet and indolence. In the eighteenth and nineteenth centuries, some physicians attributed cancer — notably of the breast and the ovaries — to psychological and behavioral causes. William Buchan's wildly popular eighteenth-century text "Domestic Medicine" judged that cancers might be caused by "excessive fear, grief, religious melancholy". In the nineteenth century, reference was repeatedly made to a "cancer personality," and, in some versions, specifically to sexual repression. As Susan Sontag observed, cancer was considered shameful, not to be mentioned, even obscene. Among the Romantics and the Victorians, suffering and dying from tuberculosis might be considered a badge of refinement; cancer death was nothing of the sort. "It seems unimaginable," Sontag wrote, "to aestheticize" cancer.

6. According to the passage, the ancient Egyptians _____.

    A. called cancer the crab

B. were able to distinguish benign tumors and malignant ones

C. found out the cause of cancer

D. knew about a lot of malignant tumors

7. Which of the following statements about the cancers of the past is best supported by the passage?

A. Ancient people did not live long enough to become prone to cancer.

B. In the past, people did not fear cancer.

C. Cancer death might be considered as a badge of refinement.

D. Some physicians believed that one's own behavioral mode could lead to cancer.

8. Which of the following is the reason for cancer to be called "the modern disease"?

A. Modern cancer care is very effective.

B. There is a lot more cancer now.

C. People understand cancer in radically new ways now.

D. There is a sharp increase in mortality in modern cancer world.

9. "Neurasthenia" and diabetes are mentioned because _____.

A. they are as fatal as cancer

B. they were considered to be "disease of civilization"

C. people dread them very much

D. they are brought by the high pressure of modern life

10. As suggested by the passage, with which of the following statements would the author most likely agree?

A. The care and management of cancer have development over time.

B. The cultural significance of cancer shifts in different times.

C. Cancer's identity has never changed.

D. Cancer is the price paid for modern life.

Passage Three

The smell from an old lady's armpits can raise your spirits, a scientist in Pennsylvania claims. Her work also suggests that in contrast, the scent of a young child does nothing to improve your mood.

Studies using animals have shown that smell is vital for conveying information. Rodents can detect and transmit fear through smell, for instance, and animals often identify a high-ranking member of a group by its smell. A recent study has shown that people can distinguish the body odor of both happy and fearful people. But the impact of body odor on people's mood has hardly been explored at all.

Denise Chen of the Monell Chemical Senses Center in Philadelphia hoped to find out more. So she recruited 30 volunteers in six different categories: girls and boys aged between three and eight, young adult women and men in their early twenties and elderly women and men in their seventies. The volunteers all gave samples of their body odor by strapping a gauze pad under each armpit and keeping it there for 10 hours.

The participants were not allowed to use any perfumes or deodorants, or eat strong-smelling foods, in the four days before the samples were collected. They could shower, but only with unscented soap and shampoo. Odors were also collected from the homes of all the donors and combined into a neutral control smell.

Chen then asked 308 university students to complete a 36-part questionnaire that assessed how positive their mood was. Then they smelled the gauze pads from one of the gauze pads from one of the six categories of people — without being told what the smells were. After this, the students answered the questionnaire a second time, this time with the questions shuffled.

People who had inhaled the samples taken from old women's armpits respond significantly more positively, Chen found. "Old women had an uplifting effect", she says. The smell of young men, on the other hand, produced a depressive effect. In general, Chen will report in a future issue of the journal *Physiology and Behavior*.

Jeannette Haviland, of Rutgers University in New Jersey, who also worked on the project, says it's possible that hormones make the body of young people signal aggression. But hormonal changes may make the odor of older people, especially women, signal that they are approachable. Alternatively, it could be that women in their golden years are generally happy, and that their odor can transmit this mood. "The air-borne chemicals that we collected from them — l'eau de grandmere (smell of grandmother) — may indicate that state," says Haviland.

11. It can be inferred from the passage that _____.

    A. there has been little literature on the impact of body odor upon people's moods

B.　human beings can convey as much information through odor as animals

C.　the relation between odor and mood has never been explored before

D.　it is more beneficial to sniff an old lady than to smell a child

12.　Chen tried to collect the samples of body odor _____.

　　A.　among three groups of volunteers　　B.　for four consecutive days

　　C.　unaffected　　　　　　　　　　　　D.　at random

13.　The participants answered the questionnaire the second time and their answers _____.

　　A.　reflected their improved moods

　　B.　revealed alterations in their moods

　　C.　represented six categories of mood

　　D.　were scrambled so as to assure objectivity

14.　The students felt good when they sniffed the samples of body odor from _____.

　　A.　people in good mood　　　　　B.　young men

　　C.　old ladies　　　　　　　　　　D.　children

15.　Haviland tried to prove the relation between _____.

　　A.　hormones and body odors　　　B.　body odors and lifestyles

　　C.　moods and lifestyles　　　　　D.　all of the above

Passage Four

Many adults may think they are getting enough shut-eye, but in a major sleep study almost 80 percent of respondents admitted to not getting their prescribed amount of nightly rest. So, what exactly is the right amount of sleep? Research shows that adults need an average of seven to nine hours of sleep a night for optimal functionality. Read on to see just how much of an impact moderate sleep deprivation can have on your mind and body.

By getting less than six hours of sleep a night, you could be putting yourself at risk of high blood pressure. When you sleep, your heart gets a break and is able to slow down for a significant period of time. But cutting back on sleep means your heart has to work overtime without its allotted break. In constantly doing so, your body must accommodate to its new conditions and elevate your overall daily blood pressure. And the heart isn't the only organ that is overtaxed by a lack of sleep. The less sleep you get, the less time the brain has to regulate stress hormones, and over time, sleep deprivation could permanently hinder the brain's ability to regulate these hormones, leading to elevated blood pressure.

We all hang around in bed during our bouts of illness. But did you know that skipping out on the bed rest can increase your risk of getting sick? Prolonged sleep deprivation has long been associated with diminished immune functions, but researchers have also found a direct correlation between "modest" sleep deprivation — less than six hours — and reduced immune response. So try to toughen up your immune system by getting at least seven hours of sleep a night, and maintaining a healthy diet. You'll be glad you got that extra hour of sleep the next time that a bug comes around and leaves everyone else bedridden with a fever for three days.

During deep REM sleep, your muscles (except those in the eyes) are essentially immobilized in order to keep you from acting out on your dreams. Unfortunately, this effort your body makes to keep you safe while dreaming can sometimes backfire, resulting in sleep paralysis. Sleep paralysis occurs when the brain is aroused from its REM cycle, but the body remains in its immobilizing state. This can be quite a frightening sensation because, while your mind is slowly regaining consciousness, it has no control over your body, leaving some with a feeling of powerlessness, fear and panic. Most people experience this eerie phenomena at least once in their lives, but those who are sleep deprived are more likely to have panicked episodes of sleep paralysis that are usually accompanied by hallucinations, as well.

For a second, imagine all of your memories are erased; every birthday, summer vacation, even what you did yesterday afternoon is completely lost, because you have no recollection of them. It's a chilling thought, but that is what a life without sleep would be like. Sleep is essential to the cognitive functions of the brain, and without it, our ability to consolidate memories, learn daily tasks, and make decisions is impaired by a large degree. Research has revealed that REM sleep, or dream-sleep, helps solidify the "fragile" memories the brain creates throughout the day to that they can be easily organized and stored in the mind's long-term cache.

16. According to the passage, what is the meaning of "sleep deprivation"?
    A. To sleep for an average period of time.
    B. To sleep deeply without dreaming.
    C. To sleep less than needed.
    D. To sleep modestly.

17. Which of the following statements is TRUE according to Paragraph 3?
    A. When everyone else gets a fever, those with sleep deprivation will be able to sleep longer.

B. When everyone else gets a fever, those who usually have adequate sleep will be alright.

C. Only modest sleep deprivation could weaken the immune system.

D. Prolonged sleep deprivation will not have impact on the immune system.

18. Why is there the so-called "sleep paralysis"?

A. It occurs when you are unable to wake up from dreams while you are sleeping.

B. It occurs when your brain immobilizes your body in order to keep you from dreaming.

C. Because you are usually too frightened to move your body when waking up from deep REM sleep.

D. Because your body, immobilized when dreaming, may still be unable to move even when your brain is woken up.

19. Which of the following statements is TRUE according to the last paragraph?

A. Memories are part of the cognitive function of the brain.

B. Memories created during the daytime are usually fragile and impaired.

C. You are likely to lose your memories of yesterday after a night's sleep.

D. Long-term memory cannot be formed without dream-sleep.

20. What effects of sleep deprivation on human mind and body are discussed in this passage?

A. High blood pressure, a toughened immune system, sleep paralysis, and memory loss.

B. Blood pressure, immune system, sleep paralysis, and long term memory.

C. Blood pressure, immune system, the brain and the body, and memory.

D. High blood pressure, a weakened immune system, sleep paralysis, and memory loss.

Passage Five

Cultural norms so completely surround people, so permeate thought and action, that we never recognize the assumptions on which their lives and their sanity rest. As one observer put it, if birds were suddenly endowed with scientific curiosity they might examine many things, but the sky itself would be overlooked as a suitable subject; if fish were to become curious about the world, it would never occur to them to begin by investigating water. For birds and fish would take the sky and sea for granted, unaware of their profound influence because they comprise the medium for every fact. Human beings, in a similar way, occupy a symbolic universe governed by codes that are unconsciously acquired and automatically employed. So much so that they rarely notice that the ways they interpret and talk about events are distinctively different from the ways people conduct their affairs in other cultures.

As long as people remain blind to the sources of their meanings, they are imprisoned within them. These cultural frames of reference are no less confining simply because they cannot be seen or touched. Whether it is an individual neurosis that keeps an individual out of contact with his neighbors, or a collective neurosis that separates neighbors of different cultures, both are forms of blindness that limit what can be experienced and what can be learned from others.

It would seem that everywhere people would desire to break out of the boundaries of their own experiential worlds. Their ability to react sensitively to a wider spectrum of events and peoples requires an overcoming of such cultural **parochialism**. But, in fact, few attain this broader vision. Some, of course, have little opportunity for wider cultural experience, though this condition should change as the movement of people accelerates. Others do not try to widen their experience because they prefer the old and familiar, seek from their affairs only further confirmation of the correctness of their own values. Still others recoil from such experiences because they feel it dangerous to probe too deeply into the personal or cultural unconscious. Exposure may reveal how tenuous and arbitrary many cultural norms are; such exposure might force people to acquire new bases for interpreting events. And even for the many who do seek actively to enlarge the variety of human beings with whom they are capable of communicating there are still difficulties.

Cultural myopia persists not merely because of inertia and habit, but chiefly because it is so difficult to overcome. One acquires a personality and a culture in childhood, long before he is capable of comprehending either of them. To survive, each person masters the perceptual orientations, cognitive biases, and communicative habits of his own culture. But once mastered, objective assessment of these same processes is awkward since the same mechanisms that are being evaluated must be used in making the evaluations.

21. The examples of birds and fish are used to _____.
    A. show that they, too, have their respective cultures
    B. explain humans occupy a symbolic universe as birds and fish occupy the sky

and the sea

    C. illustrate that human beings are unaware of the cultural codes governing them

    D. demonstrate the similarity between man, birds, and fish in their ways of thinking

22. The term "parochialism" (Line 3, Para. 3) most possibly means _____.

    A. open-mindedness   B. provincialism

    C. superiority   D. discrimination

23. It can be inferred from the last two paragraphs that _____.

    A. everyone would like to widen their cultural scope if they can

    B. the obstacles to overcoming cultural parochialism lie mainly in people's habit of thinking

    C. provided one's brought up in a culture, he may be with bias in making cultural evaluations

    D. childhood is an important stage in comprehending culture

24. Which of the following statements is TRUE according to the passage?

    A. Individual and collective neurosis might prevent communications with others.

    B. People in different cultures may be governed by the same cultural norms.

    C. People's visions will be enlarged if only they knew that cultural differences exist.

    D. If cultural norms are something tangible, they won't be so confining.

25. The passage might be entitled "_____".

    A. How to Overcome Cultural Myopia

    B. Behavioral Patterns and Cultural Background

    C. Harms of Cultural Myopia

    D. Cultural Myopia — a Deep-rooted Collective Neurosis

Passage Six

When a disease of epidemic proportions rips into the populace, scientists immediately get to work, trying to locate the source of the affliction and find ways to combat it. Oftentimes, success is achieved, as medical science is able to isolate the parasite, germ or cell that causes the problem and finds ways to effectively kill or contain it. In the most serious of cases, in which the entire population of a region or country may be at grave risk, it is deemed necessary to protect the entire population through vaccination, so as to safeguard lives and ensure that the disease will not spread.

The process of vaccination allows the patient's body to develop immunity to the virus or disease so that, if it is encountered, one can fight it off naturally. To accomplish this, a small weak or dead strain of the disease is actually injected into the patient in a controlled environment, so that his body's immune system can learn to fight the invader properly. Information on how to penetrate the disease's defenses is transmitted to all elements of the patient's immune system in a process that occurs naturally, in which genetic information is passed from cell to cell. This makes sure that, should the patient later come into contact with the real problem, his body is well equipped and trained to deal with it, having already done so before.

There are dangers inherent in the process, however. On occasion, even the weakened version of the disease contained in the vaccine proves too much for the body to handle, resulting in the immune case of the smallpox vaccine, designed to eradicate the smallpox epidemic that nearly wiped out the entire Native American population and killed massive numbers of settlers. Approximately 1 in 10,000 people who receives the vaccine contract the smallpox disease from the vaccine itself and dies from it. Thus, if the entire population of the United States were to receive the Smallpox Vaccine today, 3,000 Americans would be left dead.

Fortunately, the smallpox virus was considered eradicated in the early 1970s, ending the mandatory vaccination of all babies in America. In the event of a reintroduction of the disease, however, mandatory vaccinations may resume, resulting in more unexpected deaths from vaccination. The process, which is truly a blessing, may indeed hide some hidden cures.

26. How do vaccines protect humans from diseases according to Paragraph Two?

    A. By passing information on how to fight the disease to the disease.

    B. By passing information on how to fight the disease to the immune system.

    C. By weakening the disease so that the immune system can defeat it.

    D. By introducing the disease to the body.

27. What does the example of the smallpox vaccine illustrate?

    A. The way that vaccines protect people from diseases.

    B. The effectiveness of vaccines in eradicating certain diseases.

    C. The practical use of a vaccine to control an epidemic disease.

    D. The possible negative outcome of administering vaccines.

28. The author argues that vaccinations are both a blessing and a curse because _____.

    A. saving the many would not necessarily justify the death of the few

    B. some vaccines, such as the smallpox vaccine, have negative side effects

    C. they don't always work

    D. while many lives are saved, some are actually killed by the vaccine

29. The best title for the passage would be _____.

    A. The Smallpox Vaccine: an Analysis

    B. How Vaccines Work

    C. Vaccines: Methods and Implications

    D. A Warning on the Negative Side Effects of Vaccines

30. The main purpose of the passage is to _____.

    A. convince the readers that vaccines are not as safe as many think

    B. educate the readers on how vaccines are used and some of their dangers

    C. educate the readers on the circumstances that would necessitate widespread vaccinations

    D. present the method by which vaccines are used through the case of the smallpox vaccine

Model Test 4

Passage One

When most people think about changing their body shape, they usually focus on just losing weight. Books and magazines about dieting are among the most popular in the world. Dieting is an important part of staying fit and healthy, but losing weight by means of dieting takes time; losing weight too fast can cause great health problems. Dieting means changing one's eating habits to a healthier pattern, but many women mistake the concept of dieting and think that the less one eats, the better. As a result, they lose health as well as weight.

Aerobic exercise is a moderate intensity workout that, over a certain period of time, will improve the body's use of oxygen. Nowadays, aerobic exercise has become a very trendy workout among youths. Not only is performing aerobic exercise interesting, but it is also very beneficial for health. There are different types of aerobics like jogging, swimming, kickboxing, fitness walking, inline skating, bicycling, etc. Aerobics strengthens the heart and lungs. It is also especially popular with women.

But neither of these two methods, dieting and aerobics can help shape the body. To do this, you need to build muscles. So, if a firmer and shapelier body is your goal, 60 percent of your exercise routine should involve strengthening moves, and only 30 percent should be aerobic exercises.

For a proper body-shaping routine, you should plan three strength-training sessions a week with weights. Use weights which are as heavy as possible while still allowing you to do 8 to 12 reps of each exercise. Do one to three exercises for each muscle groups — for example, chest and biceps, or back, shoulders and triceps.

You should combine this with fast-paced aerobics activities, like swimming, cycling, walking, running, or inline skating. Plan three to four workouts a week, 15 to 20 minutes each, increasing the pace each week.

As you build muscle, you may find that you gain weight in spite of all of your calorie-burning exercise. Don't worry. It's probably muscle, which is denser than fat. And muscle is also a calorie-burning tissue. With more muscle, you can burn more calories, even when you are not exercising.

When you are trying to build muscle, you need two to three servings of protein a day, but the main part of your diet should be carbohydrates. And in order to get the energy you need for a high-intensity workout, you should eat something, especially carbohydrates, an hour or so before your workout.

While weight training will firm and shape your body, it has other benefits too. It improves bone and muscle strength and burns calories, leading to improved health and a higher quality of life.

1. Which of the following is NOT true about dieting?

    A. Dieting is about changing one's eating habits.

    B. Dieting does not necessarily mean eating less than one used to.

    C. Dieting does not necessarily mean losing weight.

    D. Losing weight is bound to cause great health problems.

2. "Workouts" include all the following EXCEPT _____.

    A. bicycling   B. dieting

    C. weight training   D. aerobic exercise

3. Which of the following is NOT one of the suggestions given in the passage?

   A. Exercise should be done for each major group of muscles.

   B. When you do weight-training, the weights you have should be as heavy as possible.

   C. Go on a proper diet for muscle-building.

   D. Muscle-building exercise should be combined with aerobic activities.

4. Which of the following is NOT true?

   A. Muscle-building exercise results in weight gain, but that is not a problem to worry about.

   B. Muscle helps one keep fit.

   C. Improved muscle strength can lead to a higher quality of life.

   D. Weight training helps shape your body.

5. What's the ultimate purpose of strength-training with weights?

   A. To increase the pace of your aerobic exercise.

   B. To burn more calories and lose weight.

   C. To build muscle and lose weight.

   D. To shape your body and make your life more enjoyable.

Passage Two

Got milk? Be very afraid. Or preferably, a bit skeptical. Some folks are about to try to convince you that milk is toxic. But the real question is, what's more dangerous to your health: milk, or celebrities and activists embarked on the latest trendy crusade（改革）? This month marks the publicity-pumped debut of the Anti Dairy Coalition, a band of physicians, self-described "Hollywood personalities" and others who decry what they call "the health and nutritional risks of consuming dairy products".

The coalition, including its spokes—Jeremiah, writer George Plimpton, would have you believe that milk causes heart disease, cancer, infections, asthma, allergies and tuberculosis. Robert Cohen, founder of the ADC (and author of milk: The Deadly Poison), writes: "The Fountain of Youth and cure to illness can be obtained by giving up milk."

Hyperbole aside, the ADC is spotlighting a question hotly debated by everyone from nutritionists to parents. Many patients ask doctors whether they should give up milk, like that supermodel they saw interviewed on TV. And to be sure, the ADC's overwrought claims do have some scientific basis.

Take heart disease. Foods like butter, cheese, ice cream and whole milk are packed with saturated fat（饱和脂肪）, which blocks arteries（动脉）and can lead to heart attacks. That's why most nutritionists advise switching to low-fat or skim milk and eating more yogurt and cottage cheese than Haagen-Dazs and Bric. Even skim milk, though, can trigger allergies in some people, including infants, who in any case will get more iron and other key nutrients from breast milk or formula.

So must you flee from milk entirely? Yes, says Cohen, who holds that skim milk is the devil's brew. It's full of — are you sitting down — protein. And here's where the ADC starts twisting the facts to reach wild conclusions. Allergies are frequently triggered by proteins (true); asthma is an allergic condition (true); it's been increasing dramatically (true); doctors don't know the cause (true); therefore, the protein in milk must be the culprit（罪魁祸首）?

A similar leap of illogic assumes that because women in the Netherlands, Denmark, Norway and Sweden consume lots of milk and also suffer high rates of breast cancer; the former must cause the latter. Another clunker is Cohen's claim that widespread lactose intolerance（乳糖不耐症）— the inability to digest dairy products — means milk is of little use as a source of calcium. In fact, many cases of lactose intolerance are mild and interfere only slightly with calcium uptake. Many people intolerant of milk can easily digest yogurt. And lactase tablets（乳糖分解酵素片）can make dairy products digestible even in severe cases.

If milk isn't the perfect food, it's still got some big things going for it. It's an inexpensive source of calcium, protein, potassium and other vitamins and minerals. And unlike other sources of calcium, such as, say, steamed kale, milk is a food kids will eat. The ADC feels that milk is the root of most human maladies（疾病）, but I can point to other single-issue obsessive who insist the villain is meat or wheat or sugar or some other substance that our species has long and happily consumed. I often learn something by examining their claims. But I keep coming back to the mainstream nutritionists, who emphasize a balanced diet and advise moderation in all things.

6. The ADC holds that drinking milk will cause the following diseases EXCEPT _____.

   A. breast cancer   B. diabetes   C. heart disease   D. lung disease

7. The writer thinks that milk _____.

   A. is toxic and we should give it up

   B. is very nutritious and we should consume it as much as possible

C. is the most ideal food

D. has its pluses and minuses and we should consume it sensibly

8. It is clear from the passage that _____.

A. the writer is of the same opinion about milk with the ADC

B. the writer regards milk as the root of most human diseases

C. the writer advises people to stay out of trouble with milk

D. the writer's opinion about milk differs greatly from the ADC's

9. According to the passage, if you suffer from lactose intolerance _____.

A. you had better give up milk entirely

B. you should have less milk every day

C. you can take lactase tablets which catalyze（催化）lactose into glucose（葡萄糖）and galactose（半乳糖）

D. you must see a doctor at once

10. We can conclude from the passage that the writer is _____.

A. an unprejudiced person   B. an opinionated person

C. a worldly person   D. a wise but peculiar person

Passage Three

Joy and sadness are experienced by people in all cultures around the world, but how can we tell when other people are happy or despondent? It turns out that the expression of many emotions may be universal. Smiling is apparently a universal sign of friendliness and approval. Baring the teeth in a hostile way, as noted by Charles Darwin in the nineteenth century, may be a universal sign of anger. As the originator of the theory of evolution, Darwin believed that the universal recognition of facial expressions would have survival value. For example, facial expressions could signal the approach of enemies (or friends) in the absence of language.

Most investigators concur that certain facial expressions suggest the same emotions in all people. Moreover, people in diverse cultures recognize the emotions manifested by the facial expressions. In classic research Paul Ekman took photographs of people exhibiting the emotions of anger, disgust, fear, happiness, and sadness. He then asked people around the world to indicate what emotions were being depicted in them. Those queried ranged from European college students to members of the Fore, a tribe that dwells in the New Guinea highlands. All groups, including the Fore, who had almost no contact with Western culture, agreed on the portrayed emotions. <u>The Fore also displayed familiar facial expressions when asked how they would respond if they were the characters in stories that called for basic emotional responses.</u> Ekman and his colleagues more recently obtained similar results in a study of ten cultures in which participants were permitted to report that multiple emotions were shown by facial expressions. The participants generally agreed on which two emotions were being shown and which emotion was more intense.

Psychological researchers generally recognize that facial expressions reflect emotional states. In fact, various emotional states give rise to certain patterns of electrical activity in the facial muscles and in the brain. The facial-feedback hypothesis argues, however, that the causal relationship between emotions and facial expressions can also — work in the opposite direction. According to this hypothesis, signals from the facial muscles ("feedback") are sent back to emotion centers of the brain, and so a person's facial expression influences that person's emotional state. Consider Darwin's words: The free expression by outward signs of an emotion intensifies it. On the other hand, the repression, as far as possible, of all outward signs softens our emotions. Can smiling give rise to feelings of good will, for example, and frowning to anger?

Psychological research has given rise to some interesting findings concerning the facial-feedback hypothesis. Causing participants in experiments to smile, for example, leads them to report more positive feelings and to rate cartoons (humorous drawings of people or situations) as being more humorous. When they are caused to frown, they rate cartoons as being more aggressive.

Ekman's observation may be relevant to the British expression "keep a stiff upper lip" as a recommendation for handling stress. It might be that a "stiff" lip suppresses emotional response — as long as the lip is not quivering with fear or tension. But when the emotion that leads to stiffening the lip is more intense, and involves strong muscle tension, facial feedback may heighten emotional response.

11. According to the passage, which of the following effects may stiffening the upper lip have?

   A. It first suppresses stress, and then intensifies it.

   B. It may cause fear and tension in those who see it.

C. It can damage the lip muscles.

D. It may either heighten or reduce emotional response.

12. The author mentions "Baring the teeth in a hostile way" in order to _____.

A. differentiate one possible meaning of a particular facial expression from other meanings of it

B. support Darwin's theory of evolution

C. contrast a facial expression that is easily understood with other facial expressions

D. provide an example of a facial expression whose meaning is widely understood

13. Which of the sentences below best expresses the essential information in the highlighted sentence in the second paragraph?

A. The Fore were asked to display familiar facial expressions when they told their stories.

B. The Fore exhibited the same relationship of facial expressions and basic emotions that is seen in western culture when they acted out stories.

C. The Fore's facial expressions indicated their unwillingness to pretend to be the characters in stories.

D. The Fore were familiar with the facial expressions and basic emotions of the characters in stories.

14. According to the passage, what effect did Darwin believe repression of all outward signs would have on humans' emotions?

A. They would become less intense.

B. They would last longer than usual.

C. They would become more negative.

D. They would cause problems later.

15. According to the passage, research involving which of the following supported the facial-feedback hypothesis?

A. The long-term effects of repressing emotions.

B. The release of neurotransmitters by people during experiments.

C. The reactions of people in experiments to cartoons.

D. The tendency of people in experiments to cooperate.

Passage Four

It was a big week for Alzheimer's disease, and not just because PBS aired *The Forgetting*, a first-rate documentary about Alzheimer's worth catching in reruns if you missed it the first time. There was also a flurry of scientific news that offered hope to the families already struggling with Alzheimer's, as well as to the baby-boom generation that's up next. Unless something dramatic happens, the number of Americans living with this terrifying brain disease could triple, to about 16 million, over the next 50 years. There's still no cure in sight, but there is progress on several fronts. Among them:

MEGADOSE VITAMINS. Doctors knew vitamins E and C, both antioxidants, help **stave off** Alzheimer's, at least in folks who haven't already developed the disorder. What they didn't know — but a big study involving 4,740 participants published in the Archives of Neurology showed — was that the two vitamins taken together in huge daily doses (at least 400 IU of E and more than 500 mg of C) could reduce the risk of Alzheimer's a remarkable 78%.

COMBINATION THERAPY. A yearlong study of more than 400 Alzheimer's patients showed that two drugs that work differently on the brain's chemistry act well together to help slow down the disease. Patients who were being treated with donepezil (sold as Aricept), an older drug that preserves the neurotransmitter acetylcholine, were also given memantine (Namenda), a new drug approved by the FDA last October that blocks overproduction of a harmful brain chemical called glutamate. The two drugs worked even better in combination than they did alone, providing substantial benefit for patients with moderate to severe Alzheimer's, according to a report in the *Journal of the American Medical Association*.

BRAIN IMAGING. Finally, scientists at the University of Pittsburgh announced that they had successfully developed a procedure that allows them to peer into the brains of Alzheimer's patients with positron emission tomography (PET) scans to see telltale plaque deposits. Before now, doctors could not track the progress of these plaques until after the patient died, when the brain could be autopsied. Using the new technique, doctors may be able to begin treatment long before the first symptoms appear.

None of these advances is a magic bullet for Alzheimer's disease. If you or your loved ones are concerned, the first step is careful evaluation by your doctor. Not all memory lapses are Alzheimer's, and there are reversible causes of forgetfulness that can be treated if caught early. Also, remember the old adage "use it or lose it". Mental exercise — reading, doing crossword puzzles, playing chess or Scrabble — is as good for preserving your mind as physical exercise is for your body.

16. From the first paragraph, we learn that _____.

    A. the baby-boom generation will not suffer from Alzheimer's disease

    B. recent progress brings hope for Alzheimer victims

    C. the week was very important for Alzheimer's because a documentary about it was shown on PBS

    D. the new achievements made on several fronts show that Alzheimer's disease can be cured

17. The phrase "stave off" (Paragraph 2) most probably means "_____".

    A. get   B. treat   C. cure   D. prevent

18. The report in the *Journal of the American Medical Association* shows that _____.

    A. combination therapy refers to combining two different ways of treatment

    B. donepezil helps block overproduction of a harmful brain chemical called glutamate

    C. combination therapy is of great benefit to all patients with Alzheimer's

    D. Aricept and Namenda have better effect when used together than used separately

19. Why is brain imaging considered progress in treating Alzheimer's?

    A. Because it helps doctors diagnose and treat the disease in an early phase by tracking the progress of plaques in the brain.

    B. Because it helps doctors autopsy the brains of the patients after they died.

    C. Because it helps doctors see the plaque clearly so that they can operate on the brain.

    D. Because it helps doctors develop a new procedure of tracking the progress of the disease.

20. To which of the following is the author likely to agree?

    A. Alzheimer's disease can be cured thanks to the new advances.

    B. Forgetfulness can be cured by doing mental exercise.

    C. Careful evaluation is important because it can tell Alzheimer's from curable memory lapses, which can be treated if found in an early phase.

    D. Mental exercises do good only to forgetfulness caused by reversible causes.

Passage Five

Any fair-minded assessment of the dangers of the deal between Britain's National Health Service (NHS) and DeepMind must start by acknowledging that both sides mean well. DeepMind is one of the leading artificial intelligence (AI) companies in the world. The potential of this work applied to healthcare is very great, but it could also lead to further concentration of power in the tech giants. It is against that background that the information commissioner, Elizabeth Denham, has issued her damning verdict against the Royal Free hospital trust under the NHS, which handed over to DeepMind the records of 1.6 million patients in 2015 on the basis of a vague agreement which took far too little account of the patients' rights and their expectations of privacy.

DeepMind has almost apologized. The NHS trust has mended its ways. Further arrangements — and there may be many — between the NHS and DeepMind will be carefully scrutinised to ensure that all necessary permissions have been asked of patients and all unnecessary data has been cleaned. There are lessons about informed patient consent to learn. But privacy is not the only angle in this case and not even the most important. Ms. Denham chose to concentrate the blame on the NHS trust, since under existing law it "controlled" the data and DeepMind merely "processed" it. But this distinction misses the point that it is processing and aggregation, not the mere possession of bits, that gives the data value.

The great question is who should benefit from the analysis of all the data that our lives now generate. Privacy law builds on the concept of damage to an individual from identifiable knowledge about them. That misses the way the surveillance economy works. The data of an individual there gains its value only when it is compared with the data of countless millions more.

The use of privacy law to curb the tech giants in this instance feels slightly maladapted. This practice does not address the real worry. It is not enough to say that the algorithms DeepMind develops will benefit patients and save lives. What matters is that they will belong to a private monopoly which developed them using public resources. If software promises to save lives on the scale that dugs now can, big data may be expected to behave as a big pharm has done. We are still at the beginning of this revolution and small choices now may turn out to have gigantic consequences later. A long struggle will be needed to avoid a future of digital feudalism. Ms. Denham's report is a welcome start.

21. What is true of the agreement between the NHS and DeepMind?

    A. It caused conflicts among tech giants.

    B. It failed to pay due attention to the patient's rights.

    C. It fell short of the latter's expectations

    D. It put both sides into a dangerous situation.

22. The NHS trust responded to Denham's verdict with _____.

    A. empty promises   B. tough resistance

    C. necessary adjustments   D. sincere apologies

23. The author argues in Paragraph 2 that _____.

    A. privacy protection must be secured at all costs

    B. leaking patients' data is worse than selling it

    C. making profits from patients' data is illegal

    D. the value of data comes from the processing of it

24. According to the last paragraph, the real worry arising from this deal is _____.

    A. the vicious rivalry among big pharmas

    B. the ineffective enforcement of privacy law

    C. the uncontrolled use of new software

    D. the monopoly of big data by tech giants

25. The author's attitude toward the application of AI to healthcare is _____.

    A. ambiguous   B. cautious

    C. appreciative   D. contemptuous

Passage Six

After years of defensiveness, a siege mentality and the stonewalling of any criticism, a quiet revolution is under way in animal research.

What has triggered this change of heart? It's partly down to the economic climate plus fewer new medicines and the removal of much of the threat from animal rights extremism, in the UK at least.

Until recently the only criticism of animal research came from antivivisection groups who persistently complained about a lack of transparency. Now criticism is coming from researchers too, with the recognition that not all aspects of animal experimentation are as robust as they should be and that something needs to change.

That is why we have published new guidelines aimed at improving the quality of reporting on animal experiments in research papers. These have been met with support, notably from the major funding bodies and many international journals. This is indicative of the new climate in which we operate.

Five years ago the guidelines would have been met with skepticism and accusations of increased bureaucracy from some within the scientific community.

The difference is that these guidelines come in the wake of recent studies, which reveal serious shortcomings in animal research. One by my own organization, the UK's NC3Rs, found that key information was missing from many of the 300 or so publications we analyzed that described publicly funded experiments on rodents and monkeys in the UK and the US.

The new guidelines should ensure the science emerging from animal research is maximized and that every animal used counts. Better reporting will allow greater opportunity to evaluate which animal models are useful and which are not. One way of doing this is through the systematic reviews that are the gold standard in clinical studies but rarely undertaken for animal studies due to the lack of information published.

Animal research has been a thorn in the side of researchers for many years. We can't afford to get this wrong, scientifically, ethically or financially. Failings in reporting animal data properly can be perceived as an attempt to hide something, either about the quality or value of what is being done. When animal research is funded from the public purse a public mandate is essential. There is much scope for improvement. It is time for scientists — funders, researchers and editors — to use the new guidelines to put our house in order.

26. According to the passage, those who had long blamed animal research are _____.

    A. those ignorant of science

    B. government officials

    C. some of the researchers' colleagues

    D. antivivisection groups

27. The passage suggests that the change of heart among animal researchers refers to _____.

    A. their reconsideration of their research

    B. their resistance to their greater enemies

C. their giving in to animal right groups

    D. their confession to their failures in work

28. The new guidelines mostly stress that the report on animal research needs to be
    _____.

    A. directive   B. comprehensive

    C. affirmative   D. authoritative

29. The UK's NC3Rs research is mentioned to illustrate that animal research _____.

    A. needs government funding

    B. needs publishing guidelines

    C. involves some serious problems

    D. involves analyses and variations

30. For animal researchers, to put their work under the systematic reviews would be
    something _____.

    A. new   B. hard   C. pleasant   D. unthinkable

Model Test 5

Passage One

Directions：*Read the following passage on Alzheimer's lost memories. Five sentences have been removed from the passage. Choose from sentences (A-F) the one which best fits each blank (1-5). There is one extra sentence you do not need to use.*

Memory loss is one of the symptoms of Alzheimer's and heartbreaking for loved ones to watch progress. Gone are the details of a first love or a child's first steps. The memory of the achievements of a distinguished 30-year career and the tales of traveling the globe that once had everyone rolling on the floor with laughter are also gone. __1__. But what if they weren't actually one-just inaccessible?

A new paper published Wednesday by the Massachusetts Institute of Technology's Nobel Prize-winning Susumu Tonegawa provides that first strong evidence of this possibility and raises the hope of future treatments that could reverse some of the destructive actions of the disease on memory. "The important point is, this is a proof of concept," Tonegawa said. "That is, even if a memory seems to be gone, it is still there. It's a matter of how to retrieve it."

The research, described in the journal *Nature*, involved two groups of mice. __2__. Both groups were given a mild electric shock to their feet. The first group appeared to remember the trauma of the incident by showing fear when placed back in the box where they had been given the shock. The Alzheimer's mice, on the other hand, seemed to quickly forget what happened and did not have an upset reaction to the box.

Their reaction changed dramatically when the scientists stimulated tagged cells in their brains in the hippocampus—the part of the brain that encodes short-term memories—with a special blue light. __3__.

Tonegawa and his colleagues wrote that the treatment appears to have boosted neurons to regrow small buds called dendritic spins that form connections with other cells. The findings have "shattered a 20-year paradigm of how we're thinking about the disease," Rudy Tanzi, a Harvard neurology professor who is not involved in the research, told the *Boston Herald*. He said that since the 1980s, researchers believed the memories just weren't getting stored properly.

The technique used in the study—optical stimulation of brain cells involves the insertion of a gene into parts of a brain to make them sensitive to blue light and then stimulate them with the light. In a commentary accompanying the paper, Eric Klann of the Center for Neural Science at New York University said that the research employed a "clever strategy" and that "the potential to rescue long-term memory in dementia is exciting. __4__ While interesting," he told the *Guardian*, "the practicalities of this approach—using a special blue light to stimulate memory—mean that we're still many years away from knowing if it would be possible to restore lost memories in people."

__5__ *Nature* reported that early trials showed that deep-brain stimulation of the hippocampus may improve memory in some Alzheimer's patients.

A. When they were put back in the box following the procedure, their memories of the shock appeared to have returned, and they displayed the same fear as their healthy counterparts.

B. Researchers believe they can identify early stages of dementia in observing eye movement patterns and brain activity.

C. One was a normal control and the other was genetically engineered to have Alzheimer's-like symptoms.

D. However, Doug Brown cautioned that the technique cannot be translated into a procedure that is safe for people worldwide with dementia just yet.

E. Scientists had assumed for a long time that the disease destroys how those memories are encoded and makes them disappear forever.

F. Electrical stimulation of the brain may be one alternative scientists can pursue, according to Christine Denny, a neurobiologist at Columbia University.

Passage Two

Directions: *The following paragraphs are given in a wrong order. For Questions 6-10, you are required to reorganize these paragraphs into a coherent article by choosing from the list A-G and filling them into the numbered boxes. Paragraphs C and F have been correctly placed. Mark your answers on the ANSWER SHEET.*

[A] These tools can help you win every argument—not in the unhelpful sense of beating your opponents but in the better sense of learning about the issues that divide people. Learning why they disagree with us and learning to talk and work together with them. If we readjust our view of arguments—from a verbal fight or tennis game to a reasoned exchange through which we all gain mutual respect, and understanding—then we change the very nature of what it means to "win" an argument.

[B] Of course, many discussions are not so successful. Still, we need to be careful not to accuse opponents of bad arguments too quickly. We need to learn how to evaluate them properly. A large part of evaluation is calling out bad arguments, but we also need to admit good arguments by opponents and to apply the same critical standards to ourselves. Humility requires you to recognize weakness in your own arguments and sometimes also to accept reasons on the opposite side.

[C] None of these will be easy but you can start even if others refuse to. Next time you state your position, formulate an argument for what you claim and honestly ask yourself whether your argument is any good. Next time you talk with someone who takes a stand, ask them to give you a reason for their view. Spell out their argument fully and charitably. Assess its strength impartially. Raise objections and listen carefully to their replies.

[D] Carnegie would be right if arguments were fights, which is how we often think of them. Like physical fights, verbal fights can leave both sides bloodied. Even when you win, you end up no better off. Your prospects would be almost as dismal if arguments were even just competitions—like, say, tennis games. Paris of opponents hit the ball back and forth until one winner emerges from all who entered. Everybody else loses. This kind of thinking is why so many people try to avoid arguments, especially about politics and religion.

[E] In his 1936 work *How to Win Friends and Influence People*, Dale Carnegie wrote: "There is only one way to get the best of an argument and that is to avoid it." This aversion to arguments is common, but it depends on a mistaken view of arguments that causes profound problems for our personal and social lives—and in many ways misses the point of arguing in the first place.

[F] These views of arguments also undermine reason. If you see a conversation as a fight or competition, you can win by cheating as long as you don't get caught. You will be happy to convince people with bad arguments. You can call their views stupid, or joke about how ignorant they are. None of these tricks will help you understand them, their positions or the issues that divide you, but they can help you win—in one way.

[G] There is a better way to win arguments. Imagine that you favor increasing the minimum wage in our state, and I do not. If you yell, "Yes." and I yell, "No." neither of us learns anything. We neither understand nor respect each other, and we have no basis for compromise or cooperation. In contrast, suppose you give a reasonable argument: that full-time workers should not have to live in poverty. Then I counter with another reasonable argument: that a higher minimum wage will force businesses to employ fewer people for less time. Now we can understand each other's positions and recognize our shared values, since we both care about needy workers.

6. ____ → 7. ____ → F → 8. ____ → 9. ____ → C → 10. ____

Passage Three

Directions: *Choose a heading from the list A-F that best fits the meaning of each numbered part of the text (11-14).*

A. CPR is of great help on any condition.

B. Traditional CPR is good, but some people struggle with its application.

C. The hands-only method has effect similar to traditional CPR.

D. How do people put a hands-only CPR into practice?

E. Doctors suggest all people use traditional CPR.

F. Traditional CPR has obvious advantages in saving persons who are already unconscious and not breathing normally.

11. _____

Cardiopulmonary resuscitation, or CPR, is help for a stopped heart. It increases the chances of survival and reduces the danger of brain damage. With traditional CPR, you push hard on the chest thirty times, then stop to give two breaths to force air into the lungs. You repeat the steps until the victim can get medical treatment. But people may worry about getting sick from blowing into a stranger's mouth. Also, the training is easy to forget, especially in a crisis. And those without training may be afraid to do anything for fear they will do something wrong.

12. _____

Now, the American Heart Association has simplified CPR's guidelines and is calling for hands-only CPR. Here is how it works. A person has collapsed and is unconscious. The victim has lost color in the face and does not appear to be breathing. These are signs of cardiac arrest and this is the time to begin CPR. Place your hands, one on top of the other, on the center of the chest. Push hard and fast, aim for a rate of about one hundred presses in a minute. Chest compressions keep the blood flowing to the brain, heart and other organs.

13. _____

The American Heart Association says everyone should use hands-only CPR unless they feel strong about their ability to do rescue breathing. The organization says the hands-only method was just as effective as traditional CPR in several studies. Scientists say there is enough oxygen remaining in a person's system for several minutes after breathing stops. They also say people need less oxygen when the heart is at rest.

14. _____

The American Heart Association says traditional CPR with a combination of breaths and compressions should be used for babies and children, and also adults who are found already unconscious and not breathing normally. And it should be used for any victims of drowning or collapse from breathing problems. These are all examples of cases where CPR with mouth-to-mouth breathing may be more helpful than hands-only CPR. The American Heart Association says because there are many such cases, people should still learn CPR that includes mouth-to-mouth.

Passage Four

Directions: *You are going to read a passage with ten statements attached to it. Each statement contains information given in one of the paragraphs. Identify the paragraph from which the information is derived. You may choose a paragraph more than once. Each paragraph is marked with a letter. Answer the questions by marking the corresponding letter.*

[A] After years of big promises, telemedicine is finally living up to its potential. Driven by faster Internet connections, ubiquitous (无处不在的) smartphones and changing insurance standards, more health providers are turning to electronic communications to do their jobs—and it's dramatically changing the delivery of healthcare.

[B] Doctors are linking up with patients by phone，email and webcam (网络摄像头). They're also consulting with each other electronically—sometimes to make split-second decisions on heart attacks and strokes. Patients, meanwhile, are using new devices to relay their blood pressure, heart rate and other vital signs to their doctors so they can manage chronic conditions at home. Telemedicine also allows for better care in places where medical expertise is hard to come by. Five to ten times a day, Doctors Without Borders relays questions about tough cases from its physicians in Niger South Sudan and elsewhere to its network of 280 experts around the world, and back again via the Internet.

[C] As a measure of how rapidly telemedicine is spreading, consider: More than 15 million Americans received some kind of medical care remotely last year, according to the American Telemedicine Association, a trade group, which expects those numbers to grow by 30% this year.

[D] None of this is to say that telemedicine has found its way into all corners of medicine. A recent survey of 500 tech-savvy (精通技术的) consumers found that 39% hadn't heard of telemedicine, and of those who haven't used it, 42% said they preferred in-person doctor visits. In a poll of 1,500 family physicians, only 15% had used it in their practices—but 90% said they would if it were appropriately reimbursed (补偿).

[E] What's more, for all the rapid growth, significant questions and challenges remain. Rules defining and regulating telemedicine differ widely from state to state. Physicians groups are issuing different guidelines about what care they consider appropriate to deliver and in what form.

[F] Some critics also question whether the quality of care is keeping up with the rapid expansion of telemedicine. And there's the question of what services physicians should be paid for: Insurance coverage varies from health plan to health plan, and a big federal plan covers only a narrow range of services. Telemedicine's future will depend on how—and whether—regulators, providers, payers and patients can address these challenges. Here's a closer look at some of these issues.

[G] Do patients trade quality for convenience? The fastest-growing services in telemedicine connect consumers with clinicians they've never met for a phone, video or email visit—on-demand, 24/7. Typically, these are for nonemergency issues such as colds, flu, earaches and skin rashes, and they cost around $45, compared with approximately $100 at a doctor's office，$160 at an urgent-care clinic or $750 and up at an emergency room.

[H] Many health plans and employers have rushed to offer the services and promote them as a convenient way for plan members to get medical care without leaving home or work. Nearly three-quarters of large employers will offer virtual doctor visits as a benefit to employees this year, up from 48% last year. Web companies such as Teladoc and American Well are expected to host some 1.2 million such virtual doctor visits this year, up 20% from last year, according to the American Telemedicine Association.

[I] But critics worry that such services may be sacrificing quality for convenience. Consulting a random doctor patients will never meet, they say, further fragments the health-care system, and even minor issues such as upper respiratory infections can't be thoroughly evaluated by a doctor who can't listen to your heart or feel your swollen glands. In a recent study, researchers posing as patients with skin problems sought help from 16 telemedicine sites—with unsettling results. In 62 encounters, fewer than one-third disclosed clinicians' credential or let patients choose; only 32% discussed potential side effects of prescribed medications. Several sites misdiagnosed serious conditions, largely because they failed to ask basic follow-up questions, the researchers said. "Telemedicine holds senormous promise，but these sites are just not ready for prime time," says Jack Resneck, the study's lead author.

[J] The American Telemedicine Association and other organizations have started accreditation (鉴定) programs to identify top-quality telemedicine sites. The American Medical Association this month approved new ethical guidelines for telemedicine, calling for participating doctors to recognize the limitations of such services and ensure that they have sufficient information to make clinical recommendations.

[K] Who pays for the services? While employers and health plans have been eager to cover virtual urgent-care visits, insurers have been far less willing to pay for telemedicine when doctors use phone, email or video to consult with existing patients about continuing issues. "It's very hard to get paid unless you physically see the patient," says Peter Rasmussen，medical director of distance health at the Cleveland Clinic. Some 32 states have passed "parity" (等同的) laws requiring private insurers to reimburse doctors for services delivered remotely if the same service would be covered in person, though not necessarily at the same rate or frequency. Medicare lags further behind. The federal health plan for the elderly covers a small number of telemedicine services—only for beneficiaries in rural areas and only when the services are received in a hospital, doctor's office or clinic.

[L] Bills to expand Medicare coverage of telemedicine have bipartisan (两党的) support in Congress. Opponents worry that such expansion would be costly for taxpayers，but advocates say it would save money in the long run.

[M] Experts say more hospitals are likely to invest in telemedicine systems as they move away from fee-for-service payments and into managed-care-type contracts that give them a set fee to provide care for patients and allow them to keep any savings they achieve.

[N] Is the state-by-state regulatory system outdated? Historically, regulation of medicine has been left to individual states. But some industry members contend that having 50 different sets of rules, licensing fees and even definitions of "medical practice" makes less sense in the era of telemedicine and is hampering its growth. Currently, doctors must have a valid license in the state where the patient is located to provide medical care, which means virtual-visit companies can match users only with locally licensed clinicians. It also causes administrative hassles (麻烦) for world-class medical centers that attract patients from across the country. At the Mayo Clinic, doctors who treat out-of-state patients can follow up with them via phone, email or web chats when they return home, but they can only discuss the conditions they treated in person. "If the patient wants to talk about a new problem, the doctor has to be licensed in that state to discuss it. If not, the patient should talk to his primary-care physician about it," says Steve Ommen, who runs Mayo's Connected Care program.

[O] To date, 17 states have joined a compact that will allow a doctor licensed in one member state to quickly obtain a license in another. While welcoming the move, some telemedicine advocates would prefer states to automatically honor one another's licenses, as they do with drivers' licenses. But states aren't likely to surrender control of medical practice, and most are considering new regulations. This year，more than 200 telemedicine-related bills have been introduced in 42 states, many regarding what services Medicaid will cover and whether payers should reimburse for remote patient monitoring. "A lot of states are still trying to define telemedicine," says Lisa Robbin, chief advocacy officer for the Federation of State Medical Boards.

15. An overwhelming majority of family physicians are willing to use telemedicine if they are duly paid.

16. Many employers are eager to provide telemedicine services as a benefit to their employees because of its convenience.

17. Different states have markedly different regulations for telemedicine.

18. With telemedicine，patients in regions short of professional medical services are able to receive better medical care.

19. Unlike employers and health plans, insurers have been rather reluctant to pay for some telemedicine services.

20. Some supporters of telemedicine hope states will accept each other's medical practice licenses as valid.

21. The fastest growing area for telemedicine services is for lesser health problems.

22. As telemedicine spreads quickly, some of its opponents doubt whether its service quality can be guaranteed.

23. The results obtained by researchers who pretended to be patients seeking help from telemedicine providers are disturbing.

24. Some people argue that the fact that different states have different regulations concerning medical services hinders the development of telemedicine.

答案与解析

Model Test 1

Passage One

1. C。本题目为首段例证题，首段例证主要为了引出全文讨论的主题（introduce the topic）。第一段引用玛丽·雪莱创作了《弗兰肯斯坦，或现代的普罗米修斯》这部作品。第一段最后一句，甚至在电灯发明之前，作者创作了这部举世瞩目的科幻小说 "that would

foreshadow many ethical questions to be raised by technologies yet to come"（这部小说预示了很多即将到来的技术所带来的很多道德伦理方面的问题），这句话对应了选项 C "involves some concerns raised by AI today"，即涉及一些今天AI人工智能带来的担忧。A，B选项都未提及。选项D "has sparked serious ethical controversies" 是说已经引发了严重的伦理方面的争议。"已经引起了严重的"这个现在完成时表达得不准确，文中只提及人们现在提出了关于伦理方面的一些问题。故C选项正确。

2. D。细节题。根据题干中的David Eagleman定位至第四段第二行："We are just in a situation where there are no good theories explaining what consciousness actually is and how you could ever build a machine to get there." 即我们仍然处在没有确凿的理论解释"意识"是什么的情况下，而且也不能发明机器实现这一点。从这句话就能知道选项D "对于我们来说去再次创造它能力太有限"。

3. B。细节题。根据题干中的autonomous vehicles定位至第五段第二行，这段一直在讲述自动驾驶汽车和人驾驶汽车的区别，最后总结 "AI 'vision' today is not nearly as sophisticated as that of humans. And to anticipate every imaginable driving situation is a difficult programming problem." 即今天人工智能的这种 "vision想象力" 还不能像人类一样复杂。并且去预测每一个可能的驾驶情形仍然是一个很难的编程问题。这句话对应了选项 B "is still beyond our capacity"，即仍然超越了我们的能力。C和D选项没有提及，A选项与原文中的But that doesn't mean crucial ethical issues involving AI aren't at hand（这句话表达了伦理问题即将到来）不符，所以A选项是错的。选项C "几乎没有引起公众关注" 以及选项D "已经引起了大量的好奇" 都没有提及，属无中生有。

4. A。细节题。 根据题干中的Google's pledges找到第七段，但是题目问的是作者的观点，可以进一步定位至第八段中的 "While the statement is vague, it represents one starting point"，意为 "虽然这个陈述是有点模糊的，但是它代表了一个开始"。从这句话就能判定出作者对谷歌的承诺是认可的，故对应选项affirmation。

5. C。主旨题。判断中心思想第一步要确定全文中心词：conscience，ethical issue of AI，所以根据这些主题词我们就可以选择出 "The Conscience of AI: Complex But Inevitable"，意为 "人工智能的道德问题：复杂但是不可避免"，该问题一直贯穿全文并和ethical issue对应。A选项 "AI的未来，在科技巨头的手中"，文中说到目前我们尚没有能力解决AI的道德意识方面的问题，所以和主旨相悖。B选项 "《弗兰肯斯坦》，一本预测了人工智能时代的小说"，只是文章的引入，并没有提及文中的核心问题ethical issue，故是片面信息，不可做全文主旨。D选项 "人工智能一旦失控，将会成为杀手"，这一点并未在文中提及。故本题选C。

Passage Two

6. B。细节题。从首段的第一句 "It was the worst tragedy in maritime history, six times more deadly than the Titanic." Wilhelm Gustloff的沉没带来的伤亡是泰坦尼克号的6倍。可知它造成了最大数量的伤亡，因此本题正确答案为B。

7. B。细节题。从第一段中的 "An ice storm had turned the decks into frozen sheets that sent hundreds of families sliding into the sea as the ship tilted and began to go down." 可知强烈的冰雹使船倾斜，正确答案为B。

8. D。细节题。从第二段中的 "Because the crimes we Germans are responsible for were and are so dominant, we didn't have the energy left to tell of our own sufferings." 可知，他们对自己在第二次世界大战中犯下的罪行深感惭愧。

9. D。细节题。从第二段中可知，Gunter Grass写了一本书，描述了一名当时怀孕的幸存者的故事，才将Wilhelm Gustloff的沉没昭告于天下。

10. C。推理题。从最后一段可知，最具有政治正确性意识的德国人都相信，他们现在有权充分讨论历史了；不是把德国人遭遇的苦难与纳粹受害者的遭遇相提并论，而只是承认一段可怕的灾难而已。由此可知德国人已经不再认为讲自己的遭遇会被误解了。因此本题正确答案为C。

Passage Three

11. D。细节题。根据题干信息定位到文中第一段与第二段。文章第一段提到在美国超过2/3的年轻人反对总统特朗普使用推特。接着提到美国公民更希望从别的渠道获得白宫的信息，而不是从总统的社交平台。第二段第二句指出由于美国人越来越不信任媒体，他们可能会想办法提高自身的媒体文化素养。由此可见，很多美国年轻人怀疑社交媒体是否值得信任。因此D选项符合文意。

12. A。猜词题。根据题干定位到第二段第二句。上文提到大部分美国人依靠社交媒体来查看每日头条。第二句紧接着指出 "由于美国人越来越不信任媒体，他们开始beef up自身的媒体文化素养"。由此推测，美国人开始对媒体产生怀疑，所以是想办法强化自身的知识来辨别媒体可不可靠。选项中只有A项有 "强化，加强" 的含义。故A选项为正确答案。

13. B。细节题。根据survey将本题定位至第三段第二句话的位置，原句指出："A knight foundation focusgroup survey of young people... found they use distributed trust to verify stories." 他们是使用distributed trust来verify stories的。而且下一句又详细指出，they cross-check sources and prefer news from different perspectives。结合选项可知B选项verify与原文一致，news对应原文中的stories，referring to diverse resources即distributed trust，

故B选项为正确答案。

14. C。细节题。从题干中的The Barna survey以及fake news可得出，本题目定位到倒数第二段的位置。该段后半部分提到了Barna survey也提到了fake news，可以定位到About a third这一句："About a third say the problem of fake news lies in misinterpretation or exaggeration of actual news via social media."。题干中的a main cause刚好对应了lie in，所以答案就是misinterpretation，对应选项C。

15. A。主旨题。通过题目中反复出现的信息看出文章与什么话题有关，题目出现了young Americans，并指出了doubts，fake news problem等负面色彩，因此，整篇文章的倾向是负面的。文章主旨一般出现在文章的第一段和第二段开头的位置，第一段是通过survey引出了文章要讨论的话题，说出了news和source的话题，第二段第二句通过yet引出要讨论的distrust等内容。总结得出，文章讲述的话题是news online，倾向态度是distrust在rise，对应就是A选项：A Rise in Critical Skills for Sharing News Online。

Passage Four

16. D。推理题。第二段中提到，该研究发现实施"行星健康"项目的中学女孩服用泻药或减肥药的概率是没有实施该项目的学校的女孩的一半，她们之所以不服用泻药就是因为她们不胖，再结合上面提到的"行星健康"是防止肥胖的，可以推断，接受了这种锻炼的女孩子们控制体重的方式更加健康和积极，因此D选项是正确答案。

17. B。细节题。第三段提到用红绿灯系统来标示食物，前面的两种食物为"通行""减速"，分别是绿灯、黄灯表示的意思，那么剩下的就应该是红灯了，红灯意为"停止"，因此，选项B为正确答案。

18. D。推理题。第三段提到，比萨饼是用黄灯来标示的，黄灯的意思是"减速"，说明该食物不像健康食物那么有利于人的身体，但也不至于是不健康的食品，选项中D最为符合。B是干扰选项，考生不能看到就立刻选择该选项，而是要加以分析。

19. C。推理题。第四段提到，一般从三年级到五年级学生超重的数量会上升，但该项目却制止了这种上升，而"hold the line"意思为"保持不变"，可以推断，实施了该项目的学校从3年级到5年级超重学生的数量没有增加，也就是说他们的体重在增长，但是却没有向着超重的方向发展，而是正常的增长。因此选项C最为符合这个意思，其余三个选项都与这个意思不符合。

20. D。细节题。最后一段提到在该小学实施了CATCH后，家长们也在孩子的带动下开始健康饮食和多做运动了，学校还另外举行了带动家长的活动。但是该学校采取CATCH面向的还是学生，因此选项中D是正确的陈述。

Passage Five

21．D。推理题。根据全文提到的这两个实验都在空气污染不是很严重的情况下测到了污染对人身体的影响，可见这里的low levels是指污染程度小，Ursula Ackermann-Liebrich博士整句话是说即使空气质量只改善一点，即使在污染很轻微的地方人们的健康也得到了提高。因此，D选项最为符合题意。

22．C。细节题。从第二段可知，柴油发动汽车的典型城市空气污染水平对人体有一定的影响，因此，C选项最为符合这点。

23．D。细节题。第三段提到，在牛津街肺功能减弱的程度要比那些在海德公园散步回来的人检测的情况"大得多"，而且牛津街的人还伴有炎症生物指标增加的状况。故答案为D。

24．A。推理题。从第四段可知，他认为柴油排放的气体污染好像要比其他形式的气体污染更为有影响力，而他前面提到了这种污染是空气颗粒，结合来看就是本段开头提到的柴油排放物中的微粒。因此只有选项A符合题意。

25．C。细节题。根据文章内容可知，两项研究都是为了测量柴油排放气体对人体健康的危害，因此A，D选项不正确；对于B选项，虽然第四段提到了这一点，但是说空气微粒减少，不是人主动暴露在空气中，所以该陈述不对；C选项的内容在第一段有所提及，因此是正确答案。

Passage Six

26．D。细节题。文章第一段在介绍这种新型减肥药C75的特点时，将新药的特点与传统上通过节食减肥（a starvation diet）对代谢率的影响进行了比较，"Scientists…results in a dramatic loss of weight without any apparent ill effects"指出由于后者使代谢速度减慢而引起疲劳、无力（causing tiredness and lethargy）等症状。故正确答案为D项。

27．A。细节题。文章第二段开头便表明了人们可使用C75来减肥的原因，即"because appetite control in the brain…as those in mice"，因为在大脑中食欲控制跟在老鼠大脑中的化学路径一致，这正是选项A所表达的意思。

28．C。细节题。文章第三段中第二句话"Research on leptin, a hormone produced in fatty tissue for controlling fat deposits, has so far failed to produce the expected slimming drug break-through"对leptin的解释是：它是脂肪组织中分泌的一种可以控制脂肪的激素（a hormone produced in fatty tissue for controlling fat deposits）。故正确答案为C项。

29．C。细节题。根据文章第四段，可知这种新型减肥药之所以可以有效地控制食欲是因为人体中被称为"脂肪酸和酶"的一种酶参与将过量摄取的食物转化成脂肪的过程。而C75可与这种酶结合，并且抑制其作用于大脑，从而抑制食欲。因此，C项符合题意。

30．D。细节题。文章在第一段"More importantly, the drug appears to prevent a serious decline in metabolic rate..." 和最后一段中 "...that C75 has no effect on metabolic rate is one of the most significant findings of the study" 都提到这种新型减肥药对新陈代谢不产生影响。故正确答案为D项。

Model Test 2

Passage One

1. C。细节题。根据题干定位于第一段。文中提到，玩暴力游戏会对人的想法和行为产生即时和持久的影响。暴力游戏的互动型和越来越逼真的场景会使它比暴力电视、暴力电影更危险，可直接选出选项C。选项A，B，D的说法不准确，排除。

2. A。细节题。根据题定位于第三段。文中提到，有侵略性性格和常玩暴力游戏的学生在现实生活中更有暴力倾向。可以选出选项A。选项B和C体现的不是因果关系。选项D说法不正确。

3. D。细节题。根据题定位于第四段。文中提到，研究人员让学生玩暴力游戏后待在一个小房间里，与一个假想对手对战，胜者可以用响亮的噪声公示输的一方。研究者们则会观察他们的行为。可以直接选出选项D。选项A，B，C表述错误。

4. A。细节题。根据题定位于最后一段。文中提到，暴力游戏影响行为，并不是激发人的激进的情绪，而是教会人用暴力的方式处理问题。可直接选出选项A。选项B，C，D的表述是正确的。

5. A。主旨题。结合文章大意可知，文章主要讲述的是暴力游戏的影响。选项B，C，D不是全文的侧重点，故排除。

Passage Two

6. D。推理题。根据文中第二段可知，新的分子和药理学工具使我们能够证实存在于免疫系统和大脑之间的复杂网络，这个网络可以让免疫系统和大脑相互迅速地发出连续的信号。再根据最后一段的信息可知，我们刚刚开始了解大脑和免疫系统相互依赖的多种途径，它们是如何相互帮助调节和反调节的，以及它们本身如何发生故障并引发疾病。据此可知，D选项（人们对大脑和免疫系统之间的信息传输有了新的理解）是正确的。

7. A。归纳题。根据文中第二段可知，新的分子和药理学工具使我们能够证实存在于免疫系统和大脑之间的复杂网络，这个网络可以让免疫系统和大脑相互迅速地发出连续的信号。免疫细胞所产生的化学物质向大脑发出信号，大脑反过来发送化学信号来抑制免疫系统。这些相同的化学信号也影响了人们的行为和对压力的反应。任何方式造成的信息网络中断，无论是遗传还是药物、有毒物质或手术，都会使由防御系统预防的下列病症恶化：感染、发炎、自体免疫和相关的情绪障碍。据此可知，A选项（免疫系统和大脑相互发出信号）是正确答案，这充分说明了它们在疾病方面的相互作用。

8. C。细节题。根据文中第三段的内容可知，这些研究成果的临床意义可能已经得到证实。它们有望扩大各种疾病的治疗范围，因为人们以前认为药物主要是在神经系统的医治方面具有疗效，如今表明医治免疫疾病也同样有效，而且反之亦然。它们还帮助证实了普遍持有的想法（在某些医学界仍然存在疑虑），即我们的精神状态可以影响我们抵抗感染或炎症性疾病或从中恢复的程度。据此可知，C选项（对精神有影响的药物在某些情况下可以用于治疗炎症性疾病）是文中支持的观点。故选C。

9. D。推理题。本文第一句就指出，精神在身体疾病治疗方面起着重要作用。第二段又说，新的分子和药理学工具使我们能够证实存在于免疫系统和大脑之间的复杂网络，这个网络可以让免疫系统和大脑相互迅速地发出连续的信号。免疫细胞所产生的化学物质向大脑发出信号，大脑反过来发送化学信号来抑制免疫系统。这些相同的化学信号也影响了人们的行为和对压力的反应。任何方式造成的信息网络中断，无论是遗传还是药物、有毒物质或手术，都会使防御系统预防的下列病症恶化：感染、发炎、自体免疫和相关的情绪障碍。最后一段又说，大脑和免疫系统在许多方面都是相互依赖的，它们相互帮助调节和反调节，以及它们本身会发生故障并引发疾病。据此可推理得知，抑郁症也与炎症性疾病有关，故D项正确。

10. B。细节题。根据文中最后一段可知，当体内平衡受到扰乱或遇到危险分子时，细胞和行为反应全都开始发挥作用。这些反应试图抵消那些干扰力量，以恢复稳定的状态。这些反应可能仅限于针对外来入侵者或特定的压力，当对体内平衡的威胁超越某个界限时，它们就扩大范围，不再有局限性。据此可知，B选项（为了维持人体内部的平衡，应激反应必须将外来病原体从体内消除）正确。

Passage Three

11. A。细节题。第三段提到 "The potential medical spin-offs from plant biotechnology are considerable." 后面则举例说明：一种新的更有效的疫苗例如玉米和香蕉将会在植物中成长，因此可推测出A项正确。byproduct副产品，by-work副业，side effect（药物等的）副作用，consequence结果。

12. A。细节题。文章第二段提到新种类的大米和其他庄稼可以抵御昆虫和疾病以及基因作物营养更加均衡，体现了health benefits，排除B项。第三段提到medical spin-offs，通过植入一种更有效的疫苗，玉米、香蕉等可以抵抗一些还未出现疫苗的疾病，体现了C和D项。A项"高科技"文章并未提及。

13. C。细节题。从第十一段的Genetic engineering is far more precise than the gene movements which occur in nature可直接找出答案。

14. D。细节题。A项"克隆"，B项"人工授精"，C项"体外授精"都与遗传工程有关，只有D项"心脏搭桥术"与遗传工程无关。

15. C。推理题。第八段媒体引用"opening Pandora's box"来形容the combination DNA from different sources。后面又提到 Among their horrific forecast were unstoppable epidemics and world-wide pestilence，由此根据上下文可推断出C项符合文意。即一些媒体争论从不同根源形成的DNA将会引发大量问题与从未存在或从不知道的灾害。

Passage Four

16. D。细节题。答案在第二段。该段讲到Vega的研究发现一些精神性疾病在美国出生的墨西哥裔美国人中的发生率比较高。

17. A。细节题。第五段讲到专家小组讲到这些移民不愿采纳美国的生活方式。

18. D。推理题。第五段讲到Vega的研究与专家小组结论一致，由于Kleinman是专家小组的一员，可以推断他们两人的看法是相同的。

19. C。细节题。答案在第六段最后一句。由该句中的"health issues"可知这个采访是针对健康问题的。

20. D。细节题。文章最后一段讲到在那些13年内进行移民的人群中，精神病的患病率最低。

Passage Five

21. D。推理题。本题答案参见第一段，说和写是人类交际的特别手段，即语言手段。人类交际还有其他手段，例如身体位置、行为、气味、目光交流等非言语手段。故选D。

22. C。细节题。第二段讲了人类通过感官和个人生物节奏体系来接受外部和内部信息，这一过程有些是有意识的，有些是无意识的，但都是心理处理过程。故选C。

23. B。细节题。本题答案参见第三段第四句，行为紊乱的人头脑混乱，不能表达个人感情和需要，不为人所理解。所以这些人受内部问题困扰，故选B。

24. D。细节题。本题答案参见第五段第一句，情感困扰在某种程度上发生在所有人身上。故选D。

25. C。细节题。本题答案参见最后一段，本文结束时讲到了消除早期情感困扰的意义。故选C。

Passage Six

26. D。细节题。本题答案参见第二段，尽管人人都会有悲伤的时刻，但是通过休息、饮食、交谈等都会恢复。但是长期处于悲伤状态就会得抑郁症。故选D。

27. D。细节题。本题答案参见第三段第一、二句，本段告诉我们在某个严重疼痛疾病带给一些家庭成员上的死亡，诸如此类情况下，即使是抑郁也是很正常的。故选D。

28. C。细节题。本题答案参见第四段倒数第一、二句，抑郁的人需要重塑自我形象成为有用的人，心理治疗在恢复自信和能力方面通常很有帮助。故选C。

29. D。推理题。第五段提到了A，B，C三个方面。故选D。

30. B。细节题。本题答案参见第六段第一句，抑郁症患者只有找到替代想法才会忘记令人不安的想法。故选B。

Model Test 3

Passage One

1. B。细节题。根据第一段内容"Behaviors that we do not understand often become nearly invisible — even when, in retrospect, we see how truly strange they are"可知，我们常常忽视这些我们不能理解的行为——甚至当我们回想时会发现那些行为有多奇怪，作者接着举例子来说明此观点。由此可知，B项符合题意。

2. B。细节题。根据第四段第四句话"Currently, depression has moved to center stage"可知，现如今抑郁症已经来到了中央舞台。由此可知，B项"depression抑郁、沮丧"符合题意，而A项"hysteria歇斯底里"、C项"messiness脏乱"、D项"obsessive compulsive disorder强迫症"均不正确。

3. B。细节题。根据第六段第一句话"In moderation, the symptoms seemed to fit right in with our workaholic culture — perhaps explaining the low profile of the diagnosis"可知，如果能适度控制，症状似乎恰好符合我们工作狂的文化精神——可能这样就解释了诊断结果被轻视。由此可知，B项符合题意。

4. A。推理题。根据第八段第三句"For such people, rules of all kinds are a godsend — they represent premade decisions"可知，对于这样的人来说，所有规则都是天赐之物—— 它们代表预先做好的决定。由此可知，A项符合题意。

5. D。归纳题。根据最后一段内容"For such a patient or for a psychiatrist, understanding a cluster of diagnostic symptoms can be a revelation"可知，对于这样的病人

或者精神病医生来说，理解一组诊断性的症状可以是一种借鉴；根据"But undoubtedly, at times we can become too reductionistic"可知有时我们可以变得简单些。根据这几句话可知，作者认为医生既要有给病人看病的本领，熟悉各种病症，以便诊断，也不能过于多虑，把所有行为都看成一种病症。由此可知，D项符合题意。

Passage Two

6. D。细节题。根据文章第一段中的"The ancient Egyptians knew about many tumors that had a bad outcome, and the Greeks made a distinction between benign tumors (oncos) and malignant ones (carcinos)."可知，古埃及人知道许多种带来恶果的肿瘤，而希腊人已经区分出良性肿瘤和恶性肿瘤了，所以答案为D。

7. D。推理题。文章中共有三处提及恐惧，但和癌症并提则在最后一段，威廉·巴契南认为过度恐惧会导致癌症，但这并不等于说人们惧怕癌症，故不选B。根据最后一段中的"Among the Romantics and the Victorians, suffering and dying from tuberculosis might be considered a badge of refinement; cancer death was nothing of the sort"可知，在浪漫主义时期和维多利亚时期，受肺结核折磨甚至死于肺结核被当成是文雅的标志；患癌死亡那就完全不同了，排除C；通读全文，A项文中没有提到；根据最后一段中的"In the eighteenth and nineteenth centuries, some physicians attributed cancer — notably of the breast and the ovaries — to psychological and behavioral causes."可知，在18和19世纪，一些医生将癌症——尤其是乳腺癌和子宫癌——的产生归咎为心理或行为方面的原因，所以D项正确。

8. C。推理题。根据文章第二段最后两句话可知，癌症致死的痛苦令人畏惧，但是恐惧并没有成为公众意识中的关注焦点，而现在不同了。医学史家罗伊·波特将其说成是"最卓越的现代病"，慕克吉称其为"现代性最典型的产物"，这就是其中一方面的原因。所以C项"现在，人们以全新的方式理解癌症"正确。

9. D。推理题。根据文章最后一段第一、二句话可知，人们曾经认为癌症是一种"文明病"，病因与神经衰弱症和糖尿病类似；前者是因现代生活的压力而产生，后者是因饮食不良和懒惰而产生。在18和19世纪，一些医生将癌症——尤其是乳腺癌和子宫癌——的产生归咎到心理或行为方面。这里提到神经衰弱症和糖尿病是为了说明癌症和它们类似，和心理及行为有关，故选D。

10. A。推理题。根据文章第一段第一、二句可知，癌症始终如影随形，但是纠缠的方式却有变化。诊治处理方法当然也随着时代进步有变化，而其存在性质、表现和意义也发生了改变。作者在这两句话中隐藏了自己的观点，所以选A。

Passage Three

11. A。推断题。答案在第二段的最后一句话。A项和C项都与原文有关，但C项的说法太绝对，而且原文中没有呈现比较关系；A项中的little更趋同于原文中hardly的意思；B项和D项虽都与原文有一点关联，但文章中的内容并不能推导出该结论，故选A。

12. C。细节题。文章第三、四段介绍了采集的方法：将志愿者分为6个组，采集每人的体味样本 10小时，样本采集前四天内不能使用香水或除臭剂，也不能吃味道很浓的食物等。A、B和D都与原文不符；C项"不受影响"符合第四段中提到的"not allowed to use any perfumes or deodorants, or eat strong-smelling foods in the four days before"，是对原文这段话的总结，故选C项。

13. B。细节题。答案在第六段。这一段表示变化的词语和句子很多。如"significantly more positively, an uplifting effect, a depressive effect, the smell of older people improved mood"。A项只表明部分正确，第六段中反映出的情绪与六种moods毫无关系；D不符合题意。故选B。

14. C。细节题。答案在第六段第一、二句话。A、B和D都与原文不符，C项"老年妇女"，是对第六段第一句 respond significantly more positively 的同义替换或诠释，故选C。

15. A。细节题。答案在最后一段，即"可能是激素（hormones）使年轻人的体味显示出攻击性，而老年人特别是女性体内激素的变化使得她们的体味显示出她们可亲近"。A"激素和体味"符合原文上述的说法；B"体味和生活方式"和C"情绪和生活方式"都与题干不符；D不符合逻辑，故选A。

Passage Four

16. C。推理题。根据文章第三段中的"Prolonged sleep deprivation has long been associated with diminished immune functions, but researchers have also found a direct correlation between 'modest' sleep deprivation—less than six hours—and reduced immune response."可知，"modest" sleep deprivation指少于六个小时的睡眠，文中说成人每天需要七到九个小时的睡眠，sleep deprivation应该指睡眠少于需要的量，故选C。

17. B。推理题。根据第三段"You'll be glad you got that extra hour of sleep the next time that a bug comes around and leaves everyone else bedridden with a fever for three days."可知，下次你会庆幸多睡了一个小时，因为别人一旦感冒，就要发烧睡上三天。所以当其他所有人发烧时，那些睡眠充足的人通常没事，故选B。

18. D。细节题。根据文章第四段中的"Sleep paralysis occurs when the brain is aroused from its REM cycle, but the body remains in its immobilizing state."可知，当大脑

从快速眼动周期被唤醒时，但身体仍然保持不动状态，这样大脑睡眠瘫痪就发生了，故选D。

19. B。推理题。根据文章最后一段最后一句话可知，研究显示，快速眼动睡眠或睡眠梦期有助于巩固大脑一天产生的脆弱记忆，这些记忆便于在大脑中长期组织和储存。所以B项"白天产生的记忆是脆弱易受损的"正确。

20. D。归纳题。第二段最后一句提到睡眠不足会导致血压升高；第三段中间提到睡眠不足与免疫功能下降有关；第四段主要讨论睡眠瘫痪；最后一段主要介绍睡眠不足导致记忆丧失。概括全文，D项符合题意。

Passage Five

21. C。细节题。根据文章第一段首句"Cultural norms so completely surround people, so permeate thought and action, that we never recognize the assumptions on which their lives and their sanity rest."可知，文化规范完全包围在人们的周围，因此渗透到思想和行动中，我们从没有意识到人们生活和理智所基于的种种假设。接着以birds和fish例子来说明这个观点。所以答案为C。

22. B。词汇题。根据题干定位到文章第三段第二句"Their ability to react sensitively to a wider spectrum of events and peoples requires an overcoming of such cultural parochialism."上一句提到"…break out of the boundaries of their own experiential worlds（要打破他们经验的限制）"，所以就要"overcoming of such cultural parochialism（克服文化的狭隘性）"。所以答案为B。"provincialism"一词意为"地方偏狭观念"。

23. C。推理题。根据文章第三段可知，要打破人们经验的限制需要克服文化的狭隘性，后面又转折说"But, in fact, few attain this broader vision.（但是很少有人能打破这种局限）"。根据第四段可知，文化短视的现象不仅是因为惯性和习惯，主要的原因是它如此难以克服。为了生存，每个人需要掌握自己的文化感知取向、认知偏见和交际习惯。但一旦掌握，对这些就很难客观评估了，这是因为被评估的机制同时需要做出评估。所以答案为C。

24. A。细节题。根据文章第二段"Whether it is an individual neurosis that keeps an individual out of contact with his neighbors, or a collective neurosis that separates neighbors of different cultures, both are forms of blindness that limit what can be experienced and what can be learned from others."可知，个人过分焦虑和集体过分焦虑可能防止与别人交流，与A选项说法一致。所以答案为A。

25. D。主旨题。文章主要讲的是文化短视，这主要是由于一种根深蒂固的集体神经症导致的，所以答案为D。

Passage Six

26．B。细节题。根据文章第二段第三句"Information on how to penetrate the disease's defenses is transmitted to all elements of the patient's immune system in a process that occurs naturally, in which genetic information is passed from cell to cell."可知，关于如何抵抗疾病的信息被传递到免疫系统的各个部位，这个过程由基因信息在细胞间传递而自然实现。所以答案为B。

27．D。推理题。此题可定位于第三段，且第三、四段的主题就是使用疫苗可能会带来负面效果，因此选项D"使用疫苗可能会带来负面结果"为正确选项。而选项A"疫苗对付疾病所使用的方法"，选项B"疫苗在于消除某些疾病的有效性"和选项C"疫苗的实际使用以控制传染病"都不是这个举证所谈论的观点。

28．D。推理题。此题可定位于第二、三段，第二段最后一句说"可以肯定，万一该病人以后再碰上这类病毒，他的身体已全副武装并且训练有素，足以对付这一现实问题，因为已经有经验了。"第三段前两句说"但是整个过程还有隐患。有时，即使疫苗中含有的病菌是弱化了的菌种，人体也接受不了，导致免疫系统失效，以致病人死亡。"由此可见，疫苗具有两面性，所以D项"许多生命被挽救的同时，也有生命因此而死亡"正确。

29．B。归纳题。根据全文可知，只有B选项能概括说明文章的中心。而选项A"天花疫苗"，漏掉了关于接种疫苗的过程，是对中心的部分概括。选项C"接种所用的原理"，这是第二段的话题。选项D"需要警惕的、有负面影响的疫苗"只涉及最后两段。

30．B。归纳题。综观全文可知，本文的中心讲的是免疫系统可以得到特殊的训练以应对疾病的较弱形式，以及疫苗有时会存在一些危险，因此选项B为正确选项。而选项A"疫苗使用不安全"，选项C"这将需要广泛的疫苗接种情况"和选项D"以天花疫苗为例说明目前疫苗被使用的方式"都不能说明原文的主题。所以选B。

Model Test 4

Passage One

1．D。细节题。由关键词dieting可定位到原文第一段，此段提到节食的作用，由此段中的"Dieting is an important part of staying fit and healthy…losing weight too fast can cause great health problems… As a result, they lose health as well as weight."可知，节食不当可引起健康问题。选项D认为节食必定会引发严重的健康问题，这种说法过于绝对，因而不正确。

2．B。细节题。由关键词workout可定位到第二段中的"Aerobic exercise is a moderate intensity workout that…"，第五段中的"You should combine this with fast-paced aerobics activities, like swimming, cycling, walking, running, or in line skating.", 文章最后一段的 "While weight training will firm and shape your body…", 由此可确定B是正确答案。

3. A。细节题。通读四个选项可知，本题考查考生对muscle-building的理解，第四段提到 "Do one to three exercises for each muscle groups — for example, chest and biceps, or back, shoulders and triceps.", 由此可确定A正确。

4. C。细节题。倒数第三段讲到 "As you build muscle, you may find that you gain weight in spite of all of your calorie-burning exercise. Don't worry. It's probably muscle, which is denser than fat. And muscle is also a calorie-burning tissue.", 由此可确定A和B正确。文章的最后一段讲到 "While weight training will firm and shape your body, it has other benefits too.", 由此可知D正确。用排除法可确定答案为C。

5. D。推理题。文章的第四段提到 "For a proper body-shaping routine, you should plan three strength-training sessions a week with weights.", 最后一段提到 "While weight training will firm and shape your body, it has other benefits too. It improves bone and muscle strength and burns calories, leading to improved health and a higher quality of life.", 这两处分别讲述力量训练的好处，由此可判断出D正确。

Passage Two

6. B。细节题。第二段提到 "… would have you believe that milk causes heart disease, cancer, infections, asthma, allergies and tuberculosis", 喝牛奶可引起心脏病、癌症、传染病、哮喘、过敏以及肺结核。倒数第二段指出 "Denmark, Norway and Sweden consume lots of milk and also suffer high rates of breast cancer…", 喝牛奶也可能患乳腺癌。综上可知B项正确。

7. D。推理题。通读全文可知，作者对牛奶有毒这一论点持质疑的态度，本文的最后一句提到 "But I keep coming back to the mainstream nutritionists, who emphasize a balanced diet and advise moderation in all things." 作者引用主流营养学家的观点：平衡饮食并适度调节饮食结构，由此可推断出作者建议理智地饮用牛奶，故D项正确。

8. D。推理题。由最后一段的 "The ADC feels that milk is the root of most human maladies（疾病）, but I can point to other single-issue obsessive…I often learn something by examining their claims." 可知，作者与ADC的观点截然相反，故D项正确。

9. C。细节题。根据关键词lactose intolerance可找到倒数第二段的对应原句 "And lactase tablets（乳糖分解酵素片）can make dairy products digestible even in severe cases.", 由此可知C项正确。

10. A。推理题。本题考查考生对作者的评价，通读全文以及根据作者对ADC观点的反驳，可判断出作者是耿直的人，选项A"无偏见的人"符合题意。B项"固执己见的人"；C项"世俗的人"；D项"聪明但奇怪的人"。

Passage Three

11．A。细节题。文章最后两句提到：只要嘴唇不因为恐惧和紧张而颤抖，那么保持嘴唇不动可能会压抑情感反应。然而，当保持嘴唇不动的情感更强烈并涉及强烈的肌肉紧绷时，面部反馈或许会强化情感反应。由此可知A选项（首先压制紧张，然后强化压力）最符合文意。

12．D。推理题。文章第一段的主旨在于说明某些表情具有普适的意义，例如微笑被普遍视为友好和赞同的意思，相反，"带着敌意咬牙"则被普遍视为愤怒的表达，文章接下来的两段也正是在说明某些表情的普适意义。由此可知D选项（提供一个面部表情具有普适意义的例子）正确。

13．B。细节题。联系上下文意可知画线处的意思是：当佛尔人处于这些会引发最基本情感反应的相同境况时，他们也会做出相似的面部表情。由此可知，文章是想说明某些面部表情具有普适意义。故B选项符合文意。

14．A。细节题。文章第三段结尾处引用达尔文的话说："通过外在形式对情感的自由表达会加强这种情感。相反，对外在表达的压抑会尽可能地缓解我们的情感。"文章后半部分正是在介绍面部表情反应对情感的反作用。由此可知，A选项（它们会变得不太强烈）符合文意。

15．C。细节题。文章第四段介绍了用来证实"面部反馈假说"的实验，实验表明微笑的人会把卡通画面看作更积极的反应，而相反，皱眉的人会把卡通画面看得更具有侵犯性。因此C选项符合文意。

Passage Four

16．B。主旨题。第一段先讲述老年痴呆症在美国社会中日益流行，患该病的概率越来越高。但最后一句but话锋一转，讲到尽管没有治愈良药，但是临床的一些进展却可能带来福音。因此B选项符合文意，其他三个选项都与第一段的细节信息有冲突。

17．D。词汇题。通过定位到第二段"...vitamins E and C, both antioxidants, help stave off Alzheimer's..."可知，维生素E和C可能都是用来在未患病时预防老年痴呆症的，所以此处近义词为prevent（阻止）。

18．D。细节题。从第三段中"The two drugs worked even better in combination than they did alone"可知，两种药一起使用时效果更好，正确答案为D。

19．A。细节题。从第四段中"Before now, doctors could not track the progress of these plaques until after the patient died, when the brain could be autopsied. Using the new technique, doctors may be able to begin treatment long before the first symptoms appear." 可知，在脑成像之前，医生只能等到病人死亡进行解剖后才能一窥究竟，但是使用新技术后，医生便可以在症状出现之前开始治疗。

20．C。判断题。A选项"老年痴呆症可以被新技术治愈"，与第一段最后一句不符；B选项"通过大脑练习便可以克服遗忘"是全文最后一句话的过度引申，最后一句讲到健脑练习对大脑有益，而不是克服健忘；C选项"详细的评估很重要，在记忆减退症状中可分辨出老年痴呆症症状，这在早期是可治愈的"与最后一段信息吻合；D选项"健脑运动只对可逆转的健忘症有好处"与最后一句相悖。因此本题最佳答案为C。

Passage Five

21．B。细节题。根据题干关键词具体定位至首段尾句，Elizabeth指控NHS旗下的一个医院，这个医院在2015年把160万病人的信息交给了DeepMind公司，基于一个模糊的协议，这个协议基本没有考虑到病人们的权利以及他们对于保护自己隐私的期望。由此可知NHS和DeepMind之间的协议没有考虑到病人的权利，故答案是B。A和D选项在文中并未提及，C选项有干扰，没能满足后者的期望，但是文中说的是没有满足病人们对保护隐私的期望，而不是没能满足DeepMind的期望，属于偷换概念。

22．C。细节题。根据关键词定位至第二段第二句，NHS已经改正错误了，短语mend one's way即"改正错误，改变习惯"的意思，接着下面就具体解释做出了哪些安排，所以答案是C。

23．D。细节题。没有具体关键词，所以要通读第二段，然后和四个选项逐一比对，选出正确选项。A选项说要不惜一切代价保护隐私，B选项说泄露病人隐私比出售隐私更糟糕，C选项说利用病人信息获利是违法的，这三个选项在第二段中并未提及。D选项来自第二段尾句，这种差别忽略了一点，即他是在加工和整合信息，不仅仅是拥有，而这给了信息以价值。说明信息的价值来自对信息的加工整合。所以答案是D。

24．D。细节题。回到原文末段，第四句话提到what matters重要的在于they belong to a private monopoly which developed them using public resources，这句话提到了真正的问题，和题干匹配，正确答案就是对这句的同义替换，故本题选D。A选项"制药公司之间的恶性竞争"来自定位句的下一句，但这句只提到制药公司，并未说他们之间存在恶性竞争；B选项"隐私法的无效实施"来自末端首句，但本句只说到the use of privacy law…feels slightly maladapted（不适应的），说成是ineffective有些程度过深；C选项"新软件的使用不受控制"来自定位句下一句，是在if条件句里面，所以也不可能成为真正的问题所在。

25．B。态度题。根据出题位置是最后一题以及定位词the application of AI to healthcare

找到最后一段的相关的词语，digital feudalism"数字化封建主义"是我们需要去avoid"避免的"，所以作者态度应该是消极的，故本题选B。最后一句还说到"Ms Denham's report is a welcome start."，说明作者对于这种报道是积极的态度，而报道在第一段中提到是against（反对）NHS和DeepMind的交易的，所以可以看出，作者是比较担心过度的人工智能化的。

Passage Six

26. D。细节题。题干关键词had long blamed animal research与原文第三段首句中的 only criticism of animal research对应，据此定位。原句中的antivivisection groups反对动物实验的倡议活动组织与选项D一致，故答案为D。

27. A。细节题。根据题干关键词change定位到原文第三段尾句。原句中的recognition 与选项A中的reconsideration对应。故答案为A。

28. B。细节题。根据题干关键词new guidelines定位到原文第四段首句。原句中的 improving the quality of reporting on animal experiments与选项B对应。故答案为B。

29. C。细节题。根据题干关键词UK's NC3Rs定位到原文第六段。原文提及the UK's NC3Rs是为了解释第六段首句提出的问题。首句中的reveal与选项C中的involves对应，serious与选项C中的serious重现，shortcomings与选项C中的problems对应。故答案为C。

30. A。细节题。根据题干关键词systematic reviews定位到原文第七段尾句。原句中的 rarely undertaken，the lack of information published与选项A对应。故答案为A。

Model Test 5

Passage One

1. E。空格前一直在讲患阿尔茨海默病的人丧失记忆的痛苦，空格后的but开启了同一个问题的不同方面：万一这些记忆没有消失，只是我们接触不到了呢？可知空格处含义应与此相反：科学家认为记忆永久消失，再也找不到了。因此，E选项（科学家长期以来一直认为阿尔茨海默病摧毁了记忆编码的方式，让记忆永远消失了）是正确答案。

2. C。空格前讲到该研究有两组mice，接下来空格后详细阐述两组mice是如何参与研究的：...involved two groups of mice...One...and the other...。因此本题正确答案为C。

3. A。空格前讲到两组老鼠（一组健康，另一组患有阿尔茨海默病）都被给予电击，健康组因为有记忆，会在电击的环境中显示出恐惧，病患组在用特殊蓝光刺激海马体区域细胞后changed dramatically，空格处应该填入这种剧烈变化的内容，可知填入A选项符合语义要求：它们消失的记忆似乎回来了，和健康组展现出同样的恐惧。

4．D。空格前讲到在老鼠试验中用到的具体技术和方式：先植入一种对蓝光敏感的基因，再用蓝光去刺激细胞，空格后讲到将这种方式用在人类身上去拯救记忆还需很长时间。中间空格的地方则需要填入人类不一定适合使用这种方式之类的语句才能让上下文通顺。因此，D选项（这种技术还无法安全转移到人类身上）是正确答案。

5．F。空格后讲到早期实验证明对海马体的刺激是会改善某些病患的记忆的，由此可推理空格前应该讲的是科学家致力于电击的治疗方式。因此F选项符合语义走向。

Passage Two

6．E。段落排序题若首段未给出，首先需要通读全部段落首句，依据每段首句与上一段末句的句间衔接关系，通过排除法选出首段。本篇文章中，A段第一句话中含有指代关系词these，作为首句的话指无可指，故根据该词直接排除，B段有of course，属于衔接上下文的词，如作为首句也是没有上文可衔接。C和G段都可用此法排除。D和E段可以作为首段的可能选项，根据D段Carnegie和E段Dale Carnegie的名称特点，考虑到首次出现人名应为全名形式，故本题答案应为E。

7．D。首段为Carnegie的观点信息，下段应为该人物的观点承接，通过扫读剩下的段落可知，只有D段合适。

8．G。F段最后一句话为：None of these tricks will help you understand them, their positions or the issues that divide you, but they can help you win—in one way. 可知these tricks是对上文信息的否定，下文应该出现win arguments肯定的表述，可知G选项首句"There is a better way to win arguments." 正好与F段尾句形成首尾衔接。

9．B。G段尾句讲述的是："Now we can understand each other's positions and recognize our shared values, since we both care about needy workers." 而根据衔接可确定，G段讲述的是成功的讨论，B段首句not so successful正好衔接上文，通过转折讲述不成功的案例。

10．A。C段末尾"Next time you talk with someone who takes a stand...Raise objections and listen carefully to their replies." 这几句话主要讲的是谈话的四种手段，正好与A段首句中的These tools 形成呼应关系，故本题答案应为A。

Passage Three

11．B。本段前面讲到如何实施CPR（心肺复苏术），但but之后讲到，虽然CPR有帮助，但是人们常常很担心和陌生人进行气息交换，同时整个步骤容易遗忘，尤其那些未经培训的人会担心自己做错了事情。因此本题选B（传统心肺复苏术虽然不错，但是人们总是对其应用比较纠结。）

12. D。第一段中讲到传统CPR有其局限性，所以AHA简化了传统方式，号召使用仅胸部按压心肺复苏的方式。该段从第二句开始，就开始讲如何实施hands-only CPR（手动心肺复苏术）。所以D选项（人们如何将手动心肺复苏术付诸实践？）是正确答案。

13. C。该段主要强调hands-only CPR的效果和传统方式相似，并且告诫人们如果对自己急救能力没有十足的把握，就应该使用新的方式。因此本题选C（手动心肺复苏术的效果和传统方式类似。）

14. F。该段讲到传统CPR因其结合呼吸和按压，对儿童和无法正常呼吸的人是有用的，对溺水者和呼吸困难的人更加有效。因此，本题正确答案为F（传统心肺复苏术在挽救昏迷和呼吸有困难的病人时有明显优势。）

Passage Four

15. D。根据题干中的overwhelming majority/family physicians/paid定位到D段最后一句"but 90% said they would if it were appropriately reimbursed（补偿）"，即90%的医生说如果有足够的补偿就可以，overwhelming majority对应90%，appropriately reimbursed对应duly paid，同义转述判定可知该句信息源自D段。

16. H。根据题干中的employers/eager to/convenience定位到H段的首句：Many health plans and employers have rushed to...without leaving home or work. 句中rushed to对应eager to，a convenient way对应题干中convenience，故该句信息源自H段。

17. E。用题干中的states/regulations定位到E段第二句：Rules defining and regulating telemedicine differ widely from state to state. 其中regulations对应句中的rules，state有复现，题干中的markedly different则对应句中的differ widely，属于非常标准的改写方式。

18. B。用题干中的regions short of professional medical service/better medical care定位到B段第四句：Telemedicine also allows for better care in places where medical expertise is hard to come by. 题干中的short of professional medical service和句中的medical expertise is hard to come by对应，better care则是直接复现。故B段为该句的信息来源。

19. K。用题干中的Unlike/insurers/reluctant/pay for定位到K段第二句：While employers and health plans have been eager...to consult with existing patients about continuing issues. 题干中用While（尽管）来对应Unlike，insurers直接复现。far less willing对应题干中的reluctant，因此本题答案为K。

20. O。用题干中的supporters/accept/practice licenses/valid定位到O段中第二句：While welcoming the move, some telemedicine advocates would prefer states to

automatically honor one another's licenses. 其中license直接复现，supporters对应原文的advocates，accept对应prefer，honor...license对应原文的valid，因此本句信息来源于O段。

21．G。用题干中的The fastest growing area/lesser health problems定位到G段的第二、三句：The fastest-growing services in telemedicine connect consumers with clinicians ...such as colds, flu, ear-aches and skin rashes. 句中的The fastest growing area对应段中的the fastest growing area，而lesser health problem则在段落中得到更长篇幅的解释：这些健康问题都是一些非紧急的情况，比如感冒、流感、耳朵疼痛和皮疹等。因此本题正确答案为G。

22．F。题干中的spreads quickly/opponents doubt/its service quality定位到F段第一句：Some critics also question whether the quality of care is keeping up with the rapid expansion of telemedicine. 题干中的spreads quickly对应段中的rapid expansion，opponents对应段中的critics，而quality部分则是同义改写：质疑服务质量对应原文中质疑质量是否能跟上发展的脚步。因此本句信息来源于F段。

23．I。根据题干中的pretended to be/seeking help/disturbing/results定位到原文I段第三句：In a recent study, researchers posing as patients with skin problems sought help from 16 telemedicine sites—with unsettling results. 其中pretended对应原文中的posing，seeking help变成sought help, disturbing results对应原文中的unsettling results。因此本句信息来源于I段。

24．N。根据题干中的different states/different regulations/hinders/development定位到N段第三句：But some industry members contend that having 50 different sets of rules, ...of telemedicine and is hampering its growth. 题干中的different states和different regulations对应段落中的having 50 different sets of rules，而hinders对应is hampering, development则对应growth。因此本题答案为N。